Regression Methods for Medical Research

T0188419

Bee Choo Tai

Saw Swee Hock School of Public Health
National University of Singapore
and National University Health System;
Yong Loo Lin School of Medicine
National University of Singapore
and National University Health System
Singapore

David Machin

Medical Statistics Unit
School of Health and Related Sciences
University of Sheffield;
Cancer Studies, Faculty of Medicine
University of Leicester
Leicester, UK

WILEY Blackwell

To

Isaac Xu-En Koh and Kheng-Chuan Koh

and

Lorna Christine Machin

Regression Methods for Medical Research

Contents

Preface

In the course of planning a new clinical study, key questions that require answering have to be determined and once this is done the purpose of the study will be to answer the questions posed. Once posed, the next stage of the process is to design the study in detail and this will entail more formally stating the hypotheses of concern and considering how these may be tested. These considerations lead to establishing the statistical models underpinning the research process. Models, once established, will ultimately be fitted to the experimental data collated and the associated statistical techniques will help to establish whether or not the research questions have been answered with the desired reliability. Thus, the chosen statistical models encapsulate the design structure and form the basis for the subsequent analysis, reporting and interpretation. In general terms, such models are termed regression models, of which there are several major types, and the fitting of these to experimental data forms the basis of this text.

Our aim is not to describe regression methods in all their technical detail but more to illustrate the situations in which each is suitable and hence to guide medical researchers of all disciplines to use the methods appropriately. Fortunately, several user-friendly statistical computer packages are available to assist in the model fitting processes. We have used Stata statistical software in the majority of our calculations, and to illustrate the types of commands that may be needed, but this is only one example of packages that can be used for this purpose. Statistical software is continually evolving so that, for example, several and improving versions of Stata have appeared during the time span in which this book has been written. We strongly advise use of the most up-to-date software available and, as we mention within the text itself, one that has excellent graphical facilities. We caution that, although we use real data extensively, our analyses are selective and are for illustration only. They should not be used to draw conclusions from the studies concerned.

We would like to give a general thank you to colleagues and students of the Saw Swee Hock School of Public Health, National University of Singapore and National University Health System, and a specific one for the permission to use the data from the Singapore Cardiovascular Cohort Study 2. Thanks are also due to colleagues at the Skaraborg Institute, Skövde, Sweden. In addition, we would like to thank the following for allowing us to use their studies for illustration: Tin Aung, Singapore Eye Research Institute; Michael J Campbell, University of Sheffield, UK; Boon-Hock Chia, Chia Clinic, Singapore; Siow-Ann Chong, Institute of Mental Health, Singapore; Richard G Grundy, University of Nottingham, UK; James H-P Hui, National University Health System, Singapore; Ronald C-H Lee, National University of Singapore; Daniel P-K Ng, National University of Singapore; R Paul Symonds, University of Leicester, UK; Veronique Viardot-Foucault, KK Women's and Children's Hospital, Singapore; Joseph T-S Wee, National Cancer Centre, Singapore; Chinnaiya Anandakumar, Camden Medical Centre, Singapore; and Annapoorna Venkat, National University Health System, Singapore. Finally, we thank Haleh G Maralani for her help with some of the statistical programming.

George EP Box (1979): 'All models are wrong, but some are useful.'

Bee Choo Tai

David Machin

1   Introduction

SUMMARY

A very large number of clinical studies with human subjects have and are being conducted in a wide range of settings. The design and analysis of such studies demands the use of statistical models in this process. To describe such situations involves specifying the model, including defining population regression coefficients (the parameters), and then stipulating the way these are to be estimated from the data arising from the subjects (the sample) who have been recruited to the study. This chapter introduces the simple linear regression model to describe studies in which the measure made on the subjects can be assumed to be a continuous variable, the value of which is thought to depend either on a single binary or a continuous covariate measure.

Associated statistical methods are also described defining the null hypothesis, estimating means and standard deviations, comparing groups by use of a z- or t-test, confidence intervals and p-values. We give examples of how a statistical computer package facilitates the relevant analyses and also provides support for suitable graphical display.

Finally, examples from the medical and associated literature are used to illustrate the wide range of application of regression techniques: further details of some of these examples are included in later chapters.

INTRODUCTION

The aim of this book is to introduce those who are involved with medical studies whether laboratory, clinic, or population based, to the wide range of regression techniques which are pertinent to the design, analysis, and reporting of the studies concerned. Thus our intended readership is expected to range from health care professionals of all disciplines who are concerned with patient care, to those more involved with the non-clinical aspects such as medical support and research in the laboratory and beyond.

Even in the simplest of medical studies in which, for example, recording of a single feature from a series of samples taken from individual patients is made, one may ask questions as to why the resulting values differ from each other. It may be that they differ between the genders

Regression Methods for Medical Research, First Edition. Bee Choo Tai and David Machin.
© 2014 Bee Choo Tai and David Machin. Published 2014 by John Wiley & Sons, Ltd.

and/or between the different ages of the patients concerned, or because of the severity of their illnesses. In more formal terms we examine whether or not the value of the observed variable, y, depends on one or more of the (covariate) variables, often termed the x's. Although the term covariate is used here in a generic sense, we will emphasize that individually they may play different roles in the design and hence analysis of the study of which they are a part. If one or more covariates does influence the outcome, then we are essentially claiming that part of the variation in y is a result of individual patients having different values of the x's concerned. In which case, any variation remaining after taking into consideration these covariates is termed the residual or random variation. If the covariates do not have influence, then we have not explained (strictly not explained an important part of) the variation in y by the x's. Nevertheless, there may be other covariates of which we are not aware that would.

Measurements made on human subjects rarely give exactly the same results from one occasion to the next. Even in adults, height varies a little during the course of the day. If one measures the cholesterol levels of an individual on one particular day and then again the following day, under exactly the same conditions, greater variation in this than that of height would be expected. Any variation that we cannot ascribe to one or more covariates is usually termed random variation, although, as we have indicated, it may be that an unknown covariate may account for some of this. The levels of inherent variability may be very high so that, perhaps in the circumstances where a subject has an illness, the oscillations in these measurements may disguise, at least in the early stages of treatment, the beneficial effect of treatment given to improve the condition.

STATISTICAL MODELS

Whatever the type of study, it is usually convenient to think of the underlying structure of the design in terms of a statistical model. This model encapsulates the research question we intend to formulate and ultimately answer. Once the model is specified, the object of the corresponding study (and hence the eventual analysis) is to estimate the parameters of this model as precisely as is reasonable.

Comparing two means

Suppose a study is designed to investigate the relationship between high density lipoprotein (HDL) cholesterol levels and gender. Once the study has been conducted, the observed data for each gender may be plotted in a histogram format as in Figure 1.1.

These figures illustrate a typical situation in that there is considerable variation in the value of the continuous variable HDL ranging from approximately 0.4 to 2.0 mmol/L. Further, both distributions tend to peak towards the centre of their ranges and there is a suggestion of a difference between males and females. In fact the mean value is higher at $\bar{y}_F =$ 1.2135 for the females compared with $\bar{y}_M = 1.0085$ mmol/L for the males.

Formal comparisons between these two groups can be made using a statistical significance test. Thus, we can regard $\bar{y}_F$ and $\bar{y}_M$ as estimates of the true or population mean values μ_F and μ_M. The corresponding standard deviations are given by $s_F=0.3425$ and $s_M=0.2881$ mmol/L, and these estimate the respective population values σ_F and σ_M. To test the null hypothesis of no difference in HDL levels between males and females, the usual procedure is to assume HDL within each group has an approximately Normal distribution of the same standard deviation. The null hypothesis, of no difference in HDL levels between

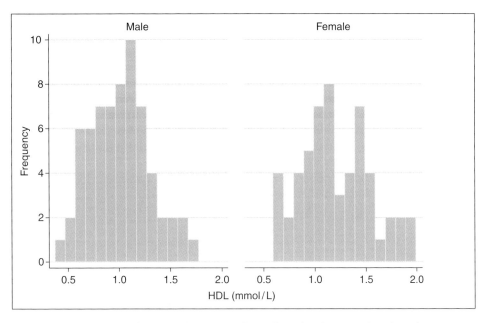

Figure 1.1 Histograms of HDL levels in 65 males and 55 females (part data from the Singapore Cardiovascular Cohort Study 2)

the sexes, is then expressed by H_0: $\mu_F = \mu_M$ or equivalently H_0: $\mu_F - \mu_M = 0$. The statistical test, the Student's t-test, is calculated using

$$t = \frac{(\bar{y}_F - \bar{y}_M) - (\mu_F - \mu_M)}{s_{Pool}\sqrt{\dfrac{1}{n_F} + \dfrac{1}{n_M}}} \qquad (1.1)$$

where $n_F = 55$ and $n_M = 65$ are the respective sample sizes, and the expression for s_{Pool} is given in *Technical details* provided at the end of this chapter on page 16. In large samples, and when the null hypothesis is true, that is if $\mu_F - \mu_M = 0$ in equation (1.1), t has a standard Normal distribution with mean 0 and standard deviation 1.

For the data of Figure 1.1, $s_{Pool} = 0.3142$ and so, if the null hypothesis is true,

$$t = \frac{(1.2135 - 1.0085) - 0}{0.3142\sqrt{\dfrac{1}{55} + \dfrac{1}{65}}} = 3.5612 \text{ or } 3.56$$

As the sample sizes are large, to determine the statistical significance this value is referred to the standard Normal distribution of Table T1 where the notation z replaces t. The value in the table corresponding to $z = 3.56$ is 0.99981. The area in the two extremes of the distribution is the p-value $= 2$ (1 − 0.99981) $= 0.00038$ in this case. This is very small probability indeed, and so on this basis we would reject the null hypothesis of no difference in HDL between the sexes. Thus, we conclude that there is a real difference in mean HDL levels between women and men estimated by 1.2135−1.0085 = 0.2050 mmol/L. These same calculations are repeated using a statistical package in Figure 1.2 in which the Student's t-test is activated by the command (**ttest**).

---

ttest hdl, by (gender)

Two-sample t test with equal variances

Group	Obs	Mean	SD
male	65	$\bar{y}_M = 1.0085$	0.2881
female	55	$\bar{y}_F = 1.2135$	0.3425

$s_{Pool} = 0.3142$ (Pooled)

diff $\bar{y}_F - \bar{y}_M = 0.2050$ 95% CI 0.0910 to 0.3190

diff = mean (female) − mean (male), t = 3.56
Ho: diff = 0, Ha: diff != 0, Pr (|T| > |t|) = 0.0005.

Note
In the main body of the text in place of Pr (|T| > |t|) = 0.0005 we use the abbreviated
notation *p*-value = 0.0005.

Figure 1.2   Edited command and annotated output for the comparison of HDL levels between 65 males and 55 females using the *t*-test (part data from the Singapore Cardiovascular Cohort Study 2)

A feature of the computer output is that a 95% confidence interval (CI) for the true difference between the means, that is for $\delta = \mu_F - \mu_M$, is given. In this situation, but only when the total study size is large, the $100\,(1 - \alpha)\%$ CI for the mean difference between the male and female populations takes the form:

$$(\bar{y}_F - \bar{y}_M) - \left[z_{\alpha/2} \times SE(\bar{y}_F - \bar{y}_M) \right] \text{ to } (\bar{y}_F - \bar{y}_M) + \left[z_{\alpha/2} \times SE(\bar{y}_F - \bar{y}_M) \right] \tag{1.2}$$

where $z_{\alpha/2}$ is taken from the z-distribution and the standard error (SE) of the difference between the means is denoted by $SE(\bar{y}_F - \bar{y}_M) = \sqrt{\dfrac{s_F^2}{n_F} + \dfrac{s_M^2}{n_M}}$.

If $\alpha = 0.05$, which corresponds to $\gamma = 0.975$ in the figure of Table T1, then $z_{0.025} = 1.96$. This value is one that is highlighted in Table T2. Equation (1.2) is adapted to the situation when the sample size is small by use of equation (1.6), see *Technical details*.

The actual 95% confidence interval quoted in Figure 1.2 suggests that, although the observed difference between the means is 0.21 mmol/L, we would not be too surprised if the true difference was either as small as 0.09 or as large as 0.32 mmol/L.

Linear regression

The object of this text is to describe statistical models so we now reformulate the above example in such terms. Consider the following equation

$$HDL = \beta_0 + \beta_1 Gender \tag{1.3}$$

where we code *Gender* = 0 for males and *Gender* = 1 for females.

For the males, equation (1.3) becomes $HDL_M = \beta_0 + \beta_1 \times 0 = \beta_0$, whereas for the females $HDL_F = \beta_0 + \beta_1 \times 1 = \beta_0 + \beta_1$. From these, the difference between females and males is

```
regress hdl gender
---------|------------------------------------------------------
    hdl |      Coef         SE        t      P>|t|        [95% CI]
---------|------------------------------------------------------
   cons |   b_0 = 1.0085
 gender |   b_G = 0.2050    0.0576    3.56    0.0005    0.0910 to 0.3190
---------|------------------------------------------------------
```

Figure 1.3   Edited commands and annotated output for the comparison of HDL levels between 65 males and 55 females using a regression command (part data from the Singapore Cardiovascular Cohort Study 2)

$HDL_F - HDL_M = (\beta_0 + \beta_1) - \beta_0 = \beta_1$. Thus, the difference in HDL between the sexes corresponds precisely to this single parameter or regression coefficient. If model (1.3) is fitted to the data, then the estimates of β_0 and β_1 are denoted by b_0 and b_1. Thus, we estimate the true or population difference between the sexes β_1 by the estimate b_1 obtained from the data collected in the study. In practice we may denote b_1 in such an example by either b_{Gender} or b_G to make the context clear.

The commands and output using a statistical package for this are given in Figure 1.3. This uses the command (**regress**) followed by the measurement concerned (**hdl**) and the name of the covariate within which comparisons are to be made (**gender**). The results replicate those of Figure 1.2, in that $b_G = 0.2050$ mmol/L exactly equals the difference between the two means obtained previously while $b_0 = \overline{y}_M = 1.0085$ mmol/L. Although this agreement is always the case, in general the approach using a regression model such as equation (1.3) is more flexible and allows more complex study designs to be analyzed efficiently.

Suppose the investigators are more interested in the relationship between HDL and body-weight of the individuals, and examine this using the scatter diagram of Figure 1.4(a). As we noted earlier, there is considerable variation in HDL ranging from 0.4 to 2.0 mmol/L. Additionally the body-weights of the individuals concerned varies from approximately 40 to 100 kg. There is a tendency for HDL to decline with increasing weight, and one objective of the study may be to quantify this in some way. This may be achieved by assuming, in the first instance, that the decline is essentially linear. In which case, a straight line may be drawn through (usually termed 'fitted to') the data in some way.

In this context, the straight line is described by the following linear equation or linear model:

$$HDL = \beta_0 + \beta_1 Weight \tag{1.4}$$

In this equation, β_0 and β_1 (in practice better denoted β_W or β_{Weight}) are constants which, once determined, position the line for the data as in the panel of Figure 1.4(b). The method of fitting the regression model to such data is given in *Technical details*. Although this fitted line suggests that there is indeed a decline in HDL with increasing weight, there are individual subjects whose HDL values are quite distant from the line. Thus, there is by no means a per-fect linear relationship and hence fitting the linear model to take account of weight has not explained all the variation in HDL values between individuals. It is usual to recognize this lack-of-fit by extending the format of equation (1.4) to add a residual term, ε, so that:

$$HDL = \beta_0 + \beta_W Weight + \varepsilon \tag{1.5}$$

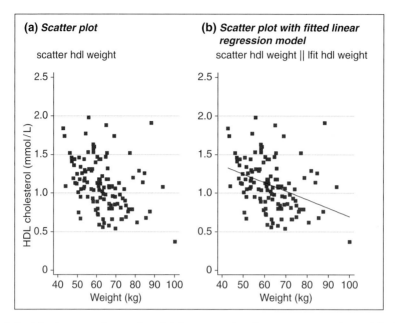

Figure 1.4   Edited command to produce (a) the scatter plot of HDL against weight, and (b) the same scatter plot with the corresponding linear regression model fitted (part data from the Singapore Cardiovascular Cohort Study 2)

Here, ε represents the residual or random variation in HDL remaining once weight has been taken into account. This noise (or error) is assumed to have a mean value of 0 across all subjects recruited to the study, and the magnitude of the variability is described by the standard deviation (SD), denoted by $\sigma_{Residual}$.

Expressed in these terms, the primary objective of the investigation will be to estimate the parameters, β_0 and β_W. In order to summarize how reliable these estimates are, we also need to estimate $\sigma_{Residual}$. Once again we write such estimates as b_0, b_W and $s_{Residual}$ to distinguish them from the corresponding parameters. For brevity, $\sigma_{Residual}$ and $s_{Residual}$ are often denoted σ and s, respectively.

The command required to fit equation (1.5) to the data is (**regress hdl weight**). This and the associated output are summarized in Figure 1.5. The fitting process estimates $b_0 = 1.7984$ and $b_W = -0.0110$, and so the model obtained is HDL = 1.7984 − 0.0110 *Weight*. This implies that for every 1 kg increase in weight, HDL declines on average by 0.0110 mmol/L. The *p*-value = 0.0001 suggests that this decline is highly statistically significant. In *Technical details*, we explain more on the Analysis of Variance (*ANOVA*) section of this output, and merely note here that $F = 18.12$ in the upper panel is very close to $t^2 = (-4.26)^2 = 18.15$ in the lower. In fact, algebraically, $F = t^2$ exactly in the situation described here—the small discrepancy is caused by rounding error in the respective calculations.

As we have seen, not all the variation in HDL has been accounted for by weight so this suggests that other features (covariates) of the individuals concerned may also influence these levels. In fact, a previous analysis suggested a difference between males and females in this respect. Figure 1.6(a) plots the data from the same 120 individuals but indicates which are male and which female. Treating these as distinct groups, then two fitted lines (one for the males and one for the females) are superimposed on the same data as illustrated in Figure 1.6(b). From this latter panel one can see that the line for males is beneath that for

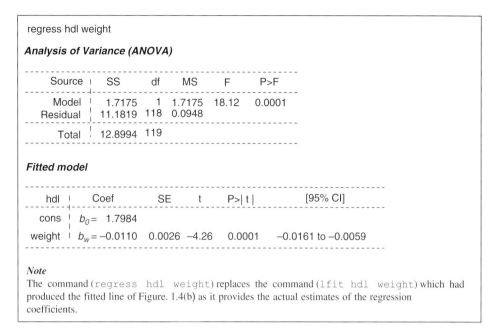

```
regress hdl weight
```

Analysis of Variance (ANOVA)

Source	SS	df	MS	F	P>F
Model	1.7175	1	1.7175	18.12	0.0001
Residual	11.1819	118	0.0948		
Total	12.8994	119			

Fitted model

hdl	Coef	SE	t	P>|t|	[95% CI]
cons	$b_0=$ 1.7984				
weight	$b_w=$ −0.0110	0.0026	−4.26	0.0001	−0.0161 to −0.0059

Note
The command (regress hdl weight) replaces the command (lfit hdl weight) which had produced the fitted line of Figure. 1.4(b) as it provides the actual estimates of the regression coefficients.

Figure 1.5 Command and annotated output for the regression of HDL on weight (part data from the Singapore Cardiovascular Cohort Study 2)

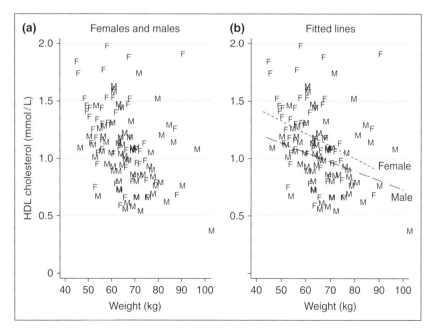

Figure 1.6 (a) Scatter plot of HDL and weight by gender in 120 individuals, and (b) the same scatter plot with linear regression lines fitted to the data for each gender separately (part data from the Singapore Cardiovascular Cohort Study 2)

females but, for both genders, the HDL declines with weight. Thus, some of the variation in HDL is accounted for by weight and some by the gender of the individuals concerned. Nevertheless, a substantial amount of the variation still remains to be accounted for.

Types of dependent variables (y-variables)

In the previous sections we have described models for explaining the variation in the values of HDL. Typically when using statistical models, HDL would be described as the dependent variable and, for general discussion purposes, it is usually termed the y-variable. However, the particular y-variable concerned may be one of several different data types with a label used for the variable name which is context specific. Thus, we refer to HDL rather than y in the above example, and note that this is a continuous variable taking non-negative values. Although we have indicated in Figure 1.1 that this may have an approximately Normal distribution form, this will not always be the case. In such a situation, a transformation of the basic variable may be considered. For a continuous variable this is often the logarithmic transformation. Thus, in a model we may consider the dependent variable as (say) $y = \log$ (HDL) rather than HDL itself.

We will see below, and in later chapters, that the underlying dependent variable may also take a binary, multinomial, ordered categorical, non-negative integer or time-to-event (survival) form. In each of these situations the y-variable for the modeling may differ in mathematical form from that of the underlying dependent variable.

SOME COMPLETED STUDIES

As we have indicated there are countless ongoing studies, and many more have been successfully completed and reported, that will use regression techniques of one form or another for analysis. To give some indication of the range and diversity of application, we describe a selection of published medical studies which span those conducted on a small scale in the laboratory to large clinical trials and epidemiological studies. These examples include some features that we also draw upon in later chapters.

Example 1.1 Linear regression: Interferon-λ production in asthma exacerbations

Busse, Lemanske Jr and Gern (2010, Figure 6) reproduce a plot of the percentage reduction in FEV_1 in individuals with asthma and in healthy volunteers against their generation of interferon-λ. These data were first described by Contoli, Message, Laza-Stanca, *et al.* (2006, Figure 2f) who state: 'Induction of IFN-λ protein by rhinovirus in BAL cells is strongly related to severity of reductions in lung function on subsequent *in vivo* rhinovirus experimental infection. IFN-λ protein production in BAL cells infected *in vitro* with RV16 was significantly inversely correlated with severity of maximal reduction from baseline in FEV_1 (forced expiratory volume in 1 s) recorded over the 2-week infection period when subjects were subsequently experimentally infected with RV16 *in vivo* ($r = 0.65$, $P < 0.03$).' Their results with the information extracted from Busse, Lemanske Jr and Gern (2010, Figure 6) are reproduced in Figure 1.7.

Expressed in terms of a regression model, using the command (`regress   FEV1 Interpgml`), the increasing slope of $b_{IFN-\lambda} = 0.1011$ per unit increase in pg/mL is statistically significant, *p*-value$= 0.017$.

We will return to this example in Chapter 2 but note here that, as there are two groups of individuals concerned (those with asthma and healthy individuals), the potential influence of this second covariate (type of subject) in addition to IFN-λ protein production must be considered.

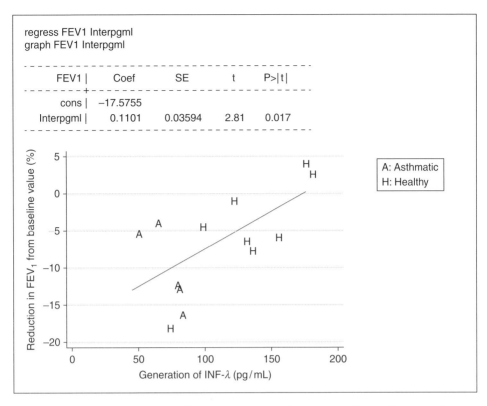

```
regress FEV1 Interpgml
graph FEV1 Interpgml

- - - - - - - - - - - - - - - - - - - - - - - - - - - - - - - -
    FEV1 |    Coef       SE        t      P>|t|
- - - - - - - - +- - - - - - - - - - - - - - - - - - - - - - - -
    cons |  −17.5755
Interpgml |   0.1101    0.03594   2.81    0.017
- - - - - - - - - - - - - - - - - - - - - - - - - - - - - - - -
```

A: Asthmatic
H: Healthy

Figure 1.7 Annotated commands and output to investigate the response to human rhinovirus infection in eight healthy individuals and five with asthma (information from Busse, Lemanske Jr and Gern, 2010, Figure 6)

	Units	Estimated regression coefficient	95% CI	p-value
Design variable				
TNF-α score	(ng/L)	0.20	0.13 to 0.27	< 0.001
Other covariates				
log(triacylglycerol)	log(mmol/L)	0.15	0.01 to 0.30	0.041
MAP	mmHg	0.01	0.002 to 0.20	0.011
Duration of diabetes	years	0.02	0.01 to 0.02	< 0.001
Total cholesterol	mmol/L	0.12	0.04 to 0.21	0.006

Figure 1.8 Association between log(ACR) and inflammatory variables in a multiple regression analysis (after Ng, Fukushima, Tai, *et al.*, 2008, Table 2)

Example 1.2 Multiple linear regression: Activation of the TNF-α system in patients with diabetes

Ng, Fukushima, Tai, *et al.* (2008) investigated whether activation of the TNF-α system may potentially exert an effect on the albumin:creatinine ratio (ACR), expressed in g/kg, in patients with type 2 diabetes. In a multiple regression equation summarized in Figure 1.8, they used the logarithm of ACR, that is log(ACR), as the *y*-variable, TNF-α score as the key covariate and log(triacylglycerol), mean arterial pressure (MAP), duration of diabetes and total choles-terol as the other covariates. They concluded that: '… log(ACR) was significantly associated with TNF-α score, with a unit change in TNF-α score resulting in a 0.20 unit change in log(ACR) … .'

As we have noted, $y=$log(ACR) rather than ACR itself was used as the dependent variable. Further, there was a principal covariate, TNF-α score, and four potentially influencing covariates: log(triacylglycerol), MAP, duration of diabetes and total cholesterol. In fact Ng, Fukushima, Tai, et al. (2008, Table 1) recorded a total of 18 potential covariates. Most of these were screened out as not influencing values of log(ACR) using a variable selection process (see Chapter 7) to leave the final model to summarize the results containing only the five covariates listed in Figure 1.8. In situations such as this when there is a principal or design covariate specified, then reporting details of the simple linear regression, here log(ACR) on TNF-α score without adjustment by the other covariates, is recommended. This information then enables the reader to judge how much the presence of the other (here four) covariates in the full model influence the magnitude of that regression coefficient (here $\beta_{TNF-\alpha}$) of principal interest.

Example 1.3 Multiple logistic regression: Intrahepatic vein fetal blood samples

Figure 1.9 includes part of the data collated by Chinnaiya, Venkat, Chia, et al. (1998, Table 6) giving the number of fetal deaths according to different puncture sites chosen for sampling from both normal and abnormal fetuses. Here the event of concern is a fetal death at some stage following the fetal blood sampling of whatever type. This is clearly a binary 0 (alive), 1 (dead) variable. There were 52 fetal deaths among the 292 sampled using the intra-hepatic vein (IHV) technique: an odds of 52:240. For percutaneous umbilical cord sampling (PUBS), the odds were 20:50. Comparing the two fetal sampling techniques gives an odds ratio: $OR = \dfrac{20/50}{52/240} = 1.85$, suggesting a greater death rate using PUBS. An even greater

Fetal loss	Intrahepatic vein (IHV)	Percutaneous umbilical cord sampling (PUBS)	Cardiocentesis	Total (%)
< 2 weeks of procedure	21	7	11	39 (10.2)
> 2 weeks of procedure	10	6	2	18 (4.7)
Postnatal death	21	7	2	30 (7.9)
Total fetal deaths (%)	52 (17.8)	20 (28.6)	15 (75.0)	87 (22.8)
Live-births	240	50	5	295
Total sampled	292	70	20	382
Odds	52:240	20:50	15:5	87:295
Odds Ratio (OR)	1	1.85	13.85	
(95% CI)	–	1.01 to 3.36	4.82 to 39.79	

Figure 1.9   Fetal loss following fetal blood sampling according to different puncture sites in both normal and abnormal fetuses (Source: Chinnaiya, Venkat, Chia, et al., 1998, Table 6. Reproduced with permission of John Wiley & Sons Ltd.)

risk is apparent when cardiocentesis is used with $OR = \dfrac{15/5}{52/240} = 13.85$ when compared with IHV.

In Figure 1.9 more detail of when the deaths occurred is given so that the y-variable of interest may be the ordered (4 – level) categorical variable fetal loss and live-birth rather than the binary variable death or live-birth. As loss following blood sampling may be influenced by gestational age of the fetus as well as clinical indications including pre-term rupture of membranes, hydrops fetalis, and the number of needle entries made, then these variables may need to be accounted for in a full analysis.

Example 1.4 Poisson regression: Hospital admissions for chronic obstructive pulmonary disease (COPD)

Maheswaran, Pearson, Hoysal and Campbell (2010) evaluated the impact of a health forecast alert service on admissions for chronic obstructive pulmonary disease (COPD) in the Bradford and Airedale region of England. Essentially, the UK Meteorological Office (UKMO) provides an alert service which forecasts when the outdoor environment is likely to adversely affect the health of COPD patients. This alert enables the patients to take appropriate action to keep themselves well, and thereby potentially avoid a hospital admission. In brief, general practitioner (GP) groups providing primary medical care chose to participate or not in the evaluation, and those that did registered their COPD patients with the UKMO. Registered patients were given an information pack which included details about the automated telephone call they would receive should bad weather trigger an alert. The number of hospital admissions was subsequently noted over the two winter periods 2006–7 and 2007–8. A summary of the study findings is given in Figure 1.10.

Winter (December to March)	Number of GP practices	Admissions		Ratio of Admissions (2007–8) / (2006–7)	
		2006–7	2007–8	R	95% CI
Exposure category					
None	51	203	195	0.96	0.79 to 1.18
Part winters	10	57	55	0.96	0.65 to 1.42
Whole winters	25	183	172	0.94	0.76 to 1.16
Total	86	443	422		
Adjusted for exposure category				$R_{Adjusted\ Category} = 0.98$	0.78 to 1.22
Exposure scale					
0	51	203	195	0.96	0.79 to 1.18
0.01 – 0.2	7	42	35	0.83	0.52 to 1.34
0.21 – 0.4	10	98	82	0.84	0.62 to 1.13
0.41 – 0.6	3	17	27	1.59	0.83 to 3.11
0.61 – 0.8	7	42	42	1.00	0.64 to 1.57
> 0.8	7	36	38	1.06	0.65 to 1.71
Total	85	438	419		
Adjusted for exposure scale				$R_{Adjusted\ Scale} = 1.11$	0.80 to 1.52

Figure 1.10 Admissions for chronic obstructive pulmonary (COPD) disease in Bradford and Airedale, England by category of general practice (GP) exposure to the Meteorological Office Forecast Alert Service (Source: Maheswaran, Pearson, Hoysal and Campbell, 2010, Table 1. Reproduced with permission of Oxford University Press.)

The GP practices concerned each comprise a very large number of patients, so that among them COPD represents a rare event. In which case, the unit for analysis is the number of hospital admissions, h, from each practice rather than the ratio of this number to the size of the practice concerned. As a consequence Poisson regression methods (see Chapter 5) were used for analysis. These models took account of the GP practice concerned as an unordered categorical variable, the particular winter (2006–7 or 2007–8) as binary, and either the exposure category or the exposure scale, both of which were treated as ordered numerical variables with equal category divisions. In Figure 1.10 the admission rate ratio adjusted for the exposure category, $R_{Adjusted\ Category}=0.98$ (95% CI 0.78 to 1.22), implies that admissions in 2007–8 were 2% lower in GP practices that participated relative to practices that did not. In contrast, the admission rate ratio adjusted for the exposure scale, $R_{Adjusted\ Scale}=1.11$ (95% CI 0.80 to 1.52) implies that admissions in 2007-8 were 11% higher in GP practices that participated and entered all their COPD patients into the forecasting system, relative to practices that did not. The wide confidence intervals, both of which cover the null hypothesis ratio of unity, indicate that the value or otherwise of the warning system has not been clearly established.

This study provides an example of a multi-level or clustered design in that the GPs agree to participate in the study but it is the admission to hospital or not of their individual patients that provides the outcome data. However, patients treated by one health care professional tend to be more similar among themselves than those treated by a different health care professional. So, if we know which GP is treating a patient, we can predict, by reference to experience from other patients, slightly better than chance, the outcome for the patient concerned. Consequently the patient outcomes for one GP are positively correlated and so are not completely independent of each other. Due note of the magnitude of this intra-cluster correlation (ICC) is required in the design and analysis processes. Multi-level designs are discussed further in Chapter 11.

Example 1.5 Cox proportional hazards regression: Nasopharyngeal cancer

Wee, Tan, Tai, *et al.* (2005) conducted a randomized trial of radiotherapy (RT) versus concurrent chemo-radiotherapy followed by adjuvant chemotherapy (CRT) in patients with nasopharyngeal cancer. The trial recruited 221 patients, 110 of whom were randomized to receive RT (the standard approach) and 111 CRT. The Kaplan-Meier estimates of the overall survival times of the patients in the two groups are given in Figure 1.11(a). The estimated hazard ratio (*HR*) of 0.50, calculated using a Cox proportional hazards regression model (see Chapter 6), indicates a survival advantage to those receiving CRT.

For nasopharyngeal cancer patients it is well known that, for example, their nodal status at the time of diagnosis has considerable influence on their ultimate survival. This is shown for those recruited to this trial in Figure 1.11(b) by a hazard ratio, *HR*=0.55, which indicates considerable additional risk for those with N3 nodal status. However, despite nodal status being an important influence on subsequent prognosis, a Cox proportional hazards regression model including the treatment received and nodal status gave a *HR*=0.51 (95% CI 0.31 to 0.85, *p*-value=0.009) in favor of CRT. All elements of which are very close to the respective components of the caption included within Figure 1.11(a). This suggests that the benefit of CRT over RT remains for all patients irrespective of their nodal status. In a final report it is not important to show Figure 1.11(b) as the considerable risk associated with N3 nodal status was known at the design stage of the trial. This is why the 95% CI and *p*-value are omitted from the caption.

In general, despite a covariate being a strong predictor of outcome, adding this to the regression model may not substantially change the estimated value of the 'key' regression coefficient, which in the case just discussed is that corresponding to the randomized

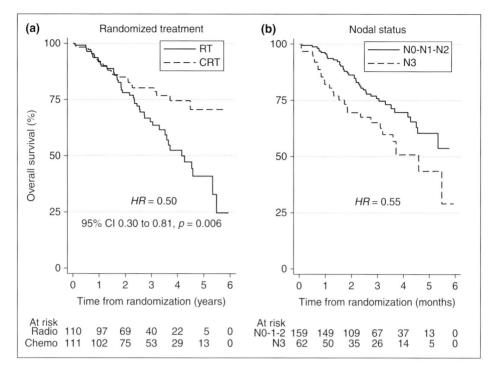

Figure 1.11   Kaplan-Meier estimates of the overall survival of patients with nasopharyngeal cancer by (a) randomized treatment received, and (b) nodal status at diagnosis (data from Wee, Tan, Tai *et al.*, 2005)

treatment given. Thus, the main concern here is the measure of treatment difference, and the role of the covariate is to see whether or not our view of this measure is modified by taking note of its presence. The aim in this situation is not to study the influence of the covariate itself.

Example 1.6 Repeated measures: Pain assessment in patients with oral lichen planus

Figure 1.12 illustrates the results from a longitudinal repeated measures design in which the pain experienced by patients with oral lichen planus (OLP) is self-recorded over time. The patients were recruited to a randomized trial conducted by Poon, Goh, Kim, *et al.* (2006) comparing the efficacy of topical steroid with topical cyclosporine for healing their OLP. In general, pain levels diminished over a 12-week period but with little difference between the treatments observed. The plots illustrate some of the difficulties with such trials. For example, although a fixed assessment schedule was described in the protocol, practical circumstances dictated that these were not strictly adhered to. Also the number of patients returning to the clinics involved declined as the period from initial diagnosis and randomization increased. Typically there are a large number of data items and considerable variation in pain levels recorded both in the same patient and between different patients. In addition, successive data points within the same patient are unlikely to be independent of each other. The use of fractional polynomials (see Chapter 11) allows flexible (not just linear) regression models to be used to describe such data.

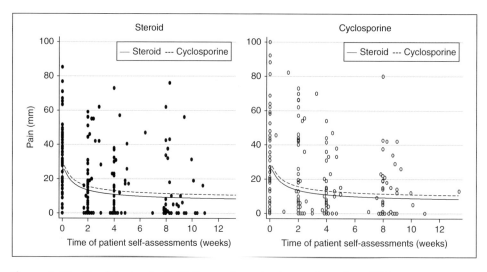

Figure 1.12 Visual Analog Scale (VAS) recordings of pain experience from OLP by treatment group. The fractional polynomial curve for the comparator treatment is added to each panel to facilitate visual comparisons between treatments (Source: Poon, Goh, Kim, *et al.*, 2006, Fig. 2. Reproduced with permission of Elsevier.)

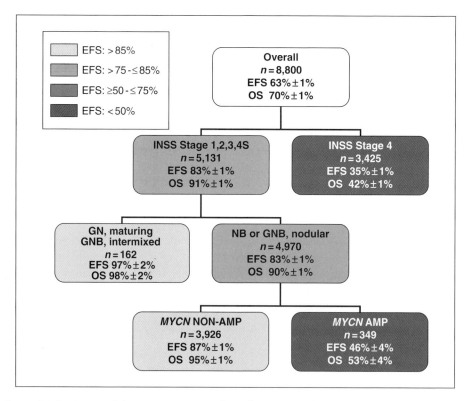

Figure 1.13 Section of the regression tree analysis of 5-year event-free (EFS) and overall (OS) survival of 8,800 young patients with neuroblastoma (Source: Cohn, Pearson, London, et al., 2009, Fig. 1A. Reproduced with permission of Springer.)

Example 1.7 Regression trees: International Neuroblastoma Risk Group

Cohn, Pearson, London, *et al*. (2009) used a regression tree approach to develop an international neuroblastoma risk group (INRG) classification system for young patients diagnosed with neuroblastoma (NB). Figure 1.13 shows their 'top-level' split which divides the 8800 patients using the International Neuroblastoma Staging System (INSS) into two quite distinct prognostic groups (Stage 1, 2, 3, and 4S versus Stage 4) with, for example, event-free survival (EFS) of 83% and 35% respectively, at five years from diagnosis. Two branches follow the first of these groups; one for the small group comprising ganglioneuroma (GN), maturing ganglioneuroblastoma (GNB), and intermixed types (EFS 97%) which is a terminal node or leaf; the other for those with neuroblastoma (NB) or GNB nodular (EFS 83%). This latter group is then further branched into those with MYCN non-amplified (EFS 87%) and amplified status (EFS 46%), which are then subsequently divided again, as is the intermediate node of INSS Stage 4 patients, until terminal nodes are reached. This branching process identified a total of 20 terminal nodes of homogeneous patient groups ranging in size from 8 to 513 with a median size of 59, and comprising 5-year EFS rates ranging from 19% to 97%, with a median of 61%.

Further reading

A general introduction to medical statistics is Swinscow and Campbell (2002), which concentrates mainly on the analysis of studies, while Bland (2000), Campbell (2006) and Campbell, Machin and Walters (2007) are intermediate texts. Altman (1991) and Armitage, Berry and Matthews (2002) give lengthier and more detailed accounts. All these books cover the topic of regression models to some extent, while Mitchell (2012) focuses specifically on using Stata for regression modeling purposes.

Machin and Campbell (2005) focus on the design, rather than analysis, of medical studies in general while Machin, Campbell, Tan and Tan (2009) specifically cover sample size issues. A useful text is that of Freeman, Walters and Campbell (2008) on how to display data.

More advanced texts which address aspects of regression models specifically include Clayton and Hills (1993), Dobson and Barnett (2008), Everitt and Rabe-Hesketh (2006) and Kleinbaum, Kupper, Muller and Nizam (2007). Collett (2002) specifically addresses the modeling of binary data, while Collett (2003) and Machin, Cheung and Parmar (2006) focus on time-to-event models. Diggle, Liang and Zeger (1994) cover the analysis of repeated measures data in detail as does Rabe-Hesketh and Skrondal (2008).

Altman DG (1991). *Practical Statistics for Medical Research*. London, Chapman and Hall.
Armitage P, Berry G and Matthews JNS (2002). *Statistical Methods in Medical Research*. (4th edn). Blackwell Science, Oxford.
Bland M (2000). *An Introduction to Medical Statistics*. (3rd edn). Oxford University Press, Oxford.
Campbell MJ (2006). *Statistics at Square Two: Understanding Modern Statistical Applications in Medicine*. (2nd edn). Blackwell BMJ Books, Oxford.
Campbell MJ, Machin D and Walters SJ (2007). *Medical Statistics: A Commonsense Approach: A Text Book for the Health Sciences*, (4th edn) Wiley, Chichester.
Clayton D and Hills M (1993). *Statistical Models in Epidemiology*, Oxford University Press, Oxford.
Collett D (2002). *Modelling Binary Data*, (2nd edn) Chapman and Hall/CRC, London.
Collett D (2003). *Modelling Survival Data in Medical Research*, (2nd edn), Chapman and Hall/CRC, London.
Diggle PJ, Liang K-Y and Zeger SL (1994). *Analysis of Longitudinal Data*. Oxford Science Publications, Oxford.
Dobson AJ and Barnett AG (2008). *Introduction to Generalized Linear Models*. (3rd edn), Chapman and Hall/CRC, London.

Everitt BS and Rabe-Hesketh S (2006). *A Handbook of Statistical Analysis using Stata*. (4th edn), Chapman and Hall/CRC, London.

Freeman JV, Walters SJ and Campbell MJ (2008). *How to Display Data*. BMJ Books, Blackwell Publishing, Oxford.

Kleinbaum G, Kupper LL, Muller KE and Nizam E (2007). *Applied Regression Analysis and Other Multivariable Methods*. (4th edn), Duxbury Press, Florence, Kentucky.

Machin D and Campbell MJ (2005). *Design of Studies for Medical Research*. Wiley, Chichester.

Machin D, Campbell MJ, Tan SB and Tan SH (2009). *Sample Size Tables for Clinical Studies*. (3rd edn). Wiley-Blackwell, Chichester.

Machin D, Cheung Y-B and Parmar MKB (2006). *Survival Analysis: A Practical Approach*. (2nd edn). Wiley, Chichester.

Mitchell MN (2012). *Interpreting and Visualizing Regression Models Using Stata*. Stata Press, College Station, TX.

Rabe-Hesketh S and Skrondal A (2008). *Multilevel and Longitudinal Modeling Using Stata (2nd edn)*, Stata Press, College Station, TX.

Swinscow TV and Campbell MJ (2002). *Statistics at Square One*. (10th edn), Blackwell, BMJ Books, Oxford.

TECHNICAL DETAILS

Student's *t*-test

For a given set of continuous data values $y_1, y_2, \ldots, y_n$ observed from n patients, the mean, $\bar{y}$, and standard deviation, s, are calculated as follows: $\bar{y} = \dfrac{\sum y_i}{n}$ and $s = \sqrt{\dfrac{\sum(y_i - \bar{y})^2}{n-1}}$.

These provide estimates of the associated parameters μ and σ.

For the data from the n_M males and n_F females of Figure 1.1, each gender provides a mean and standard deviation which we denote as $\bar{y}_M$, s_M and $\bar{y}_F$, s_F, respectively. To make a statistical comparison between these groups, it is often assumed that s_M and s_F are each estimating a common standard deviation σ estimated by s_{Pool}. In which case the two estimates

s_M and s_F are combined as follows: $s_{Pool} = \sqrt{\dfrac{(n_M - 1)s_M^2 + (n_F - 1)s_F^2}{(n_M - 1) + (n_F - 1)}}$. For the data concerned

$$s_{Pool} = \sqrt{\frac{(55-1)0.3425^2 + (65-1)0.2881^2}{(55-1) + (65-1)}} = 0.3142.$$ This is then used in equation (1.1),

which we repeat here for convenience: $t = \dfrac{(\bar{y}_F - \bar{y}_M) - (\mu_F - \mu_M)}{s_{Pool}\sqrt{\dfrac{1}{n_F} + \dfrac{1}{n_M}}}$.

As we noted previously, if the sample sizes n_M and n_F are sufficiently large then, under the assumption that the null hypothesis is true, that is H_0: $(\mu_F - \mu_M) = 0$, t can be regarded as having a Normal distribution with mean 0 and standard deviation 1. Once the value of t is calculated from the data, this can be referred to Table T1 to obtain the corresponding *p*-value.

In circumstances when the sample sizes n_M and n_F are not large, or there is some concern as to whether they are large enough, then use of Table T4, rather than Table T4, is necessary to obtain the *p*-value. Table T4 requires the degrees of freedom, *df*, which in this situation is, $df = (n_F - 1) + (n_M - 1) = n_F + n_M - 2$. In the above example, $df = (55 - 1) + (65 - 1) = 118$ is large and corresponds to the ∞ (infinity) row of Table T4. This row suggests that for a *p*-value to be less than $\alpha = 0.05$ would require t to exceed 1.960. Had the degrees of freedom been smaller, say $df=18$, then for a p-value to be less than $\alpha=0.05$ would require, from Table T4, that t exceeds 2.101. In general, as the degrees of freedom decline, more extreme values are required for t than z in order to declare statistical significance.

In the situation of small degrees of freedom, the confidence interval (CI) of equation (1.2) for the difference between two means is modified to become:

$$(\bar{y}_F - \bar{y}_M) - [t_{df,\alpha/2} \times SE(\bar{y}_F - \bar{y}_M)] \text{ to } (\bar{y}_F - \bar{y}_M) + [t_{df,\alpha/2} \times SE(\bar{y}_F - \bar{y}_M)] \quad (1.6)$$

Thus $z_{\alpha/2}$ is replaced by $t_{df,\alpha/2}$ and the necessary values are taken from Table T4 of the t-distribution with the appropriate degrees of freedom.

Linear regression

In general terms, the linear regression models of equations (1.3) and (1.4) are expressed for individual 'i' in the study as

$$y_i = \beta_0 + \beta_1 x_i + \varepsilon_i \quad (1.7)$$

where y_i is termed the dependent variable and x_i the independent variable or covariate.

Although y is a continuous variable in the case of HDL, in other circumstances the dependent variable concerned may be binary, ordered categorical, non-negative integer or a time-to-event (survival). The covariates gender and weight are respectively binary and continuous but other types of covariates such as categorical or ordered categorical variables may be involved.

In general the data of, for example Figure 1.4(a), can be regarded as a set of n pairs of observations $(x_1, y_1), (x_2, y_2), \ldots, (x_n, y_n)$. To fit the linear model to the data when y is continuous requires estimates of the regression coefficients β_0 and β_1, which are given by

$$b_0 = \bar{y} - b_1\bar{x} \text{ and } b_1 = \frac{S_{xy}}{S_{xx}} \quad (1.8)$$

where $S_{xy} = \sum(x_i - \bar{x})(y_i - \bar{y})$ and $S_{xx} = \sum(x_i - \bar{x})^2$. In addition, the residual standard deviation, $\sigma_{Residual}$ (more briefly σ) is estimated by

$$s_{Residual} = \sqrt{\frac{S_{yy} - b_1^2 S_{xx}}{(n-2)}} \quad (1.9)$$

where $S_{yy} = \sum(y_i - \bar{y})^2$. Thus, with the three equations included in (1.8) and (1.9), we have estimates b_0, b_1, and $s_{Residual}$ (or s) for the corresponding unknown parameters, β_0, β_1, and σ.

Once we have the estimates for b_0 and b_1 then, for any subject i with covariate value x_i, we could predict their y_i by $Y_i = b_0 + b_1 x_i$. Clearly, in choosing b_0 and b_1 we wish that the resulting Y_i will be close to the observed y_i and hence make our prediction error $(y_i - Y_i)$ as small as possible. The estimates of equation (1.8) result from choosing values of b_0 and b_1 which minimize the sum of squares, $\sum(y_i - Y_i)^2$. This leads b_0 and b_1 to be termed the *ordinary least-squares* (OLS) estimates of the *population* parameters β_0 and β_1.

The model of equation (1.7) once fitted to the data gives for the ith individual $y_i = b_0 + b_1 x_i + e_i = Y_i + e_i$ where the observed residual, e_i is the estimate of the true residual, ε_i. The residuals are the amount that the observed value differs from that predicted by the model, and represent (in this case) the variation not explained after fitting a straight line to the data. The e_i from all n subjects are usually assumed to have a Normal distribution with an average value of zero.

Once the problem under study is expressed by means of a statistical model, then the null hypothesis is expressed as, for example, H_0: $\beta_1 = 0$. If the null hypothesis were indeed true, then this implies that the covariate x in equation (1.7) explains none (strictly at most an unimportant amount) of the variation in y.

To test whether β_1 is significantly different from zero, the appropriate t-test is:

$$t = \frac{b_1 - 0}{SE(b_1)} \tag{1.10}$$

where $SE(b_1) = s_{Residual} / \sqrt{S_{xx}}$.

We note from Figure 1.3 that, when using (**regress hdl gender**) to test the null hypothesis of no difference in means between the genders, $b_G = 0.2050$ and this has standard error, $SE(b_G) = 0.05756$. In this case the degrees of freedom, $df = n - 2$; the '2' appears here as it is necessary to estimate 'two' parameters, β_0 and β_G, in order to fit the linear regression line. Finally, the calculated value of t is referred to Table T4 to assess the statistical significance, although in practice the p-value will usually be an integral part of the computer output.

The associated expression for $100(1 - \alpha)\%$ CI for the estimate of the regression slope β_1 is

$$b_1 - [t_{df, \alpha/2} \times SE(b_1)] \quad \text{to} \quad b_1 + [t_{df, \alpha/2} \times SE(b_1)] \tag{1.11}$$

where $t_{df, \alpha/2}$ is replaced by $z_{\alpha/2}$ in large sample situations. In practice, most computer software packages will adjust for sample size automatically.

Predicting a mean value of *y* for a particular *x*

For a specific value of an individual's weight $x = x_0$ (say) of Figure 1.5, we can obtain the estimated *mean* value of HDL for all individuals of that weight as $Y_0^{Mean} = b_0 + b_1 x_0$. This can be shown to have a standard error given by $SE(Y_0^{Mean}) = s_{Residual} \sqrt{\dfrac{1}{n} + \dfrac{(x_0 - \bar{x})^2}{S_{xx}}}$, the size

of which will increase as x_0 makes an increasing departure from $\bar{x}$. This expression can then be used to calculate the $100(1 - \alpha)\%$ CI about the regression line at x_0 given by

$$Y_0^{Mean} - [t_{df, \alpha/2} \times SE(Y_0^{Mean})] \quad \text{to} \quad Y_0^{Mean} + [t_{df, \alpha/2} \times SE(Y_0^{Mean})] \tag{1.12}$$

The resulting 95% confidence band for the regression of HDL on weight, calculated by evaluating (1.12) over the whole range of the covariate, is given in Figure 1.14(a). It

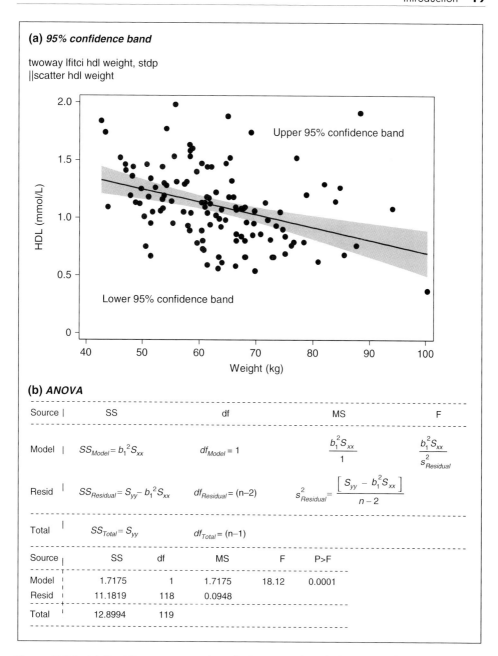

Figure 1.14 (a) Fitted linear regression line of HDL on weight with the 95% confidence band of the predicted mean values indicated by the shaded area. (b) Analysis of Variance (ANOVA) and associated output to check the goodness-of-fit of the simple linear regression model (part data from the Singapore Cardiovascular Cohort Study 2)

should be noted that the intervals bend away from the fitted line as weight moves away from about 65 kg (actually from the mean value 63.15 kg of these subjects) in either direction.

Predicting an individual's value of y for a particular x

In contrast to wanting to estimate the *mean* value of y for a particular x_0, we may wish to *predict* the HDL of an *individual* subject with that weight. Although the corresponding $Y_0^{Individual}$ is the same as the predicted mean $Y_0^{Mean} = b_0 + b_1 x_0$ in this situation, we do not require $SE(Y_0^{Mean})$ but rather the standard deviation, $SD(Y_0^{Individual})$ of the individual values $Y_0^{Individual}$ at that particular value of $x = x_0$. This is given by

$$SD(Y_0^{Individual}) = s_{Residual} \sqrt{1 + \frac{1}{n} + \frac{(x_0 - \bar{x})^2}{S_{xx}}}$$. Thus, the distribution of individuals with weight

x_0 has a mean value of $Y_0^{Individual}$ and (in broad terms) 95% of those of weight x_0 will have a HDL value which will be within the interval

$$Y_0^{Individual} - 1.96 \times SD(Y_0^{Individual}) \tag{1.13}$$

The difference between (1.12) and (1.13) lies in the use of the predicted Y_0. One purpose is to ask: What is the anticipated value of HDL for (say) a patient with weight $x_0 = 50$ kg and how precise is this estimate? The estimate is $Y_0 = 1.7984 - 0.0110 \times 50 = 1.25$ mmol/L and the 95% CI can be calculated using $SE(Y_0^{Mean})$ in equation (1.12) to give 1.16 to 1.34 mmol/L. The other is to ask: What variation about $Y_0 = 1.25$ mmol/L does one expect to see in different patients of the same 50 kg weight? The answer is provided by evaluating equation (1.13) to give the wider interval 0.64 to 1.86 mmol/L.

Analysis of Variance (ANOVA)

As we have seen in Figure 1.5, the ANOVA part of the computer output following the command (**regress hdl weight**) takes the form of Figure 1.14(b), although we have annotated this with some terminology that we have just introduced.

Essentially, ANOVA divides the total sums of squares $SS_{Total} = \sum(y_i - \bar{y})^2$, which represents the total variation of the dependent y-variable for all the subjects concerned, into a part which is explained by the linear model, $SS_{Model} = b_1^2 \sum(x - \bar{x})^2 = b_1^2 S_{xx}$, and that which remains, $SS_{Residual} = S_{yy} - b_1^2 S_{xx}$. The latter is described as the random variation component. If the null hypothesis is true, that is $\beta_1 = 0$, we would then anticipate that b_1 will be close to zero. In this situation $SS_{Model} = b_1^2 S_{xx}$ will be small. To calculate the F-statistic, the sum of squares (SS) for the model and for the residual are each divided by the corresponding degrees of freedom and their ratio obtained. Thus,

$$F = \frac{b_1^2 S_{xx} / df_{Model}}{(S_{yy} - b_1^2 S_{xx}) / df_{Residual}} = \frac{b_1^2 S_{xx} / df_{Model}}{s_{Residual}^2} \tag{1.14}$$

To ascertain the corresponding p-value, statistical tables of the F-distribution are required but these are potentially very extensive as they depend on two sets of degrees of freedom, $df_1 = df_{Model}$ and $df_2 = df_{Residual}$. Thus, only limited tabular entries are reproduced in Table T6. In the example of Figure 1.14(b), $F = \dfrac{1.7175/1}{11.1819/118} = \dfrac{1.7175}{0.0948} = 18.12$ and this has 1 and 118 degrees of freedom. As $df_2 = 118$ is large the tabular entry of infinity (∞) is used, so that with $df_1 = 1$ a value of $F = 6.66$ corresponds to $\alpha = 0.01$ so that we can conclude, as $18.12 > 6.66$, that the p-value < 0.01. However, most statistical packages output the p-value so that the statistical tables are usually unnecessary. In this case a more precise p-value $= 0.0001$ is presented.

In all situations when $df_1 = 1$, that is when only two groups are being compared, the F-test and the t-test of the null hypothesis will give precisely the same p-value. This is because, and only in this situation, the calculated F and the square of the calculated t, that is t^2, are algebraically equivalent. The corresponding t-test will have degrees of freedom equal to df_2 of the F-test. Thus, in the above example, $t = \sqrt{18.12} = 4.26$ with $df = 118$ and Table T4 can therefore in principle be used to obtain the p-value. However, as the degrees of freedom are larger than 30 there is no tabular entry available. All we can deduce from this is that the p-value is less than $\alpha = 0.001$.

In this circumstance, that is when the degrees of freedom of the t-test are large, the t-distribution approaches that of the Normal distribution. Hence the entries of Table T1 can be used to establish the p-value. The largest entry in Table T1 is for $z = 3.99$, with a corresponding two-sided $\alpha = 2(1-0.99997) = 0.00006$. Thus, for the calculated $z = 4.26$ the p-value < 0.00006.

Coefficient of determination

The coefficient of determination, R^2, measures how well a regression model performs as a predictor of y by calculating the variation accounted for by the fitted model as a proportion of the total sums of squares. In the case of a simple linear regression with a single covariate it is calculated as

$$R^2 = \frac{b_1^2 S_{xx}}{S_{yy}} \tag{1.15}$$

and which takes values between 0 and 1. For the example of Figure 1.14(b), this gives $R^2 = 1.7175/12.8994 = 0.13$ or 13%

Extending the simple linear model

Although equations (1.1) and (1.3) refer to the same two-group situation, the simple linear regression format of the latter expression can be more easily extended to describe more complex clinical study designs. Specifically, equation (1.7), the more general form of (1.3), can be extended to include other covariates by relabeling x as x_1 and then adding, for example $\beta_2 x_2$, to the right-hand side. In this extended context it often becomes necessary to use the ANOVA approach to test the relevant null hypotheses.

Correlation

In the situation where we are concerned with more than one continuous covariate, then these may not act independently of each other. For example, when examining variation in HDL one might be concerned whether both body-weight, x_1, and age, x_2, of the individuals play a role. However, the values of such variables may be associated. The strength of the linear association between them is described by the correlation coefficient, ρ, which is estimated by

$$r = \sqrt{\frac{\left[\sum (x_{1i} - \bar{x}_1)(x_{2i} - \bar{x}_2)\right]^2}{\sum (x_{1i} - \bar{x}_1)^2 \sum (x_{2i} - \bar{x}_2)^2}} \tag{1.16}$$

The corresponding test the null hypothesis, H_0: $\rho=0$, is given by

$$t = \frac{r}{\sqrt{\dfrac{1-r^2}{n-2}}} \tag{1.17}$$

If the null hypothesis is true, this has a Student's t-distribution with $df=n-2$, where n is the number of subjects concerned.

In this text we are also concerned with two other applications of the format of equation (1.16). The first is when one wishes to assess the strength of the association between the continuous dependent variable, y, and a continuous covariate x. In such a case, y replaces x_1 while x replaces x_2 in equation (1.16). This is the format which can be used for estimating the correlation between FEV_1 and IFN-λ protein production from the 13 individuals of Example 1.1. The corresponding command is (**pwcorr FEV1 Interpgml**) to give $r=0.6469$. The

test of the null hypothesis, $\rho=0$, of equation (1.17) is $t = \dfrac{0.6469}{\sqrt{\dfrac{1-0.6469^2}{13-2}}} = \dfrac{0.6469}{0.2299} = 2.81$

and use of Table T4 with $df=13-2=11$ gives the p-value<0.02. An even more precise calculation gives p-value$=0.017$.

This is the same result as that which followed the command (**regress   FEV1 Interpgml**) of Figure 1.7, where the increasing slope of $b_{IFN-\lambda}=0.1011$ per unit increase in pg/mL was found to be statistically significant, p-value$=0.017$. This is no coincidence as the test for a null correlation coefficient (H_0: $\rho=0$) is exactly equivalent to that for testing the null hypothesis: H_0: $\beta_{IFN-\lambda}=0$ in this situation.

The other application of the equation (1.16) arises when the dependent variable is measured repeatedly over time on the individuals in the study. For instance, in the clinical trial of Example 1.6, self-reported successive pain assessments are made by the patients with OLP. In this situation, the strength of the association, termed the auto-correlation, between two measures of the *same* variable on *two* occasions, y_1 and y_2, is assessed using equation (1.16) with x_1 and x_2 replaced by y_1 and y_2, respectively. We return to this second application in Chapter 8.

Logarithms and the exponential constant, e

Campbell (2006) provides a clear description of logarithms, some of their properties as well as introducing the exponential constant, and upon which we base our description.

Powers

In the simplest situation, if we define $y=x\times x$, then we can more briefly write this as x^2, which we can describe as x to the power 2 or x-squared. This can be extended to multiplying x by itself n times to give $y=x\times x\times x\times\dots\times x=x^n$.

One result that follows from this is

$$x^m \times x^n = x^{m+n} \tag{1.18}$$

and this holds for *any* values of m and n, not just whole numbers.

One important consequence is that $x^0=1$ because $x^m=x^{0+m}=x^0\times x^m$, and therefore x^0 must equal 1.

The concept of powers can be extended to allow n, m, or both to take fractional and/or negative values. Thus, $y=x^{0.5}$ is equivalent to $y = \sqrt{x}$ the square root of x. This is because $x^{0.5}\times x^{0.5}=x^{0.5+0.5}=x^1=x$ as does the product $\sqrt{x}\times\sqrt{x}=x$.

Further, if $m=1$ and $n=-1$, then $x^{m+n}=x^1\times x^{-1}=x^{1-1}=x^0=1$. Hence $x^1\times x^{-1}=x\times x^{-1}=1$ and so $x^{-1}=1/x$ or the reciprocal of x.

Logarithms

If $y=x^n$, then the definition of a logarithm of y, to what is termed the base of x, is the power that x has to be raised to in order to get y. This is written as $n=\log_x(y)$ or 'n equals the logarithm to the base x of y.'

Suppose $y=x^n$ and $z=x^m$ then $m = \log_y(z)$ and it follows that

$$\log_x(y\times z)=n+m = \log_x(y)+\log_x(z) \tag{1.19}$$

Thus, when multiplying two numbers we add their logarithms. In a similar way if we take the logarithm of a ratio of two numbers we obtain

$$\log_x(y/z)=n-m = \log_x(y)-\log_x(z) \tag{1.20}$$

Thus, when dividing two numbers we subtract their logarithms.

Choosing the base

The two most common bases for logarithms are 10 and the quantity $e=2.718281\dots$, where the dots indicate that the decimals go on indefinitely. This base has the useful property that the slope of the curve $y=e^x$ at any point (x, y) is just y itself, whereas for all other numbers the slope is proportional to y but not equal to it. The formula $y=e^x$ is often written $\exp(x)$ and we will make much use of this form in later chapters. Logarithms to the base e are often denoted '$\log_e$' or more briefly 'log' or 'ln'. We use the form 'log' throughout this book.

The log transformation and the geometric mean

In a study, conducted by Chong, Tay, Subramaniam, *et al.* (2009) of long-term residents of a psychiatric hospital, the variation in the degree of cholinergic medication (*Chol*) received by those in different diagnostic groups was recorded. As shown in Figure 1.15(a), the distribution of the dose of cholinergic medication turns out to have a rather skewed distribution with a median of 9.0 units. However, transforming the data by taking the logarithms of the individual values, so that $LChol=\log(Chol)$, results in the more symmetric distribution of Figure 1.15(b).

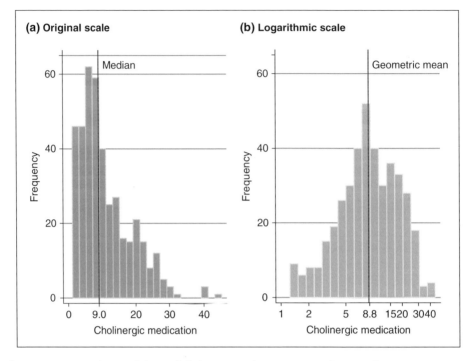

Figure 1.15 Distribution of doses of cholinergic medication given to those resident patients receiving the medication in a psychiatric hospital (a) original scale and (b) after logarithmic transformation (part data from Chong, Tay, Subramaniam, *et al.*, 2009)

It is useful to note that if the logarithm of a variable which takes positive values, $x_1, x_2, \ldots,$ x_n is taken, then the mean of $\log(x_1)$, $\log(x_2)$, ..., $\log(x_n)$ is $\overline{\log x}$, then the antilogarithm of this quantity is the geometric mean, $GM = [x_1 \times x_2 \times \ldots \times x_n]^{1/n}$. The geometric mean obtained from the transformed data of Figure 1.15(b) is 8.8 units, which is close to the median of 9.0 units on the untransformed scale.

2 Linear Regression: Practical Issues

SUMMARY

This chapter describes the different types of covariates that may arise when using regression models and how preliminary screening of these using graphical techniques may be useful. We introduced in Chapter 1 the simple linear regression model, involving a continuous dependent y-variable, and gave examples of the model being fitted to data concerned with binary and continuous covariate situations. Here we describe how an unordered categorical covariate of more than two levels is included in a model by the technique of creating dummy variables. We also include discussion of covariates of ordered categorical and numerically discrete forms. Several methods are described for verifying whether or not a chosen linear model, once fitted to the data, is appropriate for the study concerned. We caution against the use of 'in-house' statistical software and recommend that as simple a model structure as possible is used for summarizing the data collected. Aspects concerned with the choice of study design and subsequent reporting are also included.

TYPES OF COVARIATES (INDEPENDENT VARIABLES)

We indicated in Chapter 1 that the dependent, or y-variable, can take one of several different types with a label used for the variable name which is context specific. This is also the case for the independent variables or covariates (x-variables). Thus, we have introduced gender as a binary x-variable (covariate) which can take only two values usually recorded in the database as 0 or 1. We have also introduced body-weight as a continuous covariate which takes non-negative values.

A typical format when describing the results of a study is to tabulate some basic characteristics of the subjects concerned, as in Figure 2.1. This contains the variable gender which is binary, HDL and body-weight which are continuous, ethnicity (variable *Ethnic*) an unordered categorical variable, together with the ordered categorical variable alcohol consumption (*Drink*). In contrast, current smoking (*Smoke*) status is at least partially ordered as it

Regression Methods for Medical Research, First Edition. Bee Choo Tai and David Machin.
© 2014 Bee Choo Tai and David Machin. Published 2014 by John Wiley & Sons, Ltd.

		HDL (mmol/L)	Male	Female	Total
Gender		n	288	239	527
		mean	1.03	1.27	1.13
		range	0.33–2.54	0.59–2.33	0.33–2.54
Ethnicity	Chinese	n	154	123	277
		mean	1.09	1.37	1.21
		range	0.50–2.54	0.61–2.33	0.50–2.54
	Malay	n	65	55	120
		mean	1.01	1.21	1.10
		range	0.37–1.74	0.59–1.98	0.37–1.98
	Indian	n	69	61	130
		mean	0.91	1.10	1.00
		range	0.33–1.67	0.62–1.92	0.33–1.92
Weight (kg)	<49	n	15	60	75
		mean	1.22	1.48	1.43
		range	0.75–1.69	0.83–2.33	0.75–2.33
	50–74	n	210	159	369
		mean	1.04	1.20	1.11
		range	0.33–2.54	0.59–2.10	0.33–2.54
	≥75	n	63	20	83
		mean	0.93	1.12	0.98
		range	0.37–1.65	0.62–1.99	0.37–1.99
Alcohol consumption	None	n	190	211	401
		mean	1.01	1.24	1.13
		range	0.33–2.54	0.59–2.33	0.33–2.54
	Light	n	58	21	79
		mean	1.11	1.45	1.20
		range	0.57–1.77	0.88–2.10	0.57–2.10
	Moderate	n	17	0	17
		mean	1.01	–	1.01
		range	0.64–1.54	–	0.64–1.54
	Heavy	n	16	6	22
		mean	1.00	1.39	1.10
		range	0.52–1.33	1.03–1.68	0.52–1.68
	Very heavy	n	7	1	8
		mean	0.89	1.35	0.97
		range	0.43–1.44	–	0.43–1.54
Current smoking	None	n	52	38	90
		mean	0.98	1.23	1.09
		range	0.60–1.67	0.64–2.01	0.60–2.01
	Ex	n	7	8	15
		mean	1.14	1.24	1.19
		range	0.50–2.54	0.86–1.51	0.50–2.54
	Light	n	25	10	35
		mean	1.05	1.34	1.13
		range	0.59–1.67	0.97–1.99	0.59–1.99
	Moderate	n	1	4	5
		mean	0.76	1.10	1.03
		range	–	0.64–1.41	0.64–1.41
	Heavy	n	203	179	382
		mean	1.03	1.27	1.14
		range	0.33–1.93	0.59–2.33	0.33–2.33

Figure 2.1   Characteristics of individuals recruited to a study investigating risk factors associated with HDL levels (part data from the Singapore Cardiovascular Cohort Study 2)

ranges from non-smokers to heavy smokers. However, the rank position of the 'ex-smokers' is problematical as this group may comprise a range of light to heavy ex-smokers as well as those who have recently stopped to the quitters who have remained so in the long term.

Ordered categorical covariates

If we were investigating the relationship between HDL levels and self-reported alcohol consumption, one might begin by examining the data with a box-whisker plot using the command (`graph box hdl, over(Drink)`) as in Figure 2.2(a). The central horizontal line of each box represents the median, the upper closure of the box the 75th percentile of the distribution, and those within the whisker are termed adjacent values. The observations that lie beyond the whisker (and there are several in our example) are termed 'outside' values. Beneath the median the lower 25th percentile is indicated and the other values are defined in a similar way to those above the median. Both the box-whisker plot and the table of means and of medians of Figure 2.2(b) suggest a rather shallow inverted U-shaped change in HDL values across the increasing consumption categories.

Figure 2.3 shows the command (`scatter hdl Drink, jitter(5)`) used to obtain a scatter plot of the individual HDL values for each alcohol group. This makes use of the Stata command (`jitter`), which permits the individual observations for each category to be plotted around the integer values of the categorical variable – *Drink*. It does this to facilitate a better visual view of the individual data points. Otherwise, coincident points are overprinted and so cannot be distinguished. The jittering process is only for visual display purposes and plays no role in the computations for the regression equation below.

The corresponding linear model fit added to Figure 2.3 is calculated from the individual data values using the linear model command (`regress hdl Drink`) and gives $b_{Drink} = -0.01636$ with the corresponding p-value$=0.34$. This suggests that the null hypothesis of $H_0: \beta_{Drink}=0$ cannot be discounted with these data. In any event, this is of little surprise, as the fitted line suggests (on

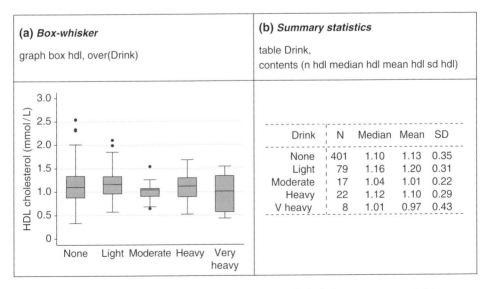

Figure 2.2 (a) Box-whisker plot of HDL levels by reported alcohol consumption and (b) summary statistics (part data from the Singapore Cardiovascular Cohort Study 2)

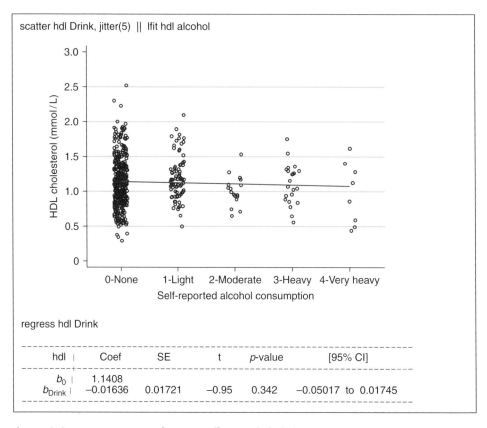

Figure 2.3   Linear regression of HDL on self-reported alcohol consumption regarded as a numerically discrete variable with equal intervals (part data from the Singapore Cardiovascular Cohort Study 2)

average) only a very small decrease in HDL of 0.01636 mmol/L for every increase in alcohol consumption level. Such a small change is unlikely to be of great clinical consequence.

Numerically discrete covariates

We have regarded alcohol consumption in Figure 2.3 as essentially a numerically discrete covariate here taking the integer values 0, 1, 2, 3, and 4. In this case, the corresponding (`lfit`) and (`regress`) commands do not differ from those for a continuous covariate so no modification to the basic command structure is required.

Unordered categorical covariates

We have discussed how to include a binary covariate, such as gender, into a regression model. Suppose, however, that we are concerned with assessing the influence of ethnicity. If only two ethnic groups are involved then the covariate is binary and we have discussed this situation previously. Nevertheless, more than two ethnic groups are possible as in the HDL study in which subjects of Chinese, Malay and Indian ethnicity are included. In many cases, as is the case for *Ethnic* here, these may be coded as '1', '2', and '3' in the database.

(a) *Summary statistics*

tabstat hdl, by(ethnic) stat(n mean sd)

ethnic	N	Mean	SD
Chinese	277	1.2122	0.3407
Malay	120	1.1024	0.3292
Indian	130	0.9975	0.2964
Total	527	1.1343	0.3392

(b) *Inappropriate commands and misleading output*

regress hdl ethnic

hdl	Coef	SE
cons	1.3194	
ethnic	−0.1076	0.0171

regress hdl Newethnic

hdl	Coef	SE
cons	1.2578	
Newethnic	−0.0726	0.0179

Figure 2.4 (a) The mean and standard deviation (SD) of HDL (mmol/L) by ethnic group and (b) inappropriate linear regression commands for analysis (part data from the Singapore Cardiovascular Cohort Study 2)

There is an indication from the corresponding mean HDL levels of Figure 2.4(a) that these differ between the ethnic groups. Superficially, the regress model describing the situation is summarized by $HDL = \beta_0 + \beta_E$ *Ethnic* with an associated command (**regress hdl ethnic**). However, we require that, in whichever way the numerical codes (labels) are chosen for the categories, the different regression analyses arising should all have the same interpretation. Nevertheless, suppose we fit the model using this command then this assumes a linear relation between the HDL and the covariate (in the chosen numerically coded form) concerned. Thus, we would expect to obtain a different answer from this had we ordered the categories alphabetically as Chinese, Indian, Malay and then allocated the codes '1', '2', and '3' to the ethnic groups in that order and used the command (**regress hdl Newethnic**) as in Figure 2.4(b). Thus, superficially, the difference Indian − Chinese = '2 units' if (**ethnic**) is used but is only '1 unit' when defined by (**Newethnic**). The difficulty here is that '1', '2', and '3' are arbitrarily assigned to the categories as convenient labels for the database and are not therefore integers that we can regard as numerically discrete and with which we can do arithmetic computations.

In order to fit a regression model including *Ethnic* as a covariate in an appropriate way, so-called dummy or indicator variables have to be generated to describe the ethnic groups. For our example there are $E = 3$ groups, so we need to construct $E − 1 = 2$ dummy variables v_1 and v_2 as in Figure 2.5(a) where the three ethnic groups correspond to different pairs of values of (v_1, v_2) in the following way. The pair $v_1 = 0$ and $v_2 = 0$ defines Chinese subjects, as the respective values of v indicate (Malay-No, Indian-No). Similarly, the pair $v_1 = 1$ and $v_2 = 0$ defines the Malay, as the v's indicate (Malay-Yes, Indian-No). Finally, the pair $v_1 = 0$ and $v_2 = 1$ defines the Indian (Malay-No, Indian-Yes) group. There is no group corresponding to $v_1 = v_2 = 1$.

The regression model for ethnicity, ignoring all other potential variables, is then written as

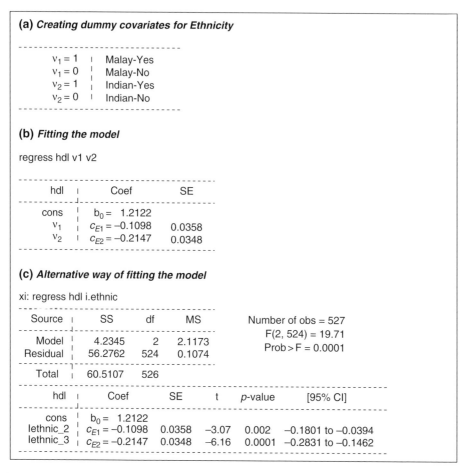

Figure 2.5 (a) Dummy variables created and (b) commands and annotated output for the regression of HDL on ethnic group using dummy variables and (c) by means of modified commands (part data from the Singapore Cardiovascular Cohort Study 2)

$$y = \beta_0 + \gamma_{E1} v_1 + \gamma_{E2} v_2 + \varepsilon \qquad (2.1)$$

In this model, besides β_0, there are two regression coefficients, γ_{E1} and γ_{E2}, and we label their estimates as c_{E1} and c_{E2}. The two coefficients are *both* concerned with describing the influence or otherwise of a *single* variable, here ethnicity.

This model can be fitted using the format of the linear model command for a single covariate by merely replacing the single covariate by two covariates, namely v_1 and v_2. The modified (**regress hdl v1 v2**) command and corresponding output to assess the influence of ethnicity (if any) on HDL levels are shown in Figure 2.5(b).

The fitted model is

$$HDL = 1.2122 - 0.1098 v_1 - 0.2147 v_2 \qquad (2.2)$$

Thus, for example, for those of Chinese ethnicity ($v_1 = 0$ and $v_2 = 0$) the model estimates the mean $HDL_{Chinese} = 1.2122 - (0.1098 \times 0) - (0.2147 \times 0) = 1.2122$ mmol/L, which confirms the mean value given in Figure 2.4(a). For the Malay ($v_1 = 1$ and $v_2 = 0$), the model estimates the mean $HDL_{Malay} = 1.2122 - (0.1098 \times 1) - (0.2147 \times 0) = 1.1024$ mmol/L, and with similar calculations for the Indian to obtain mean $HDL_{Indian} = 0.9975$ mmol/L.

In general, if a categorical variable has G categories, then $G - 1$ dummy variables need to be created for the corresponding covariate terms in a regression model and consequently these $G - 1$ regression coefficients have to be estimated.

All this is a tedious process but it can usually be done more readily in a computer package provided suitable instructions are given. Thus, in situations like this Stata uses the command (**xi:regress i.ethnic**), where (**xi**) indicates that the creation of dummy variables will be required and (**i.ethnic**) indicates that these are for the covariate *Ethnicity*. Essentially the (**i.**) device automatically creates, then uses, the indicator (dummy) variables v_1 and v_2 of Figure 2.5(a) to create the output summarized in Figure 2.5(c).

From the regression outputs of Figure 2.5(b) and (c), we can tell that both the Malays (of magnitude $c_{E1} = -0.1098$, *p*-value$=0.002$) and Indians ($c_{E2} = -0.2147$, *p*-value$=0.0001$) have significantly lower HDL levels compared with the Chinese ($b_0 = 1.2122$). These are based on the individual *t*-statistics of -3.07 and -6.16 provided for the corresponding estimated regression coefficients, but these do not evaluate the *overall* effect of ethnicity on HDL. For this, a global test is required. This is provided by the *F*-test calculated from the ratio of the mean squares (MS) of Figure 2.5(c) and takes a similar format to that described in Figure 1.14(b). Thus, $F = 2.1173/0.1074 = 19.71$.

Even though we are concerned here with the single variable *Ethnicity*, as it requires two parameters to be estimated (γ_{E1} estimated by c_{E1} and γ_{E2} by c_{E2}) for its evaluation the numerator of F has $df_1 = 2$. In such a case, and whenever the numerator $df_1 \geq 2$, tables of the *F*-distribution must be consulted to determine the corresponding *p*-value. However, the usual situation is that the computer package will output this. Thus, we have (**Prob > F = 0.0001**) or, in more familiar, terms a *p*-value$=0.0001$. Further details of the *F*-test for this situation are given in *Technical details*.

The underlying null hypothesis for the *F*-test is that the population means of HDL are the same irrespective of ethnic group. More formally, we state the null hypothesis as H_0: $\mu_{Chinese} = \mu_{Malay} = \mu_{Indian}$. However, if the resulting global test of the influence of ethnicity on HDL is statistically significant, it does not in itself give, for example, any indication of which ethnic group has the highest mean level. As we have already seen, this is found by examination of the table of means in Figure 2.4(a), which shows that the Chinese subjects have the highest and the Indians the lowest, with the Malay taking an intermediate value. In fact, we have to choose which of the following four possible alternative hypotheses reflects the actual situation: $\mu_{Chinese} \neq \mu_{Malay} \neq \mu_{Indian}$; $(\mu_{Chinese} = \mu_{Malay}) \neq \mu_{Indian}$; $\mu_{Chinese} \neq (\mu_{Malay} = \mu_{Indian})$; and $(\mu_{Chinese} = \mu_{Indian}) \neq \mu_{Malay}$.

The preceding paragraph is somewhat circular in nature, but indicates that both a global *F*-test and the individual *t*-tests of the regression coefficients involved may be necessary for a full understanding of the influence of ethnicity on HDL.

An alternative procedure for creating indicator variables such as those of Figure 2.4 is available in Stata by, in this example, using the command (**tabulate(ethnic), generate(ETHNIC)**). As ethnicity has three categories, this command generates three indicator variables ETHNIC1, ETHNIC2, and ETHNIC3 which are created with names in the same order, here Chinese, Malay and Indian, as in the database. For the subsequent regression analysis we can then use any two of these indicator variables. Thus, to produce the same output as Figure 2.5, the command is (**regress hdl ETHNIC2 ETHNIC3**) as we have chosen the Chinese individuals (ETHNIC1) as the reference group.

VERIFYING THE ASSUMPTIONS

As we will point out again, most computer packages implement the instructions given with no regard to how sensible these instructions might be. This applies to the situation of fitting a simple linear regression model for a continuous dependent variable y involving one covariate of either an ordered categorical or continuous form. However, in these cases it is usually quite straightforward to verify by graphical means whether or not the chosen model to fit is an appropriate one.

Ordered categorical covariate

When considering the potential relationship between HDL levels and self-reported alcohol consumption, we examined in Figure 2.2 the profile of change in HDL against increasing alcohol use. This was done by using both a box-whisker plot of the data and a table of median and mean values of HDL for each alcohol consumption category. Further, we then plotted in Figure 2.3 a scatter diagram of the individual HDL and alcohol values. Together, these suggested that a linear regression model seems appropriate to describe these data and consequently such a model was fitted and added to Figure 2.3. In general terms we verified that the model chosen seems reasonable for the situation concerned.

An alternative device in this situation is first to ignore the 'ordered' nature of the categorical covariate concerned. The covariate is then regarded as unordered and can now be modeled in a similar way to equation (2.1), which we used for ethnicity. As there are $G=5$ alcohol (*Drink*) categories, $G-1=4$ indicator variables are created by the computer program and as well as β_0, the regression coefficients, γ_{D1}, γ_{D2}, γ_{D3}, and γ_{D4}, have to be estimated. The corresponding command (**xi: regress hdl i.Drink**), and edited output are given in Figure 2.6. Here the computer program essentially generates the indicator variables *IDrink_1*, *IDrink_2*, to *IDrink_5*, but omits *IDrink_1* from the calculations.

From this we see that for the category 'None' the mean HDL is estimated by $b_0=1.1320$, whereas for 'Light' the mean is raised to $(b_0+c_{D1})=1.1320+0.0648=1.1968$ and for 'Very heavy' it is lower at $(b_0+c_{D4})=1.1320-0.1582=0.9738$. These are confirmed by the mean values in Figure 2.2. In general terms there appears to be no clear pattern in the estimated regression coefficients (c_{D1}, c_{D2}, c_{D3}, and c_{D4}), and, further, they seem relatively small when compared with their corresponding standard errors. Both suggest that there is unlikely to be a strong relationship between HDL and alcohol consumption, but nevertheless confirm that

```
xi: regress hdl i.Drink
```

Alcohol category		hdl Coef	SE
None	cons (b_0)	1.1320	
Light	IDrink_2 (c_{D1})	0.0648	0.0416
Moderate	IDrink_3 (c_{D2})	−0.1214	0.0838
Heavy	IDrink_4 (c_{D3})	−0.0274	0.0741
Very heavy	IDrink_5 (c_{D4})	−0.1582	0.1208

Figure 2.6 Regression of HDL on i.Drink (part data from the Singapore Cardiovascular Cohort Study 2)

a linear model may be appropriate to describe this 'weak' relation. Thus, it is reasonable to use the linear regression command (**regress hdl Drink**) to describe the relationship. As we have noted before, the output of Figure 2.3 fails to reject the null hypothesis H_0: $\beta_{Drink} = 0$ as $t = b_{Drink}/SE(b_{Drink}) = -0.01636/0.01721 = -0.95$, p-value $= 0.34$. Hence, we would conclude that alcohol consumption does not play an important role in HDL levels.

Had there been a strong but non-linear pattern in the coefficients (c_{D1}, c_{D2}, c_{D3}, and c_{D4}), perhaps markedly positive values for (c_{D1} and c_{D2}) and markedly negative for (c_{D3} and c_{D4}), then this would imply a strong inverted U-shaped relationship between HDL and increasing alcohol consumption levels. Such a pattern is clearly non-linear, and, hence, a simple linear regression model would not be appropriate to describe such a situation.

Continuous covariate

Residuals

One method of checking whether or not a linear regression model is appropriate is first to fit the model and then examine if there are any patterns in the residuals about the fitted line. In general, the residuals, ε, of equation (1.5) are defined by $\varepsilon = y - (\beta_0 + \beta_1 x_1)$. Thus, from the n subjects concerned, the residual for an individual subject i, with observation values (x_{1i}, y_i), is the vertical distance between y_i and the predicted value ($\beta_0 + \beta_1 x_{1i}$). In practice, as we do not know β_0 and β_1, but only their estimates b_0 and b_1, we can only estimate the residual by $e_i = y_i - Y_i$ where $Y_i = (b_0 + b_1 x_{1i})$.

A useful initial check for linearity is to fit a linear regression model and superimpose this fit onto a scatter diagram of the data as for the regression of HDL on weight (w) of Figure 1.4(b). One can then visually examine the vertical distance of each data point from the fitted line. These are the residuals as we have just defined, but the individual values are not calculated only judged by the analyst. If there appears to be a pattern in the residuals, for example, positive values occurring when the x's are small and also when they are large, with negative values in the intermediate range, then one would suspect a model with some curvature might better describe the situation. In our example, the scatter in Figure 1.4(b) about the fitted line appears about the same over the whole range of body-weights from 40 to 100 kg. There is no striking pattern in the residuals about the line HDL $= 1.7984 - 0.0110\ w$, and so this chosen model seems justified.

Rather than using visual means, the residuals, $e_i = \text{HDL}_i - 1.7984 - 0.0110\ w_i$, can be calculated for all the subjects concerned and these then plotted against w_i. The command (**pre-dict ResidWght, residual**) of Figure 2.7 calculates the residuals after fitting the linear model and saves these values (in a variable labeled *ResidWght*) in the database. If there is a discernible relationship between them then, depending on the type of pattern observed, this may indicate a lack of linearity of the relationship between *HDL* and w. The scatter plot of Figure 2.7, with a horizontal line added at $e = 0$, suggests there is no clear trend in the residuals over the whole range of weights from 40 to 100 kg. Nevertheless, there is a suggestion of more large positive residuals ($e > 0.50$) than large negative ones ($e < -0.50$).

In general, we would anticipate the distribution of the residuals to be approximately Normal and, hence, be symmetric about zero. Thus, a more extreme pattern of the type observed here would suggest that a Normal distribution may not be the case. In such a situation, and using this example for illustration only, setting $y = \log(\text{HDL})$ as the dependent variable rather than $y = \text{HDL}$ might be more appropriate for establishing a linear relation.

Although we did not specifically mention this earlier, it is assumed when fitting a linear model that the scatter, hence the standard deviation (σ) of the points y, at every value of the covariate x, has the same underlying value irrespective of the value of x. However, it

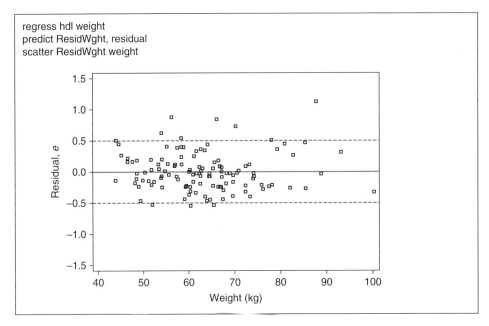

```
regress hdl weight
predict ResidWght, residual
scatter ResidWght weight
```

Figure 2.7   Scatter plot of residuals against weight; residuals obtained after fitting the regression line of HDL on weight as illustrated in Figure 1.4 (part data from the Singapore Cardiovascular Cohort Study 2)

sometimes happens that when a small x is predicting a small y, the residual is much smaller than the residual when a large x is predicting a large y. To examine if this is the case, a plot of the residuals e_i against the fitted values Y_i is made. If in this plot the residuals appear to get larger with increasing values of Y_i, then the assumption that the prediction error is unrelated to the predicted value clearly cannot hold. If this is the case, then one may attempt to remedy the situation by using a transformation of the y-variable, perhaps using the logarithm of y, and then repeat both the calculation of the regression line and the plot to see if this improves the situation. As Figure 2.8 illustrates, the command **residual versus fit plot (rvfplot)** is used to obtain the necessary scatter plot. There appears to be no consistent change in the estimated residuals, e, as the fitted values, Y, increase in this example. However, we note again the suggestion of more large positive residuals ($e > 0.5$) than large negative ones ($e < -0.5$).

We have already indicated that the residuals plotted in Figures 2.7 and 2.8 may not conform to a Normal distribution. However, the requirement of a Normal distribution for the residuals, does not imply that the y's themselves must also have a Normal distribution, or even that y must be a continuous variable. This is because even if the dependent variable is numerically discrete, perhaps a 4-point rating scale with values confined to 0, 1, 2 and 3 only to indicate the levels of pain experienced with OLP, when this y is related to some x-covariate by means of linear regression it may give residuals about that line that follow a Normal distribution. In which case, the use of linear regression for modeling purposes would be appropriate even though the y is clearly not a continuous variable and so will not itself have a Normal distribution form.

One method of checking the Normal distribution assumption of the residuals is to construct the histogram of these residuals as in Figure 2.9, and the corresponding best-fit Normal distribution is then added to this histogram. It is clear from this that the residuals are centered near 0, although their distribution is not entirely that of the idealized Normal distribution.

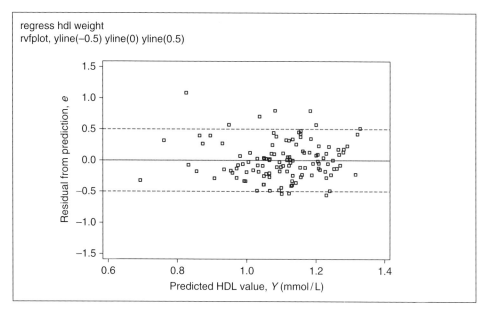

Figure 2.8 Scatter plot of residuals against Y the predicted or fitted values of HDL calculated from the regression line illustrated in Figure 1.4 (part data from the Singapore Cardiovascular Cohort Study 2)

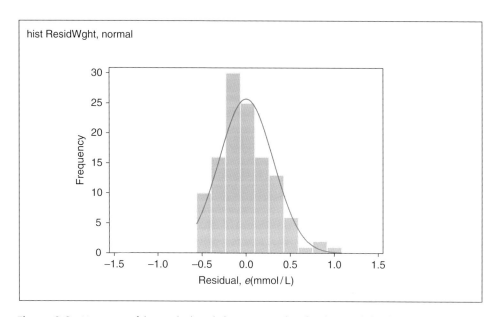

Figure 2.9 Histogram of the residuals with the corresponding fitted Normal distribution (part data from the Singapore Cardiovascular Cohort Study 2)

A further method of verifying Normality is to plot the residuals against their ordered Normal scores, which we define in *Technical details*. More commonly, this is also known as the Q-Q plot, as it compares the quantile values of one distribution against those of another. If the residual assumption with regards to Normality is valid, then we expect the points in

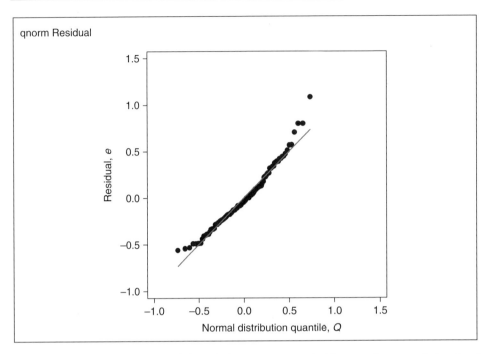

qnorm Residual

Figure 2.10   Scatter plot of residuals from the linear regression of HDL on weight against their ordered Normal scores (part data from the Singapore Cardiovascular Cohort Study 2)

the Q-Q plot to lie approximately on the line, $e=Q$. In Figure 2.10, we plot the residuals for the linear regression of HDL on weight against the standardized Normal distribution values.

It is apparent that the bulk of the points plausibly lie along the 45° straight line with some departure at each end. It is quite common to see some suggestion of a departure from linearity in these plots at the extremes but, provided the departures are not too marked and/or comprise a relatively small proportion of subjects, they can be ignored. For practical purposes we may conclude that the residuals have an approximately Normal distribution in this example.

Another concern is whether there are any 'influential' observations – essentially those which, if omitted from the calculations, fundamentally change the interpretation of the study. If we confine our attention to the eight healthy individuals without asthma included in Figure 1.7 from the data provided by Busse, Lemanske Jr and Gern (2010), then we obtain the scatter plot and fitted linear regression line of Figure 2.11(a). However, if we exclude the individual with INF-λ=68.6, and FEV$_1$ = -18.32, the corresponding fitted line in Figure 2.11(b) is somewhat different from that shown previously. This one outlier observation is certainly influential in this very small data set.

Such an extreme distortion is very unlikely when examining a larger data set, but nevertheless may arise. For example, if, for some reason, the data cluster into two or more distinct parts, that is, the scatter plot consists of separated clouds of points, then including distant clouds in the same linear model may suggest a relationship across these clouds even though no relationship between y and the covariate x is apparent within each of the clouds. In the full data described by Busse, Lemanske Jr and Gern (2010), as shown in Figure 1.7, there are essentially two clouds, although there is some overlap: one comprising the asthmatic and the other the healthy subjects. This raises further concern with respect to the final interpretation of these data.

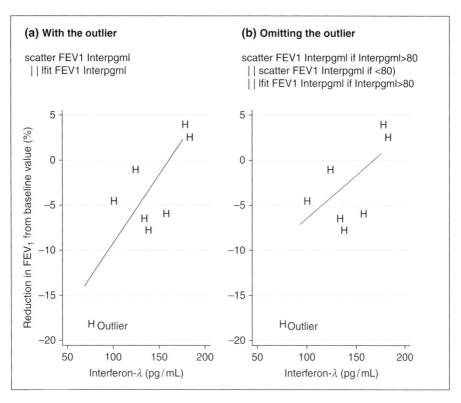

Figure 2.11 Regression of FEV$_1$ against interferon-λ in (a) eight healthy individuals and (b) excluding the outlier observation (data extracted from Busse, Lemanske Jr and Gern, 2010, Figure 6)

Another assumption made when fitting a linear regression model is that the value of an observation made on one subject does not influence that which will be reported for another. That is, we assume the observations are independent. In which case, it follows that the magnitude and sign (positive or negative) of their residuals, calculated from the eventual model fitted to all the data, will be independent also. One situation where the assumption of independence is violated is when differing numbers of observations are made on the n individuals that participate in the study, but then all the O $(>n)$ recorded observations are treated in the same way in the modeling process.

Thus, suppose one individual recruited to the study in question is inadvertently entered twice and therefore has two measurements of HDL and weight. We might not expect the exact same values of HDL and weight to be recorded on the two separate occasions (as these tend to fluctuate even on a daily basis) but one might anticipate they would not be too far distant. For example, if the subject who weighs 100.3 kg in Figure 1.4(b) with a HDL of 0.37 mmol/L and a residual of −0.33 is entered again, then we would anticipate the second assessment measure to give a HDL close to 0.37 and so again anticipate a negative value for the corresponding residual. The two sets of observations are clearly not independent.

Additionally, in the situation of repeat observations on some individuals, the study size may be regarded (incorrectly) as the larger number of observation points, O, recorded within the corresponding scatter plot, rather than the actual number of individuals, n, providing data. As $O > n$ this may then lead to incorrect estimates of the regression coefficients and their corresponding standard errors.

If repeated measurements are made on subjects as part of the study design, for example the visual analog scale (VAS) recording of pain by patients with oral lichen planus (OLP) in the clinical trial of Example 1.6, then the methods associated with Chapter 8 have to be invoked.

A further circumstance in which observations on individuals may not be independent of each other is when the observations are ordered in time in some way. For example, suppose in an investigation of the association of HDL and body-weight, blood samples are taken from the study participants and these are then sent in batches to the laboratory for HDL determination. In this case some batch-to-batch variation may be anticipated. If the residuals are then calculated from the resulting linear regression of HDL on weight of all the individuals concerned, then one might anticipate some pattern in the residuals if we noted the particular laboratory batch from which each observation arose.

In our situation, each measure of HDL, and the associated covariates, is made on individual patients. There are no data that come from measuring HDL in a patient on a subsequent occasion. In general, where we have a single y-measurement on separate individuals, then there is no problem with the lack of independence as there is no reason to suppose that measurements made on one individual are likely to affect a different individual.

Do the assumptions matter?

Some judgment is required when deciding how far the assumptions underlying the model fitted can be 'stretched' without misleading conclusions arising as a consequence. Thus, a *serious* departure from the assumptions, if ignored, has important consequences on the way we interpret the study concerned. In contrast, a departure that is *not serious* makes little or no impact on how a study is interpreted.

As we have demonstrated, and almost by definition, the presence of outliers will usually influence the final interpretation so that they are also referred to as *influential* observations. Should such a situation occur, then the report of the study must contain details of how the investigators dealt with the particular problem. Such a report might contrast the results obtained with and without the outlier(s) concerned included in the analysis.

The lack of linearity can also be serious, and its presence would suggest the need for either a transformation of y before fitting the regression equation on x, or an alternative (more complex) model possibly involving quadratic (squared) terms of x and/or possibly the need to consider the influence of other covariates.

Lack of independence of the residuals can also be serious if the data include a large proportion of individuals for whom repeated y-measures (especially those with the same fixed value of the covariate x) are included.

On the other hand, lack of Normality of the residuals is unlikely to seriously affect the estimates of the parameters of the regression model, although it may affect their standard errors and hence the size of the p-values in the associated tests of significance. Similarly, a lack of constant standard deviation of the residuals is unlikely to seriously affect the estimates, but again will have some influence on the final p-value. In either case, the advice would be to proceed with caution particularly if a marginally statistically significant or non-significant regression coefficient is obtained.

PRECAUTIONS

Computation

All the methods we describe in this text require that the associated models are fitted using a computer package of some form. Technically, some calculations could be made using only a calculating machine, but, in general, we would advise against this. Specifically, software packages should be used so as to minimize the risk of error in the calculations but also to ensure that others could easily verify the calculations if necessary. In some aspects of clinical trial work, this verification process is a regulatory requirement of the relevant supervisory authorities in any event. Further, it is usually not advisable to develop in-house programs for analysis purposes as, if for no other reason, this may take considerable time. Furthermore, such programs may also lack important features contained in the available software packages.

However, it is important to note that the software packages implement the commands of the user and will, in our context, usually fit whichever model is specified to describe the data even if totally inappropriate for the situation. Consequently, extreme care is needed in assessing what is appropriate for the study concerned.

Simple models

In general, simple models are preferable to complex ones as they are usually more straightforward to interpret. In several places we have suggested that modeling $\log(y)$ rather than y itself (although this will be very context specific) may help to linearize the relationship of the underlying dependent variable with the covariate x. If appropriate, the linear model resulting from the transformation is then easier to describe and interpret than a more complex model derived possibly using one of the methods that we introduce in Chapter 3. However, the gain achieved on the logarithmic scale is somewhat offset by greater complexity on the original measurement scale. Thus, if the fitted line is $\log_y = b_0 + b_1 x_1$ then on the original scale $y = \exp(b_0 + b_1 x_1)$, and, consequently, this is a more complex model to describe. In general, we would choose between the alternatives by examining scatter plots of the basic data and of the residuals obtained from the alternative models.

STUDY DESIGN

In the case of a simple linear regression model, the main purpose of the analysis is to test the null hypothesis, H_0: $\beta_1 = 0$. We have shown in Chapter 1, *Technical details* that this is done by using the t-test of equation (1.10) with the appropriate degrees of freedom, df. Key components of this calculation are, n, the number of subjects concerned, b_1, the estimate of β_1 obtained after fitting the model, and the standard error, $SE(b_1) = \dfrac{s_{Residual}}{\sqrt{\sum(x - \bar{x})^2}}$. The standard error has two component parts: $s_{Residual}$ and $\sum(x - \bar{x})^2$. Here $s_{Residual}$ is the estimate of the corresponding population standard deviation, σ, the value of which is, as is the case also for β_1, a feature of the study population and is not under control of the planning team.

However, at the planning stage of the study the design team will be aware that as $\sum(x-\overline{x})^2$ is in the denominator, the larger this is, the smaller will be the resultant $SE(b_1)$. Thus, in circumstances where the investigators can control the choice of the covariate, x, then, to a greater or lesser extent, they can influence the statistical efficiency of the study.

For a given number of observations, n, $\sum(x-\overline{x})^2$ is at its maximum if half the observations are taken with one value of the covariate say, x_{Low} and the other half at x_{High}. It is further increased by increasing the size of the difference $(x_{High} - x_{Low})$. This implies that the investigators should compare only two alternatives and make these as different as possible. Thus, the covariate is under the direct control of the investigating team. For example, in a clinical trial this suggests comparing a zero dose (placebo) against the highest possible dose of the drug under test. These options are then randomly allocated to the patients who are recruited to the trial. However, this design omits testing the drug at intermediate values and so prevents the possibility of investigating a dose-response profile.

In other contexts, there may be little control over the individual covariate values associated with those who are recruited to the study. Nevertheless, the design team may be able to influence the range of values in an indirect way. For example, in a study to investigate the relationship of HDL and body-weight, the investigators should avoid restricting recruitment to (say) long-distance runners but select a group to study which is likely to include individuals with as wide a range of body-weights as is reasonable.

CLINICAL AND STATISTICAL SIGNIFICANCE

In Figure 1.2 we calculated that the mean HDL was 0.2050 mmol/L greater in the females than in the males with corresponding 95% CI 0.0910 to 0.3190 mmol/L and p-value$=0.0005$, thereby demonstrating a very statistically significant result. Similarly, in Figure 1.5 the estimated regression coefficient, b_W, indicated a decline of 0.0110 mmol/L (95% CI 0.0059 to 0.0161, p-value$=0.0001$) for every 1 kg increase in body-weight of the subjects. However, it is important to determine whether a 'statistically significant' result is also clinically important and so may be described as 'clinically significant'.

A 'clinically significant' finding is one that is likely to make a real (clinical) impact. For example, if the difference in efficacy between two treatments, as established by a 'statistically significant' randomized clinical trial, is large then if the better of the two treatments is given to all future patients this will have clinical impact. It is therefore also a 'clinically significant' result.

However, differences do not necessarily have to be large to be clinically important. Thus, in certain circumstances, even small differences that are firmly established ('statistically significant') may have clinical impact. For example, the role of aspirin in reducing the risk of second attacks in patients who have suffered a myocardial infarction is not dramatic, but the modest benefit gained through its widespread use has been shown to save many lives annually as the disease is common. Hence, although the effect for an individual is small, that is proportionally few will be saved from a second attack, the result is of considerable 'clinical significance' to the population at large.

However, a 'statistically significant' result does not automatically imply a clinically important consequence of that result. For example, suppose we demonstrate that a new therapy provides a small but statistically significant improvement in survival over the standard therapy. However, the new therapy is so toxic, difficult to administer and costly that the small improvement in survival is not sufficient to make it clinically worthwhile to use the new therapy in patients. Consequently, the trial has produced a 'statistically significant' result of little 'clinical significance'.

It is also necessary to appreciate that one should not always dismiss a result that is 'not statistically significant' as therefore 'not clinically important'. A study may be too small to reliably estimate an important difference between two groups. For example, the estimate of the difference may be large, but nevertheless the 95% CI includes the null hypothesis value of no difference. In turn the p-value will be large (> 0.05) and therefore the result regarded as not statistically significant. In this situation the study may provide an estimate of the large difference, which, had it been reliably demonstrated, would have had important clinical or scientific consequences. In such circumstances a repeat of the study, perhaps in a larger group of subjects, might be undertaken to firmly establish or not this seemingly important finding.

REPORTING

It is of fundamental importance when one is reporting the completed study that this should always contain clear details of the specific objectives, the rationale for the design chosen, technical aspects of the statistical procedures used, as well as clear and unambiguous statements concerning the study outcomes and the associated conclusions. In general, the relevant details will be study specific and there may well be other issues that should be added to the list.

In the context of a study involving an investigation similar to that of the possible relationship between HDL and body-weight, whenever possible, a graphical presentation of the data should be included. If this can be in the form of a scatter plot, then the corresponding linear model (if that is the final one chosen) should be superimposed. This will facilitate understanding by the potential reader and usually ease the description of the study results for the author. In addition, the estimate of the slope of the line (b_1) together with the (conventionally) 95% confidence interval, and p-value should be reported.

However, prior to the results section of the report, sufficient detail of the chosen design should be given, and (if appropriate) a sketch of the methods used to confirm that the model chosen is justified. Particular attention should be given to how any outlier observations are dealt with. It is also important to reference the statistical software package that was used for analysis.

TECHNICAL DETAILS

Global tests

The F-test is commonly used as a global test to see if the fitted statistical model accounts for an important part of the variation in y. In the case of simple linear regression, it does this by comparing the residual variation obtained after fitting the chosen model containing a single covariate with that obtained from the null model omitting the covariate. If the model helps to describe the pattern in the data, then less (residual) variation should be apparent than for the null model.

In Figure 1.14(b) we described the situation when the covariate model involves only two parameters, β_0 and β_1, and consequently for which $df_{Model} = 1$, and $df_{Residual} = n - 2$. More generally, $df_{Model} = q$ and $df_{Residual} = n - q - 1$, where q corresponds to the number of extra parameters additional to β_0 that have to be estimated in the covariate model.

In the example of Figure 2.5(b), the dummy variable for ethnicity, v_1 and v_2, and the associated parameters γ_{E1} and γ_{E2} hence $q = 2$. Further, the degrees of freedom for the residual equal the number of observations concerned minus the number of parameters of the covariate model, here β_0, γ_{E1} and γ_{E2}. Thus, $df_{Residual}=n-2-1=524$. The corresponding p-value can be obtained directly from tables of the F-distribution. However, the nearest entry in Table T6 for $df_{Model}=2$ and $df_{Residual}=524$ is $df_1=2$ and $df_2=\infty$, which gives for $\alpha=0.01$, $F=4.63$. As the observed $F=19.71$ is much greater than this, all we can say by using the table is that the p-value <0.01. However, the computer output indicates the actual p-value $=0.0001$.

Ordered Normal scores

The Normal scores are the hypothetical values that one would anticipate if the study involved a sample from a mathematically defined standard Normal distribution with mean 0 and standard deviation 1. For example, if the study size was $n=9$ subjects with observations (x_1, y_1), (x_2, y_2), ... (x_9, y_9), then, after the regression line is fitted, the residuals e_1, e_2, ... e_9 can be calculated. These are then placed in numerical order (ranked) from smallest to largest and redenoted $e_{(1)}$, $e_{(2)}$, ... , $e_{(9)}$.

Following this, the successive values of $z_{(i)}=\Phi^{-1}[i/(n+1)]$ are obtained from the Normal distribution of Table T1. The superscript '–1' here indicates finding the value of z for which the probability is $q_i=[i/(n+1)]$. These are determined by setting $\gamma=q_i$ in Table T1. For example, if $i=9$, $q_9=0.9$, then the nearest entries in Table T1 to 0.9 are 0.89973 and 0.90147 when z is 1.28 and 1.29, respectively. More precisely, $z_{(9)}=1.2816$. Working in a similar way gives $z_{(8)}=0.8416$, $z_{(7)}=0.5244$, $z_{(6)}=0.2533$, $z_{(5)}=0$. As the Normal distribution is symmetric about 0, it follows that $z_{(4)}=-0.2533$, $z_{(3)}=-0.5244$, $z_{(2)}=-0.8416$ and $z_{(1)}=-1.2816$. Each of these is then multiplied by $s_{Residual}$ obtained from the $ANOVA$ for the fitted model to give $Q_{(i)}=s_{Residual}\times z_{(i)}$. The pairs $(Q_{(1)}, e_{(1)})$, $(Q_{(2)}, e_{(2)})$, ... , $(Q_{(10)}, e_{(10)})$ are then plotted. Deviations from linearity in this plot, particularly when they are close to the centre, indicate a lack of Normality of the residuals.

3 Multiple Linear Regression

SUMMARY

This chapter extends the simple linear regression model to the situation where two or more covariates are necessary to describe the study design and the consequent analysis. In particular we depict models that may be appropriate for non-linear situations and those that allow for the possible influence of the interaction between two covariates. We describe how these models are fitted and whether they may or may not be regarded as providing an adequate description of the data. We stress the desirability of using parsimonious (those with few covariates and a simple structure) models to describe the essence of the study results. We emphasize that simple models can best be compared with more complex ones if they are nested within them. Problems associated with collinearity of covariates are detailed.

LINEAR REGRESSION: TWO COVARIATES

In Chapter 1 we introduced two simple linear regression models to test the level of HDL changes with respect to gender in equation (1.3) and body-weight in (1.4). In general such models are expressed by

$$y = \beta_0 + \beta_1 x_1 + \varepsilon \tag{3.1}$$

Plotted on a graph, β_0 is the value of the equation when $x_1 = 0$, and is termed the *intercept*. This is where the straight line cuts the y-axis. The coefficient β_1 is the *slope* of the line so that when x_1 increases by one unit, y will change by β_1 units. In the first case, x_1 of equation (3.1) was *Gender* taking the binary values 0 or 1, whereas, in the second, x_1 was the continuous variable *Weight* taking values between 40 and 100 kg. Thus, Figure 1.6(b) suggested a gradually decreasing HDL with increasing weight, but at a higher level, and a greater declining rate for females compared with males. We also showed that whether taking note of gender alone or of weight alone, each left a considerable amount of unexplained variation in HDL levels. Such considerations suggest that a model may be required that includes both *Gender* and *Weight* as covariates.

Regression Methods for Medical Research, First Edition. Bee Choo Tai and David Machin.
© 2014 Bee Choo Tai and David Machin. Published 2014 by John Wiley & Sons, Ltd.

In general, this leads us to consider a multiple linear regression equation of the form:

$$y = \beta_0 + \beta_1 x_1 + \beta_2 x_2 + \varepsilon \tag{3.2}$$

where x_1 is the first and x_2 is the second of the covariates; often called 'independent' variables, but we avoid the use of that terminology. In specific terms this equation would be expressed as:

$$HDL = \beta_0 + \beta_{Gender} Gender + \beta_{Weight} Weight + \varepsilon$$

or more succinctly by

$$HDL = \beta_0 + \beta_G G + \beta_W W + \varepsilon \tag{3.3}$$

Figure 3.1(b) gives the appropriate statistical command (**regress hdl gender weight**) required to fit model (3.3) and the corresponding output. These are preceded in Figure 3.1(a) by the command (**regress hdl gender**) to give the same output as for Figure 1.3 and (**regress hdl weight**) to give that of Figure 1.5.

As we have seen earlier, Figure 3.1(a) gives $b_G = 0.2050$ mmol/L as the difference in mean values between males and females and $b_w = -0.0110$, which corresponds to a decline

---

(a) *Linear regression – single covariates*

regress hdl gender

hdl	Coef	SE	t	P>|t|	[95% CI]
cons	$b_0 = 1.0085$	0.0390			
gender	$b_G = 0.2050$	0.0576	3.56	0.0005	0.0910 to 0.3190

regress hdl weight

hdl	Coef	SE	t	P>|t|	[95% CI]
cons	$b_0 = 1.7984$	0.1659			
weight	$b_w = -0.0110$	0.0026	-4.26	0.0001	-0.0161 to -0.0059

(b) *Multiple regression – two covariates*

regress hdl gender weight

hdl	Coef	SE	t	P>|t|	[95% CI]
cons	$b_0 = 1.6216$	0.1729			
gender	$b_G = 0.1588$	0.0563	2.82	0.0056	0.0474 to 0.2703
weight	$b_w = -0.0094$	0.0026	-3.63	0.0004	-0.0145 to -0.0043

Figure 3.1   Edited commands and output for the linear regression models of HDL on (a) individually gender and weight, and (b) the multiple regression model including gender and weight (part data from the Singapore Cardiovascular Cohort Study 2)

in HDL of 0.0110 mmol/L for every 1 kg increase in weight among the subjects. However, once both *Gender* and *Weight* are included in the multiple regression model the corresponding regression coefficients, that is $b_G = 0.1588$ and $b_W = -0.0094$, differ from their previous values. In this example the difference between the values for b_W is quite small but the estimate b_G is reduced quite considerably by almost 25% ($0.1588/0.2050 = 0.77$). There are also different estimates of b_0. There would be no change in the estimates of the regression coefficients if the 'independent' variables were truly independent. In practice there is usually some degree of association between the 'independent variables' in a multiple regression and so, as we indicated earlier, we would rather refer to such variables as covariates, although the misleading terminology 'independent variables' remains in common use.

We also note that the standard errors associated with the covariates *Gender* and *Weight* alter between the single-covariate models and the two-covariate model. These, in turn, alter the *t*-test statistics and the corresponding *p*-values to some extent.

HOW GOOD IS THE FITTED MODEL?

A critical question when fitting a statistical model is whether or not it describes the data adequately. One step that we have taken, when considering the adequacy of a model, uses the analysis of variance (*ANOVA*) as described in Chapter 1, *Technical details*, and included in Figure 1.5. We also introduced some procedures in Chapter 2 which essentially entail examining the estimated residuals obtained after fitting the model concerned. These methods are equally relevant here, although the required action, should a 'pattern' indicating non-linearity emerge, is often less clear.

In general, there is usually more to the computer output associated with each of the three fitted models of Figure 3.1 than we have actually shown. Thus, extra detail is added in Figure 3.2 for two models describing HDL; one concerned with gender alone, the second gender and weight. The extra detail enables us to assess the adequacy of, in this case, two alternative models for the same data.

As noted earlier when describing Figure 3.1, the estimated regression coefficients for b_0 and b_G differ between Figures 3.2(a) and 3.2(b). This reflects the fact that gender and body-weight are in some way associated. Nevertheless, the statistical significance of gender remains in the second model but with a *p*-value increased from 0.0005 to 0.0056, and the 'statistical significance' is thereby reduced. Further, the *t*-test for the regression coefficient for weight in the latter model, $b_W = -0.0094$, is also statistically significant, *p*-value = 0.0004. Together, these suggest that differences in gender and weight between individuals both contribute to explaining the variation in HDL.

In Figure 3.2 each of the fitted models is preceded by an analysis of variance (*ANOVA*), which is designed to test whether the model has explained an important part of the variation in HDL. As we explained earlier, this technique partitions the total variation in *y*, namely $SS_{Total} = S_{yy} = \sum (y - \bar{y})^2$, into one part, which is explained by the fitted model (SS_{Model}), and the other of what remains ($SS_{Residual}$).

The $SS_{Model} = 1.2519$ in Figure 3.2(a) has increased to $SS_{Model} = 2.4308$ in Figure 3.2(b). This latter quantity can be split into two components equal to (i) 1.2519 from the first model and (ii) 1.1789 added to this for the second model. There are now $df_1 = 2$ degrees of freedom for the second model, an increase of 1 over the first. There is a corresponding decrease of $SS_{Residual}$ from 11.6475 to 10.4686, a difference of 1.1789, and the degrees of freedom has

(a) Simple (1-covariate) linear regression

regress hdl gender

ANOVA and fitted model

Source	SS	df		MS	F	P>F
Model	1.2519	1		1.2519	12.68	0.0005
Residual	11.6475	118	$s^2_{Residual}$ = 0.0987			
Total	12.8994	119				

In the above SS represents the sum of squares. The mean square (MS) is obtained by dividing SS by the corresponding degrees of freedom, df. F is then the ratio of the MS from the Model to that of the Residual. These details repeat those given in **Figure 1.14(b)**.

hdl	Coef	SE	t	P>|t|	[95% CI]
cons	$b_0 = 1.0085$	0.0390			
gender	$b_G = 0.2050$	0.0576	3.56	0.0005	0.0910 to 0.3190

(b) Multiple (2-covariate) linear regression

regress hdl gender weight

ANOVA and fitted model

Source	SS	df		MS	F	P>F
Model	2.4308	2		1.2154	13.58	0.0001
Residual	10.4686	117	$s^2_{Residual}$ = 0.0895			
Total	12.8994	119				

hdl	Coef	SE	t	P>|t|	[95% CI]
cons	$b_0 = 1.6216$	0.1729			
gender	$b_G = 0.1588$	0.0563	2.82	0.0056	0.0474 to 0.2703
weight	$b_W = -0.0094$	0.0026	-3.63	0.0004	-0.0145 to -0.0043

(c) No covariate (null or empty model) linear regression

regress hdl

ANOVA and fitted model

Source	SS	df		MS
Residual	12.8994	119	$s^2_{Residual}$ = 0.1084	

hdl	Coef	SE
cons	1.1024	0.0301

Figure 3.2 Edited commands and output for (a) the linear regression of HDL on gender, (b) the multiple regression on gender and weight and (c) the null or empty model (part data from the Singapore Cardiovascular Cohort Study 2)

been reduced by $118 - 117 = 1$. The test, equation (3.10), of whether the 2-covariate model improves the fit to the data over the 1-covariate model is calculated as

$$F = \frac{(2.4308 - 1.2519)/(2-1)}{10.4686/(120-3)} = \frac{1.1789/1}{10.4686/117} = \frac{1.1789}{0.0895} = 13.17$$

As we explained in Chapter 1, *Technical details*, because this is based on $df_1 = 1$ in the numerator, $t = \sqrt{F} = \sqrt{13.17} = 3.63$ can be used to determine the *p*-value. In addition, as the degrees of freedom for the denominator is large, the *z*-distribution can replace that of *t*. Hence, from Table T1 with $z = 3.63$, the *p*-value $= 2\,(1 - 0.99986) = 0.00028$. This is very small indeed, and so we conclude that adding weight to the single covariate model for gender alone improves the fit to these data.

For the model with *Gender* alone, the coefficient of determination of equation (1.15) is $R^2 = 1.2519/12.8994 = 0.0971$ or 10%, whereas when *Gender* and *Weight* are both included it is increased to $R^2 = 2.4308/12.8994 = 0.1884$ or 19%. However, this still leaves 81% of the total variation in HDL levels unaccounted for.

Although we have shown that adding weight to the model for gender appears worthwhile, we should have first checked if the model with gender alone is appropriate by considering the null or no covariate model (**regress hdl**). If it is not, then we are concluding that $\beta_G = 0$ and what remains as the model to describe the data is $y = \beta_0 + \varepsilon$. In this model, the estimate of β_0 is b_0 and this is the mean value of all the observations or $\overline{y} = 1.1024$ mmol/L. The standard deviation (SD) is calculated from the Residual MS $= 0.1084$ of Figure 3.2(c) as $s_{Residual}$ (or more briefly, $s) = \sqrt{0.1084} = 0.3292$. From this, the $SE(\overline{y}) = s/\sqrt{n} = 0.3292/\sqrt{120} = 0.0301$. If this model is chosen, no covariate (at least of those considered) would appear to account for an important part of the variation in the individual levels of HDL.

However, the contrary is actually the case, as shown by the analysis of variance (*ANOVA*) for gender summarized in Figure 3.2(a). This gives $F = \dfrac{1.2519/1}{11.6475/118} = \dfrac{1.2519}{0.0987} = 12.68$, with $df_1 = 1$ and $df_2 = 118$ leading to a *p*-value$=0.005$. This indicates that gender explains an important part of the variation in HDL.

From the analysis of both gender and weight in a single model, we conclude that both are influential on HDL levels, and so our chosen multivariable model is

$$HDL = 1.6216 + 0.1588Gender - 0.0094Weight \tag{3.4}$$

This model implies that there are two situations: one for each gender. Thus, for males (*Gender* = 0) we have:

$$HDL_{Male} = 1.6216 - 0.0094Weight$$

whereas for females (*Gender* =1) we have:

$$HDL_{Female} = 1.7804 - 0.0094Weight$$

Effectively, we are summarizing these data by the two parallel lines shown in Figure 3.3.

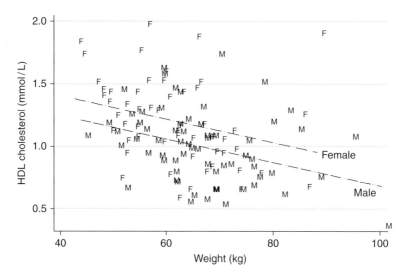

Figure 3.3 Parallel lines obtained from a multiple regression model of the dependent variable HDL on the covariates gender and weight (part data from the Singapore Cardiovascular Cohort Study 2)

This summary, which uses the data from both males and females when assessing the regression coefficient for *Weight*, and therefore is an average of that of each gender, can be contrasted with that of Figure 1.6(b). There, distinct linear regression models are fitted, one for each gender and without reference to the data from the other, to give estimates of the slope as $b_{Weight}^{Male} = -0.0082$ and $b_{Weight}^{Female} = -0.0110$, respectively. As these latter estimates of the slope differ between genders, the two regression lines fitted are not parallel to each other.

QUADRATIC MODELS

In linear regression models, when we model the *y*-variable using continuous covariates, the latter are assumed to influence *y* in a linear way. Such models imply that the effect of the *x*-covariate on *y* is linear over the whole range of possible values of the covariate concerned. So for the situation where the model for HDL includes body-weight, we anticipate that the linear effect of weight (if any) concerns individuals ranging from the lowest to the highest body-weight. This may not always be the case.

In addition to examining the residuals, another method of checking for linearity is to extend the simple model and compare the fit of the extended model with the original.

We considered the simple-linear regression fit of HDL and weight in Figure 1.4(b) and reproduce this again in Figure 3.4(a). As there is so much scatter about the fitted line, it is not immediately obvious if a linear model is, or is not, appropriate.

In such a case, one strategy is to fit the linear model in any event and then check on the goodness-of-fit using *ANOVA*. This approach is summarized in Figure 3.5(a) and establishes that weight, via the linear model, explains an important part of the variation in HDL. However, this in itself does not confirm that this is the 'best' model to describe the influence of weight on HDL.

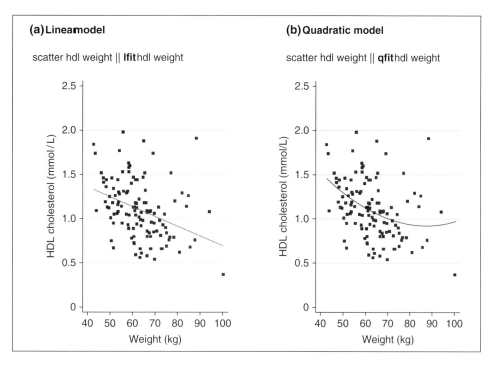

(a) Linea model

scatter hdl weight || **lfit** hdl weight

(b) Quadratic model

scatter hdl weight || **qfit** hdl weight

Figure 3.4   Scatter plot of HDL against weight in 120 individuals with fitted: (a) linear and (b) quadratic models (part data from the Singapore Cardiovascular Cohort Study 2)

A second approach is to fit a more complex model by adding a non-linear covariate and then check if this provides an improved fit to the data compared with the single-variable linear model. If it does then this implies that the variation of y with x is non-linear. Omitting the residual component, the simplest extension to the model $y = \beta_0 + \beta_1 x_1$ is to add an x_1^2 term to this expression, and so the model to fit becomes $y = \beta_0 + \beta_1 x_1 + \beta_2 x_1^2$. This, in turn, may be written in the form of equation (3.2), that is, $y = \beta_0 + \beta_1 x_1 + \beta_2 x_2$, provided we have the variable $x_2 = x_1^2$ in our database.

In the context of Figure 3.4(b) the model for weight, W, to consider is

$$y = \beta_0 + \beta_W W + \beta_{WW} W^2 + \varepsilon \qquad (3.5)$$

This type of equation is known as a polynomial of order 2 as it contains a squared (in weight) term. It is more often termed a quadratic model. The model allows us to try to describe data with a smooth 'bend' in one direction. The command for fitting the quadratic model is (**regress hdl weight ww**), where the variable WW is the square of weight. The structure of the command is the same as that used for the 2-covariate model of HDL on gender and weight of Figure 3.1(b). The resulting calculations for the quadratic model are shown in Figure 3.5(b), and the actual fit of this model to the data is illustrated graphically in Figure 3.4(b). However, it is not immediately clear if this provides an improved description of these data over that of the linear model.

The overall F-test indicates that the quadratic model explains an important part of the variation in HDL levels as $F(2, 117) = 10.70$ with associated p-value $= 0.0001$. Nevertheless,

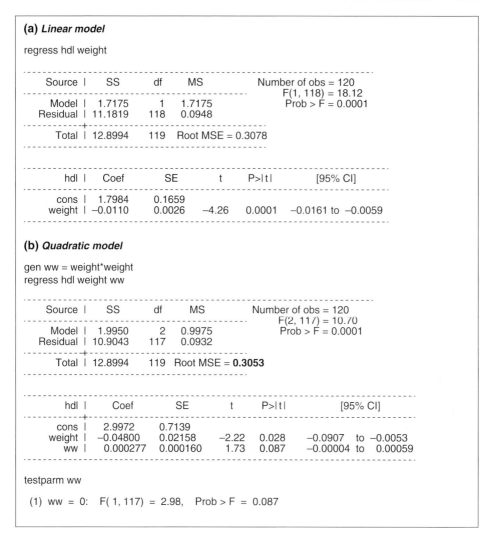

(a) Linear model

regress hdl weight

Source	SS	df	MS		Number of obs = 120
					F(1, 118) = 18.12
Model	1.7175	1	1.7175		Prob > F = 0.0001
Residual	11.1819	118	0.0948		
Total	12.8994	119	Root MSE = 0.3078		

hdl	Coef	SE	t	P>|t|	[95% CI]
cons	1.7984	0.1659			
weight	−0.0110	0.0026	−4.26	0.0001	−0.0161 to −0.0059

(b) Quadratic model

gen ww = weight*weight
regress hdl weight ww

Source	SS	df	MS		Number of obs = 120
					F(2, 117) = 10.70
Model	1.9950	2	0.9975		Prob > F = 0.0001
Residual	10.9043	117	0.0932		
Total	12.8994	119	Root MSE = **0.3053**		

hdl	Coef	SE	t	P>|t|	[95% CI]
cons	2.9972	0.7139			
weight	−0.04800	0.02158	−2.22	0.028	−0.0907 to −0.0053
ww	0.000277	0.000160	1.73	0.087	−0.00004 to 0.00059

testparm ww

(1) ww = 0:   F(1, 117) = 2.98,   Prob > F = 0.087

Figure 3.5   Comparisons of (a) linear and (b) quadratic regression models of HDL on body-weight (part data from the Singapore Cardiovascular Cohort Study 2)

the next step is to formally determine if the fit provided by this model explains, compared with the simple linear model, an important *additional* part of the total variation in HDL. This can be done by testing the null hypothesis, $\beta_{ww} = 0$. The results of such a test are given in Figure 3.5(b) where $t = 0.000277/0.000160 = 1.73$ with p-value = 0.087.

Alternatively, the extra fit obtained by adding the quadratic term to the simple linear regression model, is assessed by the methods described in *Technical details*. Thus, the amount of increase is calculated in SS_{Model} between the model involving the square of weight (*WW*) and that when weight alone (*W*) is involved. For the quadratic model $SS_{Model}(WW) = 1.9950$ and for the simple linear model $SS_{Model}(W) = 1.7175$. The corresponding increase is 0.2775 and this is attributed to the extra 1 degree of freedom involved in fitting the quadratic model. With an increase in SS_{Model} there is a corresponding decrease in Residual SS, in this case from 11.1819 to 10.9043. The latter now represents the unexplained variation in HDL with standard deviation, $s_{Residual} = \sqrt{(10.9043/117)} = \sqrt{0.0932} = 0.3053$. This is the Root MSE (Mean Square Error) of the *ANOVA* table of Figure 3.5(b).

The formal test of the 'extra' fit obtained from the quadratic model is expressed by $F = \dfrac{(1.9950 - 1.7175)/(2-1)}{10.9043/117} = \dfrac{0.2775}{0.0932} = 2.98$. Under the null hypothesis, this has an F-distribution with $df_1 = 1$ in the numerator and $df_2 = 117$ in the denominator. The closest entry to 2.98 is with $df_1 = 1$ in Table T6 is when $df_2 = 100$, $F = 2.76$ and $\alpha = 0.10$. Hence, the p-value ≈ 0.1.

However, as $df_1 = 1$ and they are large in the denominator, $z = \sqrt{2.98} = 1.73$, using Table T1 a more precise p-value $= 2(1 - 0.95818) = 0.084$ is obtained. This is similar in value to that derived when checking for linearity by testing the null hypothesis, $\beta_{ww} = 0$. The slight discrepancy in the two p-values arises by the computer package using more precision in the calculations. The same calculations can also be made using the command (**testparm ww**) to give $F(1,117) = 2.98$ and p-value $= 0.087$ as in Figure 3.5(b).

This result is not statistically significant (although marginal compared with the conventional 0.05), and therefore suggests that the extra-fit provided by adding the quadratic term to the model may not be necessary. Thus, one may cautiously conclude that the linear description cannot be improved on by this means.

The testing procedures used here are only possible as the quadratic model (a polynomial model of order 2 which includes both x_1 and x_1^2 terms) has the linear model (a polynomial model of order 1 as it includes only x_1) *nested* within it. The linear model is a special case of a quadratic model in which $\beta_2 = 0$.

Another method of checking for linearity is to divide weight (of our example) at the preliminary stage of analysis, into $G \geq 3$ categories and then fit a model assuming the categories are *not* ordered. To fit such a model requires $(G - 1)$ dummy variables to be created, as explained in Chapter 2. Once the model is fitted, and if a plot of the resulting estimated regression coefficients against the corresponding (ordered) weight category is approximately linear, then we assume that the influence of weight can be regarded as linear. This would then justify the use of *Weight* in its continuous form in the linear regression model. Should the plot suggest non-linearity of shape then, depending on the profile indicated, either a more complex model could be fitted or the covariate retained in unordered categorical form for modeling purposes. The latter option is likely to be the most useful in practice.

MULTIPLE LINEAR REGRESSION

Extending the 2-covariate model

Both the 2-covariate model of HDL on gender and age, and the quadratic model of age are special cases of a more general multiple linear regression equation. Thus, it is clear when looking at the basic structure of equation (3.2) that it is possible to add more covariate terms in addition to x_1 and x_2 and thereby extend the model $y = \beta_0 + \beta_1 x_1 + \beta_2 x_2 + \varepsilon$ to the p-covariate multiple linear regression model:

$$y = \beta_0 + \beta_1 x_1 + \beta_2 x_2 + \beta_3 x_3 + \ldots + \beta_p x_p + \varepsilon \tag{3.6}$$

```
regress hdl gender weight age

    -----------------------------------------------------
    Source |    SS       df      MS          Number of obs = 120
    -------+--------------------                F(3, 116) = 13.63
     Model |   3.3620     3    1.1207           Prob > F = 0.0001
  Residual |   9.5373   116    0.0822
    -------+--------------------
     Total |  12.8994   119
    -----------------------------------------------------


    -----------------------------------------------------------------
      hdl |   Coef      SE       t      P>|t|          [95% CI]
    ------+----------------------------------------------------------
     cons |  1.7293   0.1688
   gender |  0.1440   0.0541    2.66    0.0089     0.0368 to   0.2512
   weight | -0.0067   0.0026   -2.56    0.012     -0.0118 to  -0.0015
      age | -0.0062   0.0018   -3.37    0.0010    -0.0099 to  -0.0026
    -----------------------------------------------------------------
```

Figure 3.6 Multiple regression model for HDL on gender, weight and age (part data from the Singapore Cardiovascular Cohort Study 2)

The regression coefficients are now $\beta_0, \beta_1, \dots, \beta_p$, all of which need to be estimated from the data on y for each subject with their corresponding values of the p covariates. Such a model would allow us to explore the possibility that age, in addition to gender and weight, influences HDL. The command necessary for this calculation and the corresponding output are summarized in Figure 3.6.

The fitted model, now including gender, weight and age, is:

$$HDL = 1.7293 + 0.1440 Gender - 0.0067 Weight - 0.0062 Age$$

There is still evidence of higher HDL values in the females, decreasing values with increasing weight, and evidence now of reducing levels with increasing age. The global F-test from the ANOVA gives a value of $F = 13.63$ with $df_{Model} = 3$ and $df_{Residual} = 116$. This is statistically significant with p-value $= 0.0001$. The closest tabular entry in Table T6 is $df_1 = 3$ and $df_2 = 100$ and for $\alpha = 0.01$, $F = 3.98$, and therefore provides only a very approximate p-value < 0.01.

To see if this 3-covariate model gives a better fit to the data than the one with only *Gender* and *Weight* included, we compare $SS_{Model} = 3.3620$ of Figure 3.6 with $df = 3$ and $SS_{Model} = 2.4308$ of Figure 3.2(b) with $df = 2$. The formal test of the 'extra' fit obtained by the 3-covariate model is expressed by $F = \dfrac{(3.3620 - 2.4308)/(3-2)}{9.5373/116} = \dfrac{0.9312}{0.0822} = 11.33$. Under the null hypothesis, this has an F-distribution with $df = 1$ in the numerator and $df = 116$ in the denominator. As the numerator degrees of freedom is 1 and they are large in the denominator, $z = \sqrt{11.33} = 3.37$. Using this value in Table T1 gives the p-value $= 2 (1 - 0.99962) = 0.0008$. This is clearly statistically significant, and therefore suggests that the extra fit provided by adding the third covariate *Age* to the 2-covariate model is indeed worthwhile.

Notation

In many situations we end up with rather complex models, which then become quite complicated to describe and compare. As a consequence we introduce some notation that eases this problem. Earlier, we discussed various models to describe the variation in HDL levels, starting with the simplest linear 1-covariate model involving gender alone – for brevity we denote this model by **G**. Similarly, **W** denotes the 1-covariate model for body-weight. This notation is extended to the 2-covariate situation in a natural way by **G**+**W**, a 3-covariate by **G**+**W**+**A** and so on. Things get a little more complicated when dealing with the quadratic model for weight that we considered in equation (3.5). This is described by **W**+**W.W**; the first term of which represents the linear part of the model (the 'main' effect), and the second the weight squared or quadratic term. More briefly, this model is described by **W*W**.

Interactions

In the example of Figure 3.3 we found that both gender and weight have a significant influence on HDL values. In this investigation, we might conjecture that the slope of the linear regression relationship between HDL levels and weight may differ according to gender. There is some evidence for this in Figure 1.6(b) where the negative slope of the relationship (fitted for each gender separately) appears steeper for the females than the males. In contrast, fitting the model **G**+**W** (termed the main-effects model) to all the data forces the two slopes to be identical and the computer program fits the *best* model it can with this constraint imposed. Hence, we obtain the parallel lines of Figure 3.3.

We can check which of the 'two-parallel-lines' or the 'two-lines-of-differing-slopes' models is the better by extending the **G**+**W** model to include an 'interaction' term. This model now comprises the two main effects plus a term describing the interaction between them. We do this by fitting model **G*W**, that is model **G**+**W**+**G.W**, to the data and comparing it with model **G**+**W**, which is nested within this larger model.

The interaction model is

$$\mathbf{G} * \mathbf{W} : y = \beta_0 + \beta_G x_G + \beta_W x_W + \beta_{GW} x_G x_W + \varepsilon \tag{3.7}$$

In this equation, the covariate $x_G = 0$ for males and 1 for females, whereas x_W reflects the different body-weights of the individuals concerned. The term $x_G x_W$ represents the product of these two covariates, the value of which is calculated for each individual in the study. The values of x_G and x_W are in the database, but for our purpose one must calculate an extra variable $x_3 = x_G \times x_W$. We can then consider the right-hand side of equation (3.7) as a 3-covariate model of the form: $\beta_0 + \beta_G x_G + \beta_W x_W + \beta_3 x_3$. In this situation, a test for the presence of an interaction is equivalent to testing the null hypothesis that the regression coefficient $\beta_3 = 0$, or equivalently $\beta_{GW} = 0$. The appropriate statistical commands for calculating the interaction term (**gen gw = gender*weight**) and fitting the model for this, (**regress hdl gender weight gw**), are summarized in Figure 3.7, where (**gw**) represents x_3. Alternatively, one can avoid directly generating x_3 by using the command (**xi: regress hdl i.gender*weight**). This automatically creates, in our case, a variable, *IgenXweigh*_1, in place of the rather more elegant, *GW*, but nevertheless the numerical parts of the output remain as in Figure 3.7.

The fitted model containing the interaction term is

$$HDL = 1.5430 + 0.3323 Gender - 0.0082 Weight - 0.0028 Gender \times Weight$$

Thus, for males (*Gender* = 0) we have:

$$HDL_{Male} = 1.5430 + (0.3323 \times 0) - 0.0082\, Weight - (0.0028 \times 0 \times Weight)$$
$$= 1.5430 - 0.0082\, Weight$$

Generating the interaction

```
gen gw=gender*weight
regress hdl gender weight gw
```

```
      Source |   SS        df    MS         Number of obs = 120
-------------+---------------------          F(3, 116) = 9.09
       Model |  2.4561      3  0.8187        Prob > F = 0.0001
    Residual | 10.4433    116  0.0900
-------------+---------------------
       Total | 12.8994    119
```

```
      hdl |    Coef        SE       t     P>|t|              [95% CI]
----------+-------------------------------------------------------------------
     cons |   1.5430     0.2282
   gender |   0.3323     0.3321    1.00    0.319     -0.3256  to   0.9902
   weight |  -0.008173   0.003442 -2.37    0.019     -0.01499 to  -0.001357
       gw |  -0.002770   0.005228 -0.53    0.597     -0.01312 to   0.007583
```

Testing for interaction

```
testparm gw
```

(1) gw = 0: F(1, 116) = 0.28, Prob>F = 0.60

Figure 3.7   Generating and testing the interaction between weight and gender on levels of HDL (part data from the Singapore Cardiovascular Cohort Study 2)

whereas for females (*Gender* = 1):

$$HDL_{Female} = 1.5430 + (0.3323 \times 1) - 0.0082 \ Weight - (0.0028 \times 1 \times Weight)$$
$$= 1.8753 - 0.0110 \ Weight$$

These two linear regression equations have different slopes with a greater decline in HDL in women, as illustrated in Figure 3.8. The global $F = 9.09$ from the *ANOVA* with $df_{Model} = 3$ and $df_{Residual} = 116$ for the extended model, including the interaction term of gender by weight, is statistically significant with p-value $= 0.0001$.

A simple test of whether or not an interaction is present, when only a single additional parameter is needed to describe the interaction term, is to compare the estimated regression coefficient with its standard error. Thus, from Figure 3.7, $b_{GW} = -0.002770$, $SE(b_{GW}) = 0.005228$, so that their ratio is $z = -0.002770/0.005228 = -0.53$. From Table T1, the p-value $= 2(1 - 0.70194) = 0.60$.

Alternatively, to determine if this interaction model gives a better fit to the data than the one with only *Gender* and *Weight* included, we compare $SS_{Model} = 2.4561$ with $df = 3$ of Figure 3.7 with $SS_{Model} = 2.4308$ of Figure 3.2(b) with $df = 2$. The formal test of the 'extra' fit obtained by the 3-covariate model is expressed by $F = \dfrac{(2.4561 - 2.4308)/(3-2)}{10.4433/116} = \dfrac{0.0253}{0.0900} = 0.28.$

Under the null hypothesis, this has an F-distribution with $df_1 = 1$ in the numerator and $df_2 = 116$ in the denominator. As the numerator $df = 1$, and they are large in the denominator, $z = \sqrt{0.28} = 0.53$ and use of Table T1 gives the p-value $= 0.60$.

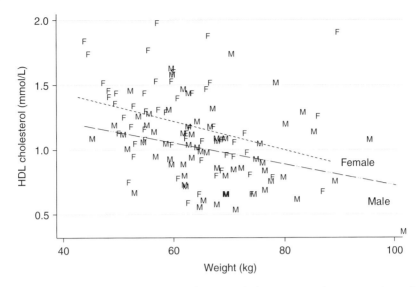

Figure 3.8   Individual lines fitted for each gender in a multiple regression of HDL on gender and weight and including a gender by weight interaction term (part data from the Singapore Cardiovascular Cohort Study 2)

The same test can be made directly using the command (**testparm gw**) shown in Figure 3.7. Whichever approach is used, the result is clearly not statistically significant and therefore suggests that the extra fit provided by including the interaction term in the model is not worthwhile. Thus, in this case, we retain the simpler parallel line model of Figure 3.3.

We note that the two parallel lines model requires three parameters $(\beta_0, \beta_G, \beta_W)$ to be estimated, the interaction model four $(\beta_0, \beta_G, \beta_W, \beta_{GW})$, and the one for two entirely separate lines also requires four $\left(\beta_0^{Male}, \beta_{Weight}^{Male}, \beta_0^{Female}, \beta_{Weight}^{Female}\right)$. Suppose the interaction model had been chosen in the above example, then would we prefer this model over that of two separate lines fitted? The answer is usually – Yes. This is because the interaction model provides a $SD = s_{Residual}$ based on all the information available. This then gives a better estimate of the population SD, $\sigma_{Residual}$, and thereby enables more reliable statistical inferences to be made.

In Figure 3.2(b) we found that both gender and weight (main effects – Model I: $G+W$) were significantly associated with HDL. This model included $p+1 = 3$ regression coefficients corresponding to β_G, β_W and β_0. However, in order not to have too many overlapping data points in the scatter plots, our analysis was confined to only 120 subjects from one of the ethnic groups recruited to the study. Thus, the model $G+W$ is fitted again in Figure 3.9, but now with the data from all the three ethnic groups concerned. The importance of both components G and W are confirmed by examining the t-tests giving 5.91 for G and −8.26 for W, with corresponding p-values<0.0001 in both instances. This analysis is supplemented by the more global F-test, which suggests that the model explains an important fraction of the total variation as $F(2, 524) = 76.12, p$-value<0.0001.

Suppose we now wish to evaluate the effect of adding ethnicity to this model. The task is then to determine if the more complex main effects model (Model II: $G+W+E$) would better explain the variation in HDL. As noted in Chapter 2, as ethnicity is an unordered categorical covariate of three categories (Chinese, Malay, Indian), it is necessary to create two indicator variables for the modeling process. Consequently we are adding a further $q = 2$ regression coefficients, γ_{E1} and γ_{E2}, to Model I to create Model II. Specifically, we then test the null hypothesis H_0: $\gamma_{E1} = \gamma_{E2} = 0$ by comparing the additional fit of Model II over that of Model I.

Figure 3.9(a) shows that the regression sum of squares for Model I, $SS_{Model}(I) = 13.6231$. In this model two explanatory variables gender and weight, each with a single regression coefficient or parameter to be estimated, are considered hence $p = 2$. Their combined effect explains $R^2 = 13.6231/60.5107 = 0.2251$, or approximately 23% of the total variation in HDL.

(a) Model I: G + W

regress hdl gender weight

Source	SS	df	MS			
Model	13.6231	2	6.8116			
Residual	46.8876	524	0.08948			
Total	60.5107	526				

Number of obs = 527
F(2, 524) = 76.12
Prob > F = 0.0001

Root MSE = 0.2991

hdl	Coef	SE	t	P>|t|	[95% CI]	
cons	1.6669	0.0796				
gender	0.1641	0.0277	5.91	0.0001	0.1096 to	0.2185
weight	−0.009635	0.001166	−8.26	0.0001	−0.0119 to	−0.0073

(b) Model II: G + W + E

xi: regress hdl gender weight i.ethnic

Source	SS	df	MS			
Model	16.2770	4	4.0693			
Residual	44.2336	522	0.0847			
Total	60.5107	526				

Number of obs = 527
F(4, 522) = 48.02
Prob > F = 0.0001

Root MSE = 0.2911

hdl	Coef	SE	t	P>|t|	[95% CI]	
cons	1.6383	0.0780				
gender	0.1780	0.0271	6.57	0.0001	0.1247 to	0.2313
weight	−0.008260	0.001162	−7.11	0.0001	−0.0105 to	−0.0060
Iethnic2	**−0.0958**	0.0319	−3.00	0.0038	−0.1585 to	−0.0331
Iethnic3	**−0.1722**	0.0317	−5.43	0.0001	−0.2345 to	−0.1100

(c) Testing the addition of E

testparm Iethnic2 Iethnic3

(1) Iethnic2 = Iethnic3 = 0:   F(2, 522) = 15.66,   Prob > F = 0.0001

Figure 3.9 Regression commands and output to explain the variation in levels of HDL for (a) Model I: G+W, (b) Model II: G+W+E and (c) testing the inclusion of E (part data from the Singapore Cardiovascular Cohort Study 2)

With the inclusion of ethnicity into the model, which requires that $q = 2$ dummy covariates are added, the regression sum of squares for Model II in Figure 3.9(b) is $SS_{Model}(II) = 16.2770$. The 3-covariates in the model now require $p+q = 4$ parameters to be estimated. The revised model now explains about 27% of the variation in HDL. The corresponding $SS_{Residual}(II) = 44.2336$, with $df_2 = 527 - (p+q) - 1 = 527 - 5 = 522$. We also note that $df_1 = (p+q) - q = 4 - 2 = 2$.

By reference to equation (3.10), to test the value of adding E to the model we calculate: $F(2,522) = \dfrac{[16.2770 - 13.6231]/2}{44.2336/522} = \dfrac{2.6539/2}{44.2336/522} = 15.66$, with an associated p-value = 0.0001.

Alternatively, the overall effect of adding E (to a model already containing G and W) may be evaluated by using the (**testparm Iethnic2 Iethnic3**) of Figure 3.9(c). In doing this we have to be sure to include both dummy variables in this expression, although use of (**i. ethnic**) in the original model command would do this automatically. This analysis also gives p-value = 0.0001 and suggests that adding E to the model is justified. The full model is shown in Figure 3.9(b) with the regression coefficients for the dummy variables highlighted.

A more technical description of how two nested models are compared in this way is given in *Technical details*. Alternatively, models may be compared using the Akaike Information Criterion (AIC), also described in *Technical details*, which is implemented by, for example, adding after the command (**regress hdl gender**) the supplementary command (**estat ic**) as in Figure 3.10. This gives values of AIC of 289.03, 226.51, and 199.81 for models for HDL of G, $G+W$, and $G+W+E$, respectively, with the lowest value indicating that the model involving all three covariates may be the most appropriate.

```
regress hdl gender
estat ic
```

Model	Obs	L(null)	L(model)	df	AIC
G	527	−177.47	−142.51	2	289.03

```
regress hdl gender weight
estat ic
```

Model	Obs	L(null)	L(model)	df	AIC
G + W	527	−177.47	−110.26	3	226.51

```
xi: regress hdl gender weight i.ethnic
estat ic
```

Model	Obs	L(null)	L(model)	df	AIC
G + W + E	527	−177.47	−94.90	5	199.81

Figure 3.10 Akaike information criterion (AIC) evaluated for three nested models (G, G+W, and G+W+E) to explain the variation in levels of HDL (part data from the Singapore Cardiovascular Cohort Study 2)

```
regress hdl gender
regress hdl weight
xi: regress hdl i.ethnic
```

hdl	Coef	SE	t	P>ltl	[95% CI]
cons	1.0255	0.0187			
gender	0.2399	0.0278	8.63	0.0001	0.1853 to 0.2945
cons	1.8852	0.0728			
weight	−0.0119	0.0011	−10.49	0.0001	−0.0141 to −0.0097
cons	1.2122	0.01969			
Iethnic2	−0.1098	0.03581	−3.07	0.0021	−0.1801 to −0.0394
Iethnic3	−0.2147	0.03484	−6.16	0.0001	−0.2831 to −0.1462

```
estat ic
```

Model	Obs	L(null)	L(model)	df	AIC
Gender	527	−177.47	−142.51	2	289.03
Weight	527	−177.47	−127.28	2	258.57
Ethnicity	527	−177.47	−158.35	3	322.70

Figure 3.11 Akaike information criterion (AIC) evaluated for comparing three non-nested models (G, W, and E) to explain the variation in levels of HDL (part data from the Singapore Cardiovascular Cohort Study 2)

Non-nested models

In some situations, one may wish to compare non-nested models and the Akaike criterion can also be used in this situation. Figure 3.11 gives a simple example in which three univariate non-nested models are compared when used to explain the variation in HDL levels. The AIC for models G, W and E are, respectively, 289.03, 258.57, and 322.70 and on the basis of this, model W would be preferred. All three models have lower log likelihood, L(Model), than for the null model of −177.47, which therefore implies that each covariate studied appears to explain (at least) some of the variation in HDL levels between patients.

PRECAUTIONS

Nested models

We indicated earlier that, for example, the linear model W for HDL on body-weight is nested within the quadratic model $W*W = W + W \cdot W$. We can best compare how well alternative regression models describe the data if one model is nested within the other. In certain situations it may not be immediately clear if models are nested or not, and so care is needed with the choice of covariates that are included in models we wish to compare. For example, when investigating the possibility of differing slopes of the regression lines of HDL on weight of the males and females, an interaction term is required. However, suppose we correctly define a new variable as the product of x_G and x_W but then label it (say) U in the database. The interaction model $G*W$ then becomes $G+W+U$. In such a situation we may be tempted to imagine that the three models $G+W$, $G+U$, and $W+U$ are all nested within this 3-covariate model. In fact, only $G+W$ is nested within model $G*W$, whereas models $G+U$ and $W+U$ are not. Of course, each of the 1-covariate models G and W remain nested within $G+W$, whereas the (apparent) model U is not one we should consider.

If the analyst uses the form $G+W+U$ without due care, then the computer will fit this model, as well as all three models we have alluded to, rather than confining the calculations to $G+W$. In general, one should not fit a model containing the interaction covariate U that does not also include both main covariates G and W. The possibility of fitting inappropriate models becomes particularly acute when using automatic variable selection methods, which we discuss in Chapter 7.

Collinearity

In one illustration, we concluded that it was worthwhile adding the third covariate *Age*, A, to the 2-covariate model of $G+W$ when describing levels of HDL. However, when *Age* is added, the estimated regression coefficients for *Weight*, $b_W = -0.0067$, and for *Gender*, $b_G = 0.1440$, obtained for Figure 3.6 have both declined in magnitude compared with the 2-covariate model values, $b_W = -0.0094$ and $b_G = 0.1588$, of Figure 3.2(b). This would not be the case if each covariate acted in a way that was independent of the other. When there are several candidate covariates to consider for a model, it is advisable to ascertain the strength of any association between them before beginning the modeling process.

In addition to gender, age and weight, among the candidate covariates in the study of HDL are waist and hip circumferences (cm). The scatter diagrams of each of the latter against the other and against weight are shown in Figure 3.12. It can be seen from these plots that, using equation (1.16), there are strong linear associations between these variables with, for example, a correlation between body-weight and waist-circumference of $r = 0.8650$. If the correlation is high between two covariates, then they are termed collinear.

Where there is evidence of collinearity in the data set, some care is required on how to proceed with the regression modeling. It is difficult to be specific, but one simple option is to ignore one of the collinear covariates involved before any regression modeling commences. However, when the study results are reported some rationale for this exclusion should be provided.

Figure 3.13 gives an example in which the relationship between HDL levels and waist and hip circumference measures are investigated. The first analyses consist of univariate regression models for *Hip* and for *Waist*, followed by a multiple regression model involving both covariates. The univariate models estimates are $b_{Uni.Hip} = -0.002300$ and $b_{Uni.Waist} = -0.01340$, whereas the corresponding estimates from the multiple regression are $b_{Mul.Hip} = +0.02121$ and $b_{Mul.Waist} = -0.02146$, which are quite different. The ratios of the two estimates of the regression coefficients $C_{Hip} = +0.02121/-0.002300 = -9.2$ and $C_{Waist} = -0.02146/-0.01340 = 1.6$ suggest that these changes are quite dramatic. Such changes may pose several challenges for the final interpretation of such a study.

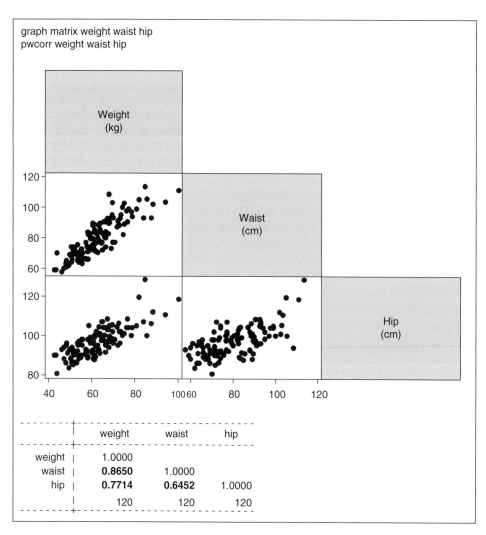

Figure 3.12 Matrix of scatter plots of body-weight, waist circumference and hip circumference in 120 subjects (part data from the Singapore Cardiovascular Cohort Study 2)

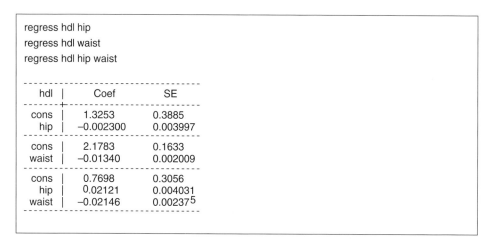

Figure 3.13 Univariate regressions of HDL on hip, and waist circumference and multiple regression of HDL on both hip and waist measures in 120 subjects (part data from the Singapore Cardiovascular Cohort Study 2)

PARSIMONIOUS MODELS

In general terms we prefer the parallel line model of Figure 3.3 to the non-parallel lines model of Figure 3.8, especially as the interaction term is not statistically significant, because the latter model is easier to describe. Specifically it is then only necessary to quote one rate of decline of HDL with body-weight as a single rate applies to both genders. Although this may be our preference, the decision as to which model is appropriate should be made on the balance between statistical and practical considerations. In our situation the decision seems clear, but this will not always be the case.

If we go a step further, our preference would be for a single linear regression line calculated from all subjects (both male and female) such as that of Figure 1.4(b). This gives a very simple model with a very easy description. However, our analyses have suggested that gender differences are important as these help to explain a lot of the variation in HDL. As a consequence, gender differences cannot be ignored.

However, had this not been the case, we would have been satisfied with the single-covariate model of Figure 1.4(b) considering weight only. Nonetheless, there is an even simpler model to potentially consider and that is one in which body-weight plays no role at all in explaining the variation observed in HDL levels from individual-to-individual. Should this be the true situation, then the mean weight of all subjects, with the corresponding 95% confidence interval, is quoted as the final summary of the study. This is the simplest situation to describe, albeit possibly a great disappointment to the study investigators concerned.

The object of the modeling process is to find the simplest (most parsimonious) model yet one that still describes the essential features of the data adequately.

VERIFYING ASSUMPTIONS

Just as indicated in Chapter 2, it is important to check as comprehensively as possible whether the chosen model is the most appropriate for the situation in hand. Thus, in the context of multiple regression, graphical plots and examination of the residuals remain important. For example, from visual inspection of Figures 3.3 and 3.8, one might conclude that the parallel line model of the first, as opposed to two lines of different slope for each gender of the second, is adequate. Additionally, one might wish to compare the residuals of each gender about the corresponding parallel lines model of equation (3.4) using Q-Q plots as indicated in Figure 3.14. These suggest a greater spread of residual values for the females, but both plots are essentially linear and so are supportive of the model chosen. More detailed examinations than we have outlined may be necessary in examples when non-linear patterns appear in such plots.

TECHNICAL DETAILS

Nested models

A regression model (Model I) is termed nested within another model (Model II) when the first of these can be obtained by setting some of the regression coefficients in Model II to be zero.

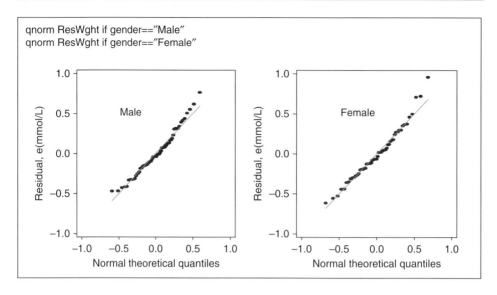

qnorm ResWght if gender=="Male"
qnorm ResWght if gender=="Female"

Figure 3.14   Scatter plots of residuals by gender from the multiple regression of HDL on weight and gender against the ordered Normal scores (part data from the Singapore Cardiovascular Cohort Study 2)

$$\text{Model II} : y = \beta_0 + \beta_1 x_1 + \ldots + \beta_p x_p + \beta_{p+1} x_{p+1} + \ldots + \beta_{p+q} x_{p+q} \tag{3.8}$$

$$\text{Model I} : y = \beta_0 + \beta_1 x_1 + \ldots + \beta_p x_p \tag{3.9}$$

Thus, the multiple regression equation (3.8) contains $k = (1+p+q)$ regression coefficients, which is reduced to equation (3.9) containing $(1+p)$ coefficients if $\beta_{p+1}, \beta_{p+2}, \ldots, \beta_{p+q}$ are all set to zero. Consequently, Model I is nested within Model II.

The F-test is used for comparing nested multiple linear regression models, where the aim is to identify the model that best describes the data. The statistic follows an F-distribution under the null hypothesis that a simpler model requiring fewer parameters (and which therefore is more parsimonious) is adequate.

As in the situation above, suppose that in addition to β_0, the simpler (null hypothesis) model has p parameters to estimate, and we wish to determine if an additional set of covariates, requiring q further parameters to be estimated, improve the fit of the model. Specifically, we wish to test the null hypothesis that including the q extra parameters does not improve the fit over equation (3.9), that is:

$$H_0 : \beta_{p+1} = \beta_{p+2} = \ldots = \beta_{p+q} = 0$$

In general, the two models may be compared by first fitting them separately and obtaining their respective model (or regression) and residual sums of squares indicated in the *ANOVA* of Figure 3.15.

Source of variation	Model I		Model II	
	Sums of squares	Degrees of freedom (*df*)	Sums of squares	Degrees of freedom (*df*)
Due to regression	$SS_{Model}(I)$	p	$SS_{Model}(II)$	$p+q$
Residual	$SS_{Residual}(I)$	$n-(p+1)$	$SS_{Residual}(II)$	$n-(p+q+1)$

Figure 3.15 ANOVA sums of squares and degrees of freedom for the comparison of two nested models in a multiple regression of *n* subjects

If H_0 is true, then under this null hypothesis

$$F = \frac{[SS_{Model}(II) - SS_{Model}(I)]/q}{SS_{Residual}(II)/[n-(p+q+1)]} \tag{3.10}$$

will follow an *F*-distribution with degrees of freedom for the numerator, $df_{Model} = (p+q) - p = q$ and for the denominator $df_{Residual} = n - (p+q+1)$.

Akaike's criterion

The Akaike criterion is calculated by

$$AIC = 2k - 2L \tag{3.11}$$

where *k* is the number of parameters estimated in the model. The expression involves the log-likelihood, $L = \log \ell$, where ℓ is termed the likelihood. We discuss the likelihood in more detail in Chapter 4, *Technical details*, in the context of estimating a proportion rather than a regression coefficient. There we show that in a study of *n* patients if *r* respond, and the remainder do not, then *r/n* is the maximum likelihood estimator of the true population proportion, π. In the context of this chapter, estimated regression coefficients like those of b_0 and b_1 calculated from equations (1.8), as well as being the least squares estimates of β_0 and β_1 they are essentially the maximum likelihood estimates also. The corresponding log likelihood, *L*, is a complex mathematical expression and is purposely omitted here.

In the example of (**xi: regress hdl gender weight i.ethnic**) in Figure 3.10, the number of parameters $k = 5$ corresponding to β_0, β_G, and β_W plus two for the dummy variables created in order to include ethnicity into the fitted model. Further, the log likelihood is given by $L(Model) = -94.90$. Hence, $AIC = 2 \times 5 - 2 \times (-94.90) = 10 + 189.8 = 199.8$. Thus, as Cassimally (2011) states: '… the Akaike information criterion … rewards hypotheses (in our case – models) for fitting the data well, but penalises them if they are too complex, with too many variables and parameters'.

4 Logistic Regression

SUMMARY

In this chapter we first describe regression models appropriate for a binary outcome variable. In this case the basic variable has to be transformed by the logit transformation before a regression model can be constructed, fitted and subsequently tested. Situations where the single covariate is binary, unordered categorical, ordered categorical or continuous are described. We show how the estimated parameters of such models can be expressed in terms of the odds ratio (OR). The 1-covariate model is then extended to the multiple logistic regression situation. Methods of investigating whether the fitted model is appropriate for the study concerned are discussed. These involve estimating standardized residuals, recognizing covariate patterns, and calculating leverages. We describe the use of conditional logistic regression, which is suitable for designs such as matched case–control studies. Ordered logistic regression which extends the binary outcome variable situation to allow more than two ordered categories is included.

THE LOGIT TRANSFORMATION

Odds ratio

If the outcome or dependent variable in a study is of binary form, then this implies that it can take only one of two values (conventionally coded 0 and 1). This enables the simplest type of summary to be obtained by merely counting the number of 1's in different groups and expressing these totals as proportions of the corresponding group sizes. For example Jackson, Gangnon, Evans, *et al.* (2008) provide the proportion of children experiencing asthma by six years of age with respect to whether or not they had been previously exposed to the human rhinovirus (HRV). The results of this study are described in the 2×2 contingency table format of Figure 4.1, where the proportions of children developing asthma are $21/45 = 0.4667$ (46.67%) in those who have been exposed to HRV wheezing illnesses, and $50/210 = 0.2381$ (23.81%) in those who have not.

Regression Methods for Medical Research, First Edition. Bee Choo Tai and David Machin.
© 2014 Bee Choo Tai and David Machin. Published 2014 by John Wiley & Sons, Ltd.

```
tabulate HRV Asthma

-----------+-------------------------+-----------|-----------------------
           | No Asthma     Asthma    |           | Proportion
   HRV     |    (0)          (1)     |   Total   | with asthma (%)
-----------+-------------------------+-----------|-----------------------
  No (0)   | 160  (a)     50  (c)    | 210 (a+c) | 50/210 (23.81%)
  Yes (1)  |  24  (b)     21  (d)    |  45 (b+d) | 21/45  (46.67%)
-----------+-------------------------+-----------|
  Total    | 184  (a+b)   71  (c+d)  | 255       |
-----------+-------------------------+-----------|-----------------------
```

Figure 4.1 Proportion of children who develop asthma by six years of age in those exposed or not to human rhinovirus (HRV) wheezing illnesses in their first year of life (data from Jackson, Gangnon, Evans, et al., 2008, TABLE 3)

The adverse influence of the exposure to HRV on the development of asthma is estimated by the difference in proportions

$$d = p_{YesHRV} - p_{NoHRV} = \frac{d}{b+d} - \frac{c}{a+c} = 0.4667 - 0.2381 = 0.2286\,(22.86\%)$$

Each of the proportions p_{YesHRV} and p_{NoHRV} is an estimate of the corresponding true or underlying population parameter π_{YesHRV} and π_{NoHRV}. The aim of the study would be to estimate these as precisely as possible, and subsequently test the null hypothesis: H_0: $\pi_{YesHRV} - \pi_{NoHRV} = 0$.

An alternative summary option is to express the results in terms of 'odds'. The odds of an event is defined as the ratio of the probability of occurrence of the event to the probability of non-occurrence of that event, that is, $p/(1-p)$. Thus, for those who have experienced a HRV episode, the odds of acquiring asthma by six years of age are $p_{YesHRV}/(1-p_{YesHRV}) = 0.4667/(1-0.4667) = 0.8751$. In contrast, for those without a HRV episode the odds are $p_{NoHRV}/(1-p_{NoHRV}) = 0.2381/(1-0.2381) = 0.3125$. From these two odds, the odds ratio (OR) is then

$$OR_{Asthma} = \frac{p_{YesHRV}/(1-p_{YesHRV})}{p_{NoHRV}/(1-p_{NoHRV})} = \frac{0.8751}{0.3125} = 2.8003$$

This can be calculated directly from the cells of Figure 4.1 using

$$OR = \frac{ad}{bc} = \frac{160 \times 21}{50 \times 24} = 2.8000 \tag{4.1}$$

As we have indicated, the null hypothesis: H_0: $\pi_{YesHRV} - \pi_{NoHRV} = 0$ implies that we are testing $\pi_{YesHRV} = \pi_{NoHRV}$, in which case the null hypothesis can be expressed in terms of the OR measure as H_0: $OR_0 = \dfrac{\pi_{YesHRV}/(1-\pi_{YesHRV})}{\pi_{NoHRV}/(1-\pi_{NoHRV})} = 1$.

The logit transformation

The potential range of values for a continuous outcome variable is from $-\infty$ to $+\infty$, and this same range applies to any summary statistic calculated, such as the mean. In contrast, a binary outcome variable is restricted to be either 0 or 1 and any resulting summary statistic must be either 0 or 1 or have a value between these two extremes. Thus, a binary outcome, leads to estimates of proportions with a particular feature, for example, 4 from 10 patients ($p=0.4$) in a particular group have the disease of interest. As we have indicated such an estimate will lie between 0 or 0% (none with the disease) and 1 or 100% (all with the disease). This restriction in the range of possible values causes technical difficulties in estimating the parameters in any associated regression model. However, if we express the proportion, p, first in terms of the odds, $p/(1-p)$, then the logarithm of the odds, $y=\log[p/(1-p)]$, also known as logit(p), can potentially lie between $-\infty$ and $+\infty$.

For example, if $p=0.4$, log $[0.4/0.6] = -0.4055$ and if 6 of 10 had the disease then logit[0.6]$=\log[0.6/0.4]=\log[1.5]=+0.4055$. In a more extreme example, if only one from 1000 has the disease, $p=0.001$ with $y=\text{logit}(p)=\log[0.001/0.999] = -6.9068$, whereas if 999 in 1000 then logit[0.999]$=+6.9068$. In all situations, logit[$1-p$]$=-\text{logit}[p]$ except if $p=0.5$ when logit[0.5]$=\log[0.5/0.5]=\log[1]=0$. Thus, the values of logit[p] can range from $-\infty$ to $+\infty$, and are symmetric about 0.

Logistic regression

In the situation of Figure 4.1, the corresponding logistic regression model is written in terms of the presence of asthma as the outcome variable and assumes that the population probability of asthma for a child with covariate HRV is π_{Asthma}. Thus, the logistic regression model for this situation is

$$\log\left(\frac{\pi_{Asthma}}{1-\pi_{Asthma}}\right) = \beta_0 + \beta_{HRV} HRV \tag{4.2}$$

In the above equation and subsequent regression models, we have omitted the residual term, ε, unless we wish to emphasise some specific comments such as those following equation (8.1). The values of the regression coefficients β_0 and β_{HRV} are chosen as the ones that give expected proportions that are closest to the observed proportions, using a technique known as maximum likelihood (ML), some details of which are explained in *Technical details*. The associated logistic regression command (`logit Asthma HRV`) and the resulting output from Stata for the data of Figure 4.1 are shown in Figure 4.2(a). The latter implies:

$$H:\log\left(\frac{p_{Asthma}}{1-p_{Asthma}}\right) = b_0 + b_{HRV} HRV = -1.1632 + 1.0296 HRV \tag{4.3}$$

where b_0 and b_{HRV} are the estimates of the parameters β_0 and β_{HRV}, respectively.

After taking the antilog, that is taking the exponential (exp), of both sides of equation (4.3) and making some rearrangement of the resulting expression, it can be rewritten as:

$$p_{Asthma} = \frac{\exp(b_0 + b_{HRV} HRV)}{1+\exp(b_0 + b_{HRV} HRV)} \tag{4.4}$$

Thus, if we then substitute the regression coefficient estimates from Figure 4.2(a) into this, we obtain

$$p_{Asthma} = \frac{\exp(-1.1632 + 1.0296 HRV)}{1+\exp(-1.1632 + 1.0296 HRV)}$$

(a) *Estimating the regression coefficients*

logit Asthma HRV

Number of obs = 255, LR chi2 (1) = 8.94, Prob > chi2 = 0.0028

```
---------------------------------------------------------------------
   Asthma |   Coef     SE      z      P>|z|          [95% CI]
----------+----------------------------------------------------------
     cons |  -1.1632
      HRV |  1.0296   0.3399   3.03   0.0024    0.3634 to 1.6958
---------------------------------------------------------------------
```

(b) *Estimating the proportions with asthma*

predict p
summarize Asthma HRV if HRV == 0
summarize Asthma HRV if HRV == 1

```
-------+------------------------------
 HRV |  Obs             p
-------+------------------------------
   0 |   210          0.2381
   1 |    45          0.4667
-------+------------------------------
```

(c) *Estimating the OR*

logistic Asthma HRV

```
---------------------------------------------------------------------
   Asthma |   OR        SE      z     P>|z|          [95% CI]
----------+----------------------------------------------------------
      HRV |   2.8     0.9517   3.03   0.002     1.4382 to 5.4511
---------------------------------------------------------------------
```

(d) *Analysis in the grouped format of the 2×2 table of Figure 4.1*

list HRV Asthma n

```
      +-----------------------------+
      | HRV     Asthma      n  |
      |-----------------------------|
   1. |  0        50       210 |
   2. |  1        21        45 |
      +-----------------------------+
```

blogit Asthma n HRV

This gives identical output to **(a)** above

Figure 4.2 Logistic regression of the proportion of children who develop asthma by six years of age in those exposed or not exposed to human rhinovirus (HRV) wheezing illnesses in their first year of life (data from Jackson, Gangnon, Evans, *et al.*, 2008, TABLE 3)

Further, if we set $HRV=0$ for those not experiencing HRV, then $P_{Asthma,NoHRV} =$ $\dfrac{\exp(-1.1632)}{1+\exp(-1.1632)} = \dfrac{0.31248}{1+0.31248} = 0.2381$ or 23.81%. In a similar way, $HRV=1$ for those experiencing HRV, and $P_{Asthma,HRV} = \dfrac{\exp(-1.1632+1.0296)}{1+\exp(-1.1632+1.0296)} = \dfrac{\exp(-0.1336)}{1+\exp(-0.1336)} = \dfrac{0.87494}{1.87494} = 0.4667$ or 46.67%. These are the exact percentages we noted in Figure 4.1. They can also be obtained by use of the (**predict**) command as in the edited output of Figure 4.2(b).

However, we are now in a position to test the null hypothesis of H_0: $\pi_{YesHRV} - \pi_{NoHRV}=0$ or equivalently expressed as: H_0: $\beta_{HRV}=0$. This is done by calculating $z=b_{HRV}/SE(b_{HRV})$. Using the values obtained from Figure 4.2(a), $z=1.0296/0.3399=3.03$ and use of Table T1 gives the p-value=0.0024. An alternative in this situation is to calculate $z^2=[b_{HRV}/SE(b_{HRV})]^2= 3.03^2=9.18$. Under the null hypothesis, z^2 follows the χ^2 (chi-squared) distribution with $df=1$, and Table T5 is then used to obtain an approximate p-value. The entry in the first row of this table for $df=1$ and $\alpha=0.01$ gives 6.63, and for $\alpha=0.001$ gives 10.83. The p-value corresponding to $\chi^2=9.18$ is therefore <0.01 but >0.001 so we may infer the p-value ≈ 0.005. More exact calculations give the p-value=0.0024.

In fact, the output in Figure 4.2(a) gives information from two different statistical tests that test the null hypothesis $\beta_{HRV}=0$. One we have just described, the second appears as (LR chi2 (1) = 8.94, Prob > chi2 = 0.0028) where (chi2) represents χ^2. This latter test is termed the likelihood ratio (LR) test. The principles on which it is based are explained in *Technical details*.

The logit transformation has the useful property that if a covariate, x, in the model is binary with values 0 or 1, and has associated regression coefficient β, then $\exp(\beta)$ is the odds ratio, *OR*. In our case we compare those exposed to HRV wheezing illness in their first year of life ($HRV=1$) with those of no exposure ($HRV=0$) by

$$OR = \exp(\beta_{HRV}) \tag{4.5}$$

Therefore, as β_{HRV} is estimated by $b_{HRV}=1.0296$, the estimated value of $OR=\exp(+1.0296)= 2.8000$ as previously noted in equation (4.1). The test of the null hypothesis: H_0: $\pi_{YesHRV} - \pi_{NoHRV}=0$ and H_0: $\beta_{HRV}=0$ are thus alternative forms of expressing: H_0: $OR=1$.

Rather than using equation (4.5), the *OR* can be obtained directly by modifying the command of Figure 4.2(a) from (**logit Asthma HRV**) to that of Figure 4.2(c) which is (**logistic Asthma HRV**). This also provides an estimate of the corresponding 95% confidence interval for the *OR* of 1.44 to 5.45. This and the p-value=0.0024 indicate that the influence of the exposure to HRV on the subsequent presence of asthma by six years in these children is statistically significant. The difference of 23% or an $OR=2.80$ both indicate a substantially increased risk of asthma development in those experiencing an HRV wheezing illness.

In these analyses we have assumed a database format in which each individual in the study has a single row in the database with one or more columns indicating the covariate values and a further column taking values of 1 or 0 depending on whether or not the individual concerned has experienced asthma. However, data may be presented in the grouped format of Figure 4.1. In this case the database will comprise only two rows as in Figure 4.2(d), and in which case the grouped form of logistic regression via the command (**blogit Asthma n HRV**) produces the same results as those of Figure 4.2(a).

CATEGORICAL AND CONTINUOUS COVARIATES

Unordered categorical covariate

Just as we have discussed with the linear regression model for a continuous dependent variable, when an unordered categorical covariate of G (> 2) levels is to be included in the logistic model then $G - 1$ dummy variables need to be created. However, as we have previously indicated, this process can often be automatically initiated using appropriate regression commands in a statistical package. Figure 4.3(a) shows the percentage of individuals in each of the three ethnic groups found to have ischaemic heart disease (IHD). The corresponding command for fitting a logistic regression is (**xi: logit**

(a) *Presence of IHD by ethnic group*

tabulate ihd ethnic

		ethnicity		
ihd	Chinese	Malay	Indian	Total
No	216	88	68	372
Yes	61	32	62	155
Total	277	120	130	527
IHD (%)	22.0	26.7	47.7	...

(b) *Estimating the regression coefficients*

xi : logit ihd i .ethnic

Number of obs = 527, LR chi2(2) = 27.33, Prob > chi2 = 0.0001
Log likelihood = –305.5899

ihd	Coef	SE	z	P>|z|	[95% CI]
b0	–1.2644				
c1	0				
c2	0.2528	0.2523	1.00	0.32	–0.2416 to 0.7472
c3	1.1720	0.2277	5.15	0.0001	0.7257 to 1.6184

(c) *Estimating the OR*

xi : logistic ihd i .ethnic

ihd	OR	SE	z	P>|z|	[95% CI]
c1	1				
c2	1.2876	0.3248	1.00	0.32	0.7854 to 2.1111
c3	3.2285	0.7352	5.15	0.0001	2.0662 to 5.0448

Figure 4.3 Proportion with ischaemic heart disease (IHD) by ethnic group and the corresponding estimated logistic regression model (part data from the Singapore Cardiovascular Cohort Study 2)

`ihd i.ethnic`) and gives the estimates of the regression parameters of Figure 4.3(b) defining the following model:

$$E : \log\left(\frac{p_{IHD}}{1 - p_{IHD}}\right) = b_0 + c_{E1}v_1 + c_{E2}v_2 = -1.2644 + 0.2528v_1 + 1.1720v_2. \qquad (4.6)$$

In this situation we have used the dummy variables of Figure 2.5(a) so that $v_1 = 1$ if the subject is Malay, otherwise $v_1 = 0$; and $v_2 = 1$ if the subject is Indian, otherwise $v_2 = 0$. Note that we have modified the labels for the estimated regression coefficients to b0, c2 and c3 and added c1 = 0 to emphasize that there are indeed three ethnic groups.

The command (`xi: logistic ihd i.ethnic`) gives the estimates of the odds ratios of Figure 4.3(c). From these panels the individual z-values of 1.00 and 5.15 associated with the corresponding estimated parameters lead to p-values of 0.32 and 0.0001, suggesting a non-significant increase in the proportion of the Malay with IHD compared with the Chinese ($OR = 1.29$), but a statistically significantly higher value in the Indians when compared with the Chinese ($OR = 3.23$).

An overall judgment of whether ethnicity plays an important part in explaining the variation in who has, and who does not have, a differing risk of IHD in the 1-covariate but 2-associated-parameters model, E, is provided by (`LR chi2 (2) =27.33, Prob > chi2 = 0.0001`) of Figure 4.3(b). This is statistically significant as the p-value=0.0001, and we would conclude ethnicity should remain in the model.

Ordered categorical covariate

No new principles are required when considering an ordered categorical variable which is to be entered into a 1-covariate logistic regression, except to consider whether the category intervals should be regarded as equal or not. This situation may be explored by examining the profile of how the proportions, on the logistic transformation scale, of the feature of concern vary as the covariate values change. For example, in Figure 4.4(a) the proportion with IHD appears to be decreasing as educational levels increase. However, the pattern may not be linear as those with 'moderate', 'high', and 'very high' educational experience have very similar rates. Despite this, a linear model of educational level, L, indicates a strongly negative and linear decline following the command (`logit ihd educ`) of Figure 4.4(b). This decline is summarized by:

$$L : \log\left(\frac{p_{IHD}}{1 - p_{IHD}}\right) = b_0 + b_{Educ} Level = 0.3383 - 0.6717 Level \qquad (4.7)$$

Further, the command (`logistic ihd educ`) provides the estimate of the corresponding $OR = 0.5108$ (95% CI 0.4072 to 0.6409, p-value=0.0001). In the calculation of the OR, those of 'very low' educational experience are used as the reference group and the OR is a measure of a single category change. So the estimated OR for the 'low' group is 0.5108 itself, whereas for the 'moderate' group it is $OR^2 = 0.5108 \times 0.5108 = 0.2609$ and, as we are assuming 'equal' intervals between the successive educational levels, that for the 'high' is $OR^3 = 0.1333$, and for the 'very high' is $OR^4 = 0.0681$. These OR estimates for each educational level are also included in Figure 4.4(a).

(a) *Presence of IHD by educational level*

tabulate ihd educ

ihd	educational level					Total
	very low	low	moderate	high	very high	
No	81	53	105	48	20	307
Yes	58	24	14	4	3	103
Total	139	77	119	52	23	410
IHD %	41.7	31.2	11.8	7.7	13.0	25.1
logit	−0.334	−0.792	2.015	−2.485	−1.897	−1.092
OR	1	0.5108	0.2609	0.1333	0.0681	

(b) *Estimating the regression coefficients and the OR*

logit ihd educ

Number of obs = 410, LR chi2(1) = 40.73, Prob > chi2 = 0.0001
Log likelihood = −210.7402

ihd	Coef	SE	z	P>|z|	[95% CI]
cons	0.3383	0.2508			
educ	−0.6717	0.1157	−5.81	0.0001	−0.8985 to −0.4449

logistic ihd educ

ihd	OR	SE	z	P>|z|	[95% CI]
educ	0.5108	0.0591	−5.81	0.0001	0.4072 to 0.6409

Figure 4.4 Logistic regression of the proportion with ischaemic heart disease (IHD) by educational experience (part data from the Singapore Cardiovascular Cohort Study 2)

The fitted model of equation (4.7) is plotted in Figure 4.5(a), whereas that for the proportion $p_{IHD,Level} = \dfrac{\exp(0.3383 - 0.6717Level)}{1 + \exp(0.3383 - 0.6717Level)}$, obtained using equation (4.4), is shown in Figure 4.5(b). These indicate a reasonable fit of the model, except for the 'very high' educational level group. However, subject numbers are small in this group so, when considered alone, the estimated proportion is $p = 3/23 = 0.13$ and has a wide 95% CI of 0.05 to 0.32 indicating that this point is not well established. Nevertheless, the model fitting process takes account of this small group size and thereby provides a smooth summary of the study results. The confidence interval quoted here is calculated using the exact approach described in Altman, Machin, Bryant and Gardner (2000, chapter 6).

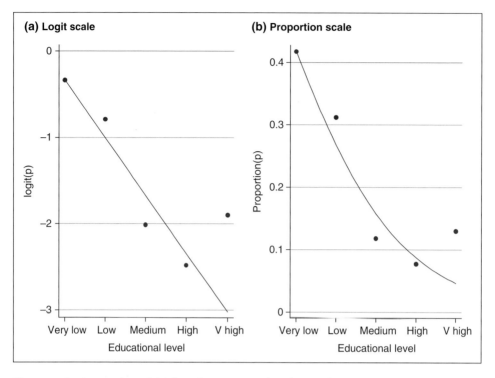

Figure 4.5 Scatter plots of (a) logit [proportion with ischaemic heart disease (IHD)] and (b) the corresponding estimated proportion itself by educational level together with the fitted logistic model added (part data from the Singapore Cardiovascular Cohort Study 2)

Continuous covariate

In the case of a continuous covariate we cannot tabulate the data as in Figures 4.1, 4.3(a), and 4.4(a), and thereby calculate the proportions of interest at each observed covariate value, x. In theory at least, every individual in the study may have a distinct value of x to which will be attached an endpoint value of either 0 or 1. Nevertheless, the logistic regression model of IHD on age in years, $Agey$, takes the same form as for the other types of covariates, thus:

$$A : \log\left(\frac{\pi_{IHD}}{1 - \pi_{IHD}}\right) = \beta_0 + \beta_A Agey \tag{4.8}$$

The value of the parameter π_{IHD} will depend on the age of the individual in the study concerned unless the null hypothesis: H_0: $\beta_A = 0$ is not rejected by the corresponding statistical test. Figure 4.6(a) shows the command and output for such a model to quantify the influence of age on the risk of developing IHD. On this basis the risk, not unexpectedly, appears to increase with age (as the estimated regression coefficient is positive) and the effect is highly statistically significant, p-value$=0.0001$. However, it is not immediately obvious how to interpret this table.

The fitted model is

$$A : \operatorname{logit}\left(p_{IHD}\right) = \log\left(\frac{p_{IHD}}{1 - p_{IHD}}\right) = b_0 + b_A Agey = -5.8097 + 0.1045 Agey \tag{4.9}$$

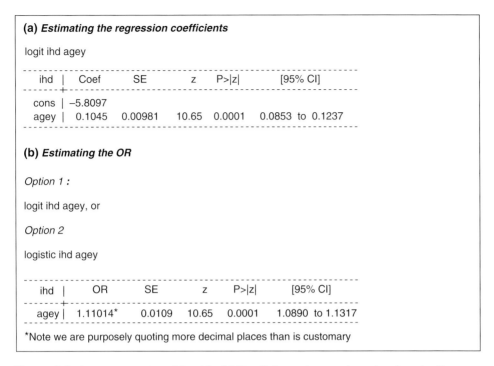

(a) *Estimating the regression coefficients*

logit ihd agey

ihd	Coef	SE	z	P>|z|	[95% CI]
cons	−5.8097				
agey	0.1045	0.00981	10.65	0.0001	0.0853 to 0.1237

(b) *Estimating the OR*

Option 1 :

logit ihd agey, or

Option 2

logistic ihd agey

ihd	OR	SE	z	P>|z|	[95% CI]
agey	1.11014*	0.0109	10.65	0.0001	1.0890 to 1.1317

*Note we are purposely quoting more decimal places than is customary

Figure 4.6 Logistic regression of the risk of IHD with increasing age (part data from the Singapore Cardiovascular Cohort Study 2)

For a continuous variable x, such as age in equation (4.9), the corresponding proportion p, in that example p_{IHD}, increases with increasing x following the general shape of the sigmoid curve of Figure 4.7.

Suppose we wish to compare two subjects whose ages are 40 and 60 years. First, dropping the subscript IHD for convenience, for someone aged 40, $\text{logit}(p_{40}) = -5.8097 + (0.1045 \times 40) = -1.6297$, from which using an equivalent expression to equation (4.4), $p_{40} = 0.1639$. Thus, the model estimates approximately 16% with IHD at age 40 years. For someone aged 60, $\text{logit}(p_{60}) = -5.8097 + (0.1045 \times 60) = 0.4603$ from which $p_{60} = 0.6131$. Thus, the model predicts approximately 61% with IHD at age 60 years. We can now compare the odds of IHD at 60 years with the odds of IHD at 40 years by means of the odds ratio $OR = [0.6131/(1 - 0.6131)]/[0.1639/(1 - 0.1639)] = 8.08$. Thus, those at 60 years have about eight times the risk of IHD compared with those at 40! This calculation can be obtained rather more easily by noting from equation (4.9) that: $\text{logit}(p_{60}) - \text{logit}(p_{40}) = [-5.8097 + 0.1045 \times 60] - [-5.8097 + 0.1045 \times 40] = 0.1045 (60 - 40) = 0.1045 \times 20 = 2.09$ and $\exp(2.09) = 8.08$.

These results can also be obtained by amending (**logit ihd agey**) to (**logit ihd agey, or**) or by using (**logistic ihd agey**) as shown in Figure 4.6(b). From this output, we can conclude that a subject 20 years older than another has an $OR = (1.11014)^{20} = 8.08$ times that of the younger.

The extra decimal places quoted for the OR are retained here so that rounding errors are reduced as we are raising this to a high power of 20. We should note too that the size of the OR given here depends directly on the units in which age is measured. Had months been used rather than years, then the OR given would have been $(1.11014)^{1/12} = (1.11014)^{0.08333} = 1.0008745$, which misguidingly appears very close to the null hypothesis value of H_0: $OR = 1$. Any change

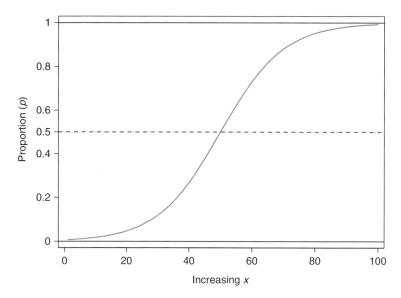

Figure 4.7 Logistic plot of increasing proportion with a particular condition as the continuous covariate x increases in magnitude

in units will change the reported OR, make appropriate changes to the size of the standard error and the 95% confidence interval, but will still give the same z (here 10.65) and p-value (here 0.0001) in the output. Importantly, any interpretation of the results remains unchanged. However, to avoid having the appearance of an OR close to 1 (unity), the scale of the continuous variable may be changed. Here, we might talk of the OR as applying to decades, hence quote: $OR_{Decade}=(1.11014)^{10}=2.84$ with 95% CI from 1.0890^{10} to 1.1317^{10} or 2.35 to 3.45.

However, such a description assumes that age (over the whole range from 18 to 79 years in this example) has a linear effect on the logit scale. This may need to be verified before firm conclusions are drawn concerning its effect on the occurrence of IHD.

If the covariate is continuous, or indeed numerical in nature, the (log) linear assumption with, for example, age in years of the participants, can be verified by fitting a quadratic model to the data. This takes the form:

$$A * A : \log\left(\frac{\pi}{1-\pi}\right) = \beta_0 + \beta_A Agey + \beta_{AA} Agey^2 \tag{4.10}$$

We then test the hypothesis, H_0: $\beta_{AA}=0$, which, if not rejected, implies that $\log\left(\frac{\pi}{1-\pi}\right) = \beta_0 + \beta_A Agey$ and we revert back to the simple model, A. In order to fit the quadratic model, the variable $AA=Agey \times Agey$ needs to be added to the database. The command (**logit ihd agey AA**) will then fit the quadratic model. It is worth noting that, and this is often the case in practice, the estimated regression coefficients corresponding to β_A are quite different in the two models.

The test of the null hypothesis $\beta_{AA}=0$ in model $A*A$ of Figure 4.8 gives $z=b_{AA}/$ SE(b_{AA}) = −4.08 and this implies, as the largest value of z in Table T1 is 3.99, that the p-value<2 $(1 - 0.99997)=0.00006$. Thus, we reject the null hypothesis and conclude that the assumption of linearity does not hold.

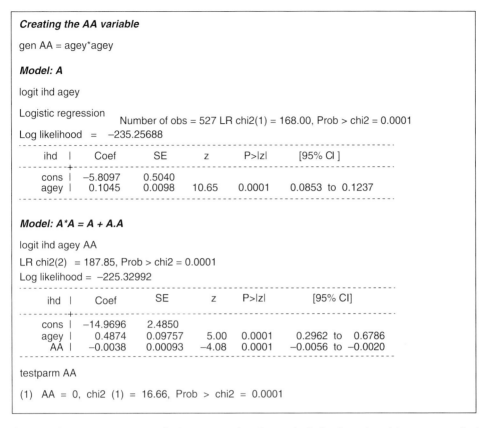

Figure 4.8 Logistic regression of IHD on age and age² to verify if a log (linear) model on age is justified (part data from the Singapore Cardiovascular Cohort Study 2)

This result is confirmed using the command (**testparm AA**), which gives a $\chi^2 = 16.66$ with $df = 1$, and p-value$= 0.0001$.

These analyses do not suggest that the relationship is *truly* quadratic, but only that it departs from (log) linearity. Further investigation may be necessary to identify the underlying pattern perhaps by dividing the continuous covariate, here age, into distinct groups to create an *ordered* categorical variable. This is then treated as an *unordered* categorical covariate in the consequent regression analysis. As an illustration, we first categorize age into the six groups (17–29, 30–39, 40–49, 50–59, 60–69, 70–79: covariate *AgeG6*), and then the profiles of the proportions with HDL and their corresponding logits, are examined. From Figure 4.9(a) one can see that the proportion with IHD increases rapidly from the youngest age group until 50–59 years, after which it tends to plateau. This plateau is confirmed when the oldest two categories are merged in Figure 4.9(b) (covariate *AgeG5*), and perhaps may be further merged into a broader 50–79 category. Moreover, as there is only one case of IHD in those aged 17–29, they too may be merged to create the wider age category 17–39 of Figure 4.9(c).

In general, such a process would precede any logistic regression analysis of such a covariate. Once decided on the appropriate form, the logistic regression of (say) *AgeG3* can then be fitted using dummy variables by the commands (**xi:logit ihd i.AgeG3**) and

(a) *Proportion with IHD in 6 age categories*

tabulate ihd AgeG6

ihd	AgeG6 (years)						Total
	17–29	30–39	40–49	50–59	60–69	70–79	
No	105	120	75	35	35	2	372
Yes	1	8	37	55	50	4	155
Total	106	128	112	90	85	6	527
p	0.0094	0.0625	0.3304	0.6111	0.5882	0.6667	0.2941
logit (p)	−4.65	−2.71	−0.71	0.45	0.36	0.69	−0.88

tabulate ihd AgeG5

(b) *Proportion with IHD in 5 age categories*

ihd	AgeG5					Total
	17–29	30–39	40–49	50–59	60–79	
No	105	120	75	35	37	372
Yes	1	8	37	55	54	155
Total	106	128	112	90	91	527
p	0.0094	0.0625	0.3304	0.6111	0.5934	0.2941
logit (p)	−4.65	−2.71	−0.71	0.45	0.38	−0.88

tabulate ihd AgeG3

(c) *Proportion with IHD in 3 age categories*

ihd	AgeG3			Total
	17–39	40–49	50–79	
No	225	75	72	372
Yes	9	37	109	155
Total	234	112	181	527
p	0.0385	0.3304	0.6022	0.2941
logit (p)	−3.22	−0.71	0.41	−0.88

Figure 4.9 Proportions with IHD when age is grouped into one of 6, 5 or 3 distinct categories (part data from the Singapore Cardiovascular Cohort Study 2)

(a) *Assuming AgeG3 is unordered categorical*

xi : logit ihd i.AgeG3

xi : logit ihd i.AgeG3, or

Logistic regression   Number of obs = 527

ihd	Coef.	SE	z	P>|z|	[95% CI]
b0	−3.2189	0.3399			
c1	0				
c2	2.5123	0.3949	6.36	0.0001	1.7384 to 3.2862
c3	3.6336	0.3723	9.76	0.0001	2.9038 to 4.3633

ihd	OR	SE	z	P>|z|	[95% CI]
c1	1				
c2	12.3333	4.8700	6.36	0.0001	5.6882 to 26.7416
c3	37.8472	14.0911	9.76	0.0001	18.2439 to 78.5144

(b) *Assuming AgeG3 as ordered categorical on an equal step numerical scale*

logit ihd AgeG3

logit ihd AgeG3, or

ihd	Coef	SE	z	P>|z|	[95% CI]
b0	−4.4223	0.3779			
AgeG3	1.6494	0.1509	10.93	0.0001	1.3536 to 1.9452

ihd	OR	SE	z	P>|z|	[95% CI]
AgeG3	5.2038	0.7854	10.93	0.0001	3.8712 to 6.9950

Figure 4.10 Logistic regression of IHD on age where the continuous variable age is categorized in three distinct groups and then regarded as an (a) unordered and (b) ordered categorical covariate in the regression model (part data from the Singapore Cardiovascular Cohort Study 2)

(**xi:logit ihd i.AgeG3, or**) of Figure 4.10(a). These regard the ordered categorical covariate *AgeG3* as if it were unordered. If the relationship was perfectly linear then, as the dummy variable regression coefficient of $c_2 = 2.5123$, we would anticipate $c_3 = 2 \times 2.5123 = 5.0246$. This is clearly not exactly the case. However, despite this, if the covariate is treated as ordered categorical (with three equally spaced numerical values, 0, 1 and 2), then the appropriate command is (**logit ihd AgeG3**). The corresponding output is shown in Figure 4.10(b) with a single regression coefficient ($b_{AgeG3} = 1.6494$) giving an $OR_{AgeG3} = \exp(1.6494) = 5.2038$. This implies that as we compare age groups 17–39 and 40–49 the $OR = 5.2$, and when comparing those who are 50-79 years with the youngest of 17–39 it is $OR^2 = 27.0$. Some judgment is required as to whether this facilitates a better description of the study results, particularly as the value just quoted is very different from that of $OR = 37.8$ calculated for this oldest age group in Figure 4.10(a). By creating *unequal* but ordered category divisions and then giving these an *equal* interval numerical scale, we have imposed a linear response. In this example, a better numerical scale might be the one provided by the mid-ages of each category, that is, 28, 45, and 65 years.

MULTIPLE LOGISTIC REGRESSION

In the same way that multiple regression is an extension of simple linear regression, we can extend logistic regression to multiple logistic regression to include more than one covariate. These covariates can be binary, unordered categorical, ordered categorical, discrete numerical or continuous in form and in any combination within the model. In general, if there are k covariates $x_1, x_2, \ldots, x_k$, then the model becomes:

$$\log\left(\frac{\pi}{1-\pi}\right) = \beta_0 + \beta_1 x_1 + \ldots + \beta_k x_k \tag{4.11}$$

Although both the quadratic model of Age and the unordered categorical model of $AgeG3$ are dealing with a single covariate, the fitting process requires a multi-variable regression model. In both situations each model involves β_0 and two additional parameters. However, in other circumstances the covariates concerned may only require a single additional parameter to be added to the model.

For example, apart from recording episodes of HRV illnesses, the study conducted by Jackson, Gangnon, Evans, *et al.* (2008) summarized in Figure 4.1 also noted whether the infants had or did not have experience of aeroallergen ($Aero$) sensitisation in their first year of life. Thus, the presence of asthma or not by six years of age can be presented by the four HRV by Aero groups as in Figure 4.11(a).

With covariates, HRV and $Aero$, there are now three different logistic models to compare. The first of Figure 4.11(b) is the univariate model, H, and concerns the presence or absence of HRV: the results of which have been summarized in Figure 4.2 and equation (4.3). The second is again a univariate model but now that for $Aero$, model Ae, and the third model combines both HRV and $Aero$, model $H+Ae$, into a multiple logistic regression.

It is clear from Figure 4.11(b) that each of the univariate models H and Ae appear to be strongly predictive of asthma by six years in these children. Of the two models, Ae appears to be the most predictive with p-value$=0.0008$ as opposed to 0.0024 for H. However, the main focus of the study is on the influence of HRV, so this poses the question: Does adding $Aero$ to the univariate model of HRV alone improve the model fit?

The log likelihood associated with $H+Ae$ is $L_{H+Ae} = -140.8757$, and that for H is $L_H = -146.3552$. Applying the likelihood ratio test of equation (4.19) in the *Technical details* section gives $LR = -2\,[L_H - L_{H+Ae}] = -2[-146.3552 - (-140.8757)] = 10.9590$. This has $df=1$ as the model $H+Ae$ has only one more parameter than H. Hence, $z = \sqrt{10.9590} = 3.31$ and Table T1 gives a p-value$=2\,(1-0.99953)=0.00094$, which is highly statistically significant. This is close to the value obtained by using the command (`testparm Aero`) as in Figure 4.11(d). Alternatively, using Table T5 with $df=1$ suggests a p-value close to 0.001. This also confirms the analysis suggested following the command (`logit Asthma HRV Aero`) of Figure 4.11(c), which gives $z=3.33$ and p-value$=0.0009$.

The analysis firmly suggests that both HRV and $Aero$ should be in the model for predicting asthma by six years of age and this is estimated by:

$$H + Ae : \text{logit}(p) = -1.3705 + 1.0452\,HRV + 1.2869\,Aero \tag{4.12}$$

If ($HRV=0$, $Aero=0$), then $\text{logit}(p) = -1.3705$ from which $p_{0,0}=\exp(-1.3705)/[1+\exp(-1.3705]=0.2025$. Similarly, if ($HRV=1, Aero=0$) then $\text{logit}(p)=-1.3705+1.0452 = -0.3253$ from which $p_{1,0} = 0.4194$, when ($HRV = 0$, $Aero = 1$) then $\text{logit}(p) = -1.3705 +$

(a) *Two binary covariates: HRV and Aero*

table Asthma Aero HRV

```
-------------------------------------------------
            |              HRV  and  Aero
            |------- No HRV -----   ------ Yes HRV -----
   Asthma |  No  Aero  Yes  Aero    No Aero  Yes  Aero
------------+------------------------------------------
No Asthma |      145          15          23          1
   Asthma |       38          12          15          6
-------------------------------------------------
Total      |      183          27          38          7
-------------------------------------------------
Asthma (%) |    20.77       44.44       39.47      85.71
-------------------------------------------------
```

(b) *Single covariate models H and Ae*

logit Asthma HRV

Logistic regression   Number of obs = 255

LR chi2 (1) = 8.94, Prob > chi2 = 0.0028, Log likelihood = −146.3552

Asthma	Coef	SE	z	P>|z|	[95% CI]
cons	−1.1632	0.1620			
HRV	1.0296	0.3399	3.03	0.0024	0.3634 to 1.6958

logit Asthma Aero

LR chi2 (1) = 11.15, Prob > chi2 = 0.0008, Log likelihood = −145.2507

Asthma	Coef	SE	z	P>|z|	[95% CI]
cons	−1.1537	0.1575			
Aero	1.2715	0.3780	3.36	0.0008	0.5306 to 2.0123

(c) *Multi-variable model: H + Ae*

logit Asthma HRV Aero

LR chi2(2) = 19.90, Prob > chi2 = 0.0001, Log likelihood = −140.8757

Asthma	Coef	SE	z	P>|z|	[95% CI]
cons	−1.3705	0.1808			
HRV	1.0452	0.3491	2.99	0.0028	0.3610 to 1.7293
Aero	1.2869	0.3862	3.33	0.0009	0.5299 to 2.0439

(d) *Comparing model H + Ae with H*

testparm Aero

(1) Aero = 0, chi2 (1) = 11.10, Prob > chi2 = 0.0009

Figure 4.11 Proportion of children who develop asthma by six years of age in those exposed or not exposed to human rhinovirus (HRV) wheezing illnesses and aeroallergen (*Aero*) sensitization in their first year of life (data from Jackson, Gangnon, Evans, *et al.*, 2008, TABLE 3)

$1.2869 = -0.0836$ from which $p_{0,1} = 0.4791$, and finally if $(HRV = 1, Aero = 1)$ then $\text{logit}(p) = -1.3705 + 1.0452 + 1.2869 = +0.9616$ from which $p_{1,1} = 0.7234$.

If we now calculate the OR of $(HRV=1, Aero=0)$ compared with $(HRV=0, Aero=0)$ we

have $OR_{1,0} = \dfrac{p_{1,0}/(1-p_{1,0})}{p_{0,0}/(1-p_{0,0})} = \dfrac{0.4194/(1-0.4194)}{0.2025/(1-0.2025)} = 2.8448$. Similarly, we can calculate

$OR_{0,1} = \dfrac{0.4791/(1-0.4791)}{0.2025/(1-0.2025)} = 3.6222$, and finally $OR_{1,1} = \dfrac{0.7234/(1-0.7234)}{0.2025/(1-0.2025)} = 10.2999$

≈ 10.30. However, we note that we can calculate the latter directly by $OR_{1,1} = OR_{1,0} \times OR_{0,1} = 2.8448 \times 3.6222 = 10.3044 \approx 10.30$ also.

Interactions

A further question before deciding on a final model for any investigation which includes two or more covariates is: Are there any interactions present between any of the covariates that are included in the model? For example, if a patient has been exposed to both risk factors, in the previous example the group $HRV=1$ *and* $Aero=1$, then the combined effect of the presence of both may give greater (or lesser) risk than would be anticipated from the sum of the effect of each factor as determined from the corresponding univariate models. However, as the logistic model is described in terms of logarithms, what is additive on a logarithmic scale is actually multiplicative on the linear scale.

As with multiple regression, the multiple logistic regression equation can investigate potential interactions arising from a particular combination of covariates. The 'interaction' covariate can be generated by the product of the two covariates concerned, for example, $x_3 = x_1 \times x_2$. We can then add this term to the 2-covariate model to give:

$$\log\left(\frac{\pi}{1-\pi}\right) = \beta_0 + \beta_1 x_1 + \beta_2 x_2 + \beta_3 x_3 \tag{4.13}$$

The magnitude of the associated regression coefficient then indicates whether the two factors interact together in an antagonistic or a synergistic (either more or less than multiplicative) way, or essentially act independently of each other. In this latter situation, the associated estimated regression coefficient for the interaction term will be close to zero.

The test of the null hypothesis of no interaction is conducted by testing the hypothesis: $\beta_3 = 0$ in equation (4.13). Such an analysis is summarized in Figure 4.12(a), which investigates the interaction between the binary covariates presence of HRV and Aero sensitization using the model: ***H*Ae: H+Ae+H.Ae.*** In this example $x_3 = HRV \times Aero$ and the corresponding regression parameter, $\beta_{HRVAero}$, is estimated by $b_3 = b_{HRVAero} = 1.1032$, with standard error, $SE = 1.2083$. From these $z = 1.1032/1.2083 = 0.91$, with associated p-value $= 0.36$. Alternatively the command (`testparm HRVAero`) can be used as in Figure 4.12(b). The result is not statistically significant so we do not need to include the interaction term in the final model, and it remains that of equation (4.12). This model, on the OR scale, is repeated in Figure 4.12(c), and we note that their product (corresponding to $HRV=1$ and $Aero=1$) is $2.84 \times 3.62 = 10.3$ as demonstrated earlier. In contrast, had the interaction term been statistically significant then the multiplicative nature of these ORs would no longer hold.

In Stata (2007b), and this is similar with other statistical programs, the command to generate *HRVAero* can be circumvented by expressing the commands of Figure 4.12(a) into a

(a) *Fitting the interaction model H*Ae*

gen HRVAero=HRV*Aero

logit Asthma HRV Aero HRVAero

Logistic regression   Number of obs = 255

LR chi2 (3) = 20.87, Prob > chi2 = 0.0001, Log likelihood = −140.39123

```
--------------------------------------------------------------------
   Asthma |   Coef      SE      z    P>|z|         [95% CI]
----------+---------------------------------------------------------
     cons |  −1.3391   0.1822
      HRV |   0.9117   0.3786   2.41  0.016    0.1696 to 1.6538
     Aero |   1.1160   0.4280   2.61  0.0091   0.2771 to 1.9549
  HRVAero |   1.1032   1.2083   0.91  0.36    −1.2651 to 3.4715
--------------------------------------------------------------------
```

(b) *Testing for the presence of an interaction*

testparm HRVAero

(1) HRVAero = 0, chi2(1) = 0.83, Prob > chi2 = 0.36

(c) *ORs for the final model: H + Ae*

logistic Asthma HRV Aero

```
--------------------------------------------------------------------
   Asthma |   OR      SE      z    P>|z|         [95% CI]
----------+---------------------------------------------------------
      HRV |  2.84   0.9927   2.99  0.0028   1.4347 to 5.6369
     Aero |  3.62   1.3988   3.33  0.0009   1.6988 to 7.7207
--------------------------------------------------------------------
```

Figure 4.12 Proportion of children who develop asthma by six years of age in those exposed or not exposed to human rhinovirus (HRV) wheezing illnesses and aeroallergen (*Aero*) sensitization or not in their first year of life: investigating the possible interaction between HRV and *Aero* (data from Jackson, Gangnon, Evans, *et al.*, 2008, TABLE 3)

single command (`xi : logit Asthma i.HRV*i.Aero`), where the (*) indicates that an interaction term is to be included in the model in addition to the covariates *HRV* and *Aero*.

MODEL CHECKING

Tabulations

An important question is whether the logistic model describes the data well. If the logistic model is obtained from grouped data, then there is no difficulty as one can compare the observed proportions in each of the groups with those that are predicted by the model. Such tabulations are a very useful preliminary *before* a model is chosen, as they will often give a strong indication of the type of model to fit.

As an example, Figure 4.13(a) tabulates the number of subjects with and without a diagnosis of IHD by gender and ethnic group and gives, for example, the observed percentage of Chinese

---

(a) Proportions with IHD in each gender by ethnic group

table ihd ethnic gender

			gender and ethnicity			
		Male			Female	
ihd	chinese	malay	indian	chinese	malay	indian
No	110	43	26	106	45	42
Yes	44	22	43	17	10	19
Total	154	65	69	123	55	61
Observed Yes(%)	28.57	33.85	62.32	13.82	18.18	31.15
Predicted Yes(%)	29.26	35.33	59.38	12.96	16.43	34.47
Obs - Pred	−0.69	−1.48	+2.94	+0.86	+1.75	−3.32

(b) Model E + G

xi: logit ihd i.ethnic gender
xi: logistic ihd i.ethnic gender

ihd	Coef	SE	OR	z	P>|z|
b_0	−0.8827	0.1612			
Chinese	0		1		
Malay	0.2781	0.2580	1.3206	1.08	0.28
Indian	1.2624	0.2361	3.5340	5.35	0.0001
Male	0		1		
Female	−1.0221	0.2122	0.3598	−4.82	0.0001

Figure 4.13   The proportion of individuals diagnosed with IHD classified by gender and ethnicity (part data from the Singapore Cardiovascular Cohort Study 2)

males with IHD as 28.57%. The corresponding logistic regression model is obtained using the command (**xi: logit ihd i.ethnic gender**) to obtain the regression coefficients and (**xi: logistic ihd i.ethnic gender**) the ORs of Figure 4.13(b) from which the predicted percentages in each of the six gender by ethnic groups can be obtained. For the Chinese males this is 29.26%, and this is quite close to that observed. The agreement is also close for the other five subject groups. In general therefore, we might conclude that the model is satisfactory.

Lack of an important covariate

In some situations the model may not fit well because an important covariate is omitted from the model. This problem can be investigated by trying all available covariates, and the possible interactions between them, to see if the model can be improved.

Outlying or influential observations

We introduced the concept of residuals in Chapter 2 in the situation where y is a continuous variable whose value will differ from subject-to-subject. In this situation, once a specific regression model is fitted, the predicted Y can be obtained. The residual for a particular observation (say) i, is then calculated as $e_i = y_i - Y_i$. For the n subjects concerned, these residuals could all have unique values. Potential patterns in the e_i observed are then used, for example, to identify influential observations among the individuals concerned and the extent of their impact on the final interpretation of the study established. However, for a binary outcome variable the situation is somewhat different.

Consider the situation in which the influence of gender and ethnicity on the probability of an individual having IHD is to be investigated. In this example, there are six covariate patterns in the data set corresponding to the 2 gender by 3 ethnic groups in the table of Figure 4.13(a). These patterns are identified using the command (`predict patGE, number`), followed by (`summarize patGE`) after the model (`xi : logistic ihd gender i.ethnic`) is fitted to the data to obtain the details given in Figure 4.14(a). Here in `patGE`, 'pat' indicates pattern and the 'GE' is added to indicate the particular model being fitted. Further, the subsequent command (`predict residGE, residuals`) of Figure 4.14(b) calculates the corresponding Pearson residuals; that is the difference between the observed and the estimated probability divided by the standard deviation of the estimated probability, whereas (`predict leverGE, hat`) calculates the Pregibon (1981) leverage of the covariate pattern which we term 'leverGE'. These are plotted in Figure 4.14(c), where the three points to the left of the vertical line correspond to the three gender by ethnicity groups whose estimated proportion with IHD predicted from the fitted model is greater than that observed, whereas for those to the right the opposite is the case.

The leverage is a measure of distance in terms of the covariates. A large value indicates a pattern distinct from the average covariate pattern and is therefore one that may have a large effect on the value of the estimates of the regression coefficients in the fitted model even if the corresponding residual is small. As might be anticipated, the largest leverage of 0.8287 is attached to the Male Chinese who are the largest group of subjects but have the smallest residual, −0.1883.

In the scatter plot of Figure 4.14(c) it is very obvious that there are 6 gender by ethnic group covariate patterns so that the pattern command is somewhat redundant in this example. In contrast, if the model (`logit ihd agey`) is fitted to the data, as in Figure 4.15(a), there are now 520 distinct patterns among the 527 subjects concerned and this would not have been easy to establish in such a large data set. Thus, as we are looking at age alone here and ignoring other covariates, virtually every subject has a different age and hence a different covariate pattern. Once again the scatter plot of `leverAge` against `residAge` (consisting of 520 distinct data points) can be divided into those patterns for which the estimated proportion with IHD predicted from the fitted model is greater than that observed, and those for which it is less. Further, patterns which are 'outside' the general behavior can be identified such as those, for example, with leverage greater than 0.012 in Figure 4.15(b). This identifies two individuals listed in Figure 4.15(c) of precisely the same age of 63.28 years, but one has IHD and the other does not. Coincidentally, they are both of Malay ethnicity and male so that even if gender and ethnicity were to be added to the model fitted they would still comprise a single covariate pattern. Despite the highest leverage of 0.0128 (range from 0.0021 to 0.0128), the corresponding residuals for the two individuals (range from −3.2699 to +3.9184) are −0.5827 and so are not extreme. One coincident point indicates that an Indian Male and a Chinese Female, both aged

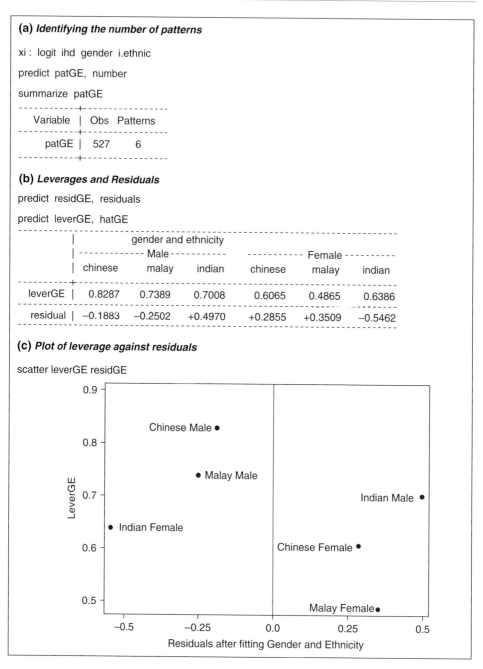

(a) *Identifying the number of patterns*

xi : logit ihd gender i.ethnic

predict patGE, number

summarize patGE

```
-----------+-------------------
 Variable |  Obs  Patterns
-----------+-------------------
   patGE |  527    6
-----------+-------------------
```

(b) *Leverages and Residuals*

predict residGE, residuals

predict leverGE, hatGE

```
-----------------------------------------------------------------------------------
         |               gender and ethnicity
         |-------------- Male ----------      ---------- Female ----------
         | chinese     malay      indian      chinese     malay      indian
---------+-------------------------------------------------------------------------
 leverGE |  0.8287     0.7389     0.7008      0.6065     0.4865     0.6386
---------+-------------------------------------------------------------------------
 residual| -0.1883    -0.2502    +0.4970      +0.2855    +0.3509    -0.5462
-----------------------------------------------------------------------------------
```

(c) *Plot of leverage against residuals*

scatter leverGE residGE

Figure 4.14 Patterns of the leverage and residuals within the six gender by ethnicity groups with respect to the probability of IHD (part data from the Singapore Cardiovascular Cohort Study 2)

39.4 years, have the same residual (1.3408) and the same leverage (0.0063) but only one exhibits evidence of IHD.

The general pattern of the residuals for age alone of Figure 4.15 (b) is somewhat difficult to interpret. However, when the model (**xi : logit agey i.ethnic**) is fitted to the

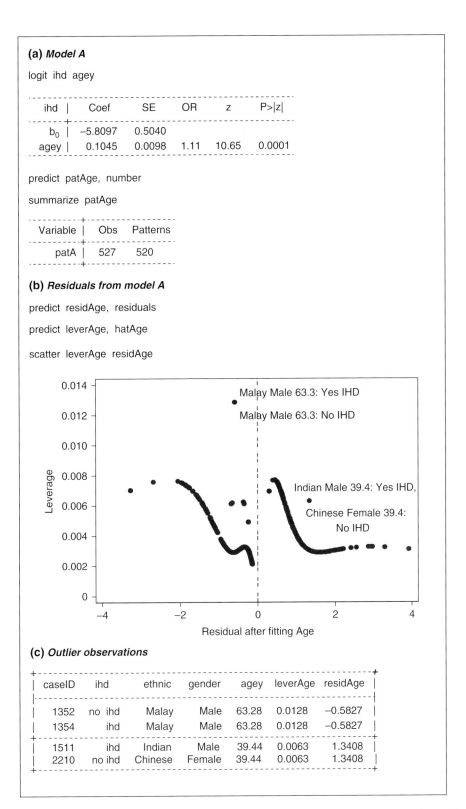

(a) *Model A*

logit ihd agey

ihd	Coef	SE	OR	z	P>|z|
b_0	−5.8097	0.5040			
agey	0.1045	0.0098	1.11	10.65	0.0001

predict patAge, number

summarize patAge

Variable	Obs	Patterns
patA	527	520

(b) *Residuals from model A*

predict residAge, residuals

predict leverAge, hatAge

scatter leverAge residAge

Malay Male 63.3: Yes IHD

Malay Male 63.3: No IHD

Indian Male 39.4: Yes IHD,

Chinese Female 39.4: No IHD

Leverage

Residual after fitting Age

(c) *Outlier observations*

caseID	ihd	ethnic	gender	agey	leverAge	residAge
1352	no ihd	Malay	Male	63.28	0.0128	−0.5827
1354	ihd	Malay	Male	63.28	0.0128	−0.5827
1511	ihd	Indian	Male	39.44	0.0063	1.3408
2210	no ihd	Chinese	Female	39.44	0.0063	1.3408

Figure 4.15 Influence of age on the probability of IHD (part data from the Singapore Cardiovascular Cohort Study 2)

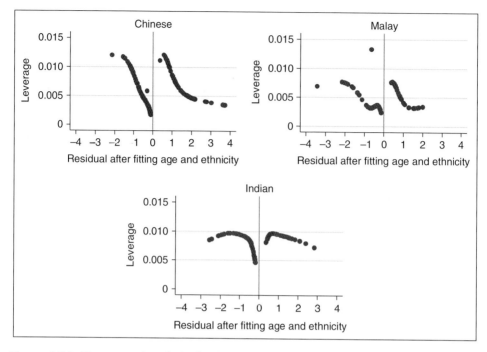

Figure 4.16 The pattern of residuals after fitting a logistic model examining the influence of age and ethnicity on the probability of IHD (part data from the Singapore Cardiovascular Cohort Study 2)

data, the corresponding plots for each ethnic group are shown in Figure 4.16. Once again outliers can be identified but, more importantly for this example, very different profiles are evident in each ethnic group. Consequently, the analyst needs to be concerned as to whether or not a single regression model is appropriate for these data or perhaps separate models for each ethnic group may be required.

We have indicated that, for the 527 subjects for which we have their IHD status (presence or absence), if we consider only the binary covariate gender and the unordered categorical covariate ethnicity then there are only $M=6$ covariate patterns associated with the corresponding model. Extending such a model to include (say) smoking status classified as heavy, moderate, light, non- or ex-smoker, increases the number of covariate patterns to: $M=2 \times 3 \times 5=30$. The associated scatter plot of leverage against residual will comprise 30 points unless there is one or more of the patterns for which there are no individuals included in the study. In general, if there are v binary and/or categorical covariates to consider making a total of (say) V patterns in all, then the covariate values for each individual subject in the study provide a point in V-dimensional space (this locates the pattern concerned) and there may be several subjects with a covariate pattern at the same point in which case $M<V$. If these coincident points are far from (say) the cloud of all other points, then the associated pattern has high leverage. On the other hand, if the pattern is within the cloud of other patterns it will have low leverage. If the leverage is low then there is likely to be minimal impact of these points on the final study interpretation, whereas if it is high the consequences may need careful examination and reporting.

Goodness-of-fit

If there are not too many patterns, the goodness-of-fit of a model can be assessed using the Pearson statistic. This compares the observed number of events in each pattern, y_j, with the number predicted by the chosen logistic model. Thus, if there are M patterns, and m_j is the number of subjects in each pattern, then the number of events predicted by the model is $m_j p_j$ where p_j is obtained from, for example, expressions such as equation (4.4). The Pearson residual compares the difference $(y_j - m_j p_j)$ with the corresponding standard deviation estimated by $\sqrt{[m_j p_j (1 - p_j)]}$. The Pearson statistic is the sum of squares of the corresponding residual and is defined by:

$$Pearson = \sum_{j=1}^{M} \frac{(y_j - m_j p_j)^2}{m_j p_j (1 - p_j)} \tag{4.14}$$

The *Pearson* statistic follows the χ^2 distribution of Table T5 with $df = M - k$, where k is the number of parameters estimated in the model concerned. However, for some situations the df will be too large for the table, where the maximum is 30, but most statistical packages will automatically provide the necessary p-value. If the test is statistically significant, then this immediately suggests that the model does not describe the data adequately.

Figure 4.17(a) tabulates IHD status within the $M = 6$ covariate patterns determined by gender and ethnicity. The corresponding model is fitted by the command (**xi: logit ihd i.ethnic gender**) and provides estimates for the corresponding $k = 4$ regression coefficients concerned. The command (**estat gof, table**) tests the goodness-of-fit of the model and indicates quite clearly with $Pearson = 0.85$, $df = 2$ and p-value $= 0.65$ that the model provides a good fit to these data. The output also provides the individual estimates of the proportions with IHD provided by the fitted model. Thus, for example, for Chinese Male the observed proportion with IHD is 0.2857 (44/154), whereas the fitted model predicts (labeled Group 3 in the output) 0.2926 (approximately 45.1/154), which is very similar.

If the model is extended to include smoking status then the command is extended to (**xi: logit ihd i.ethnic gender i.smoke**) and the number of covariate patterns is extended to $M = 18$. However, the corresponding goodness-of-fit test of Figure 4.17(b), omitting the (**table**) option, only indicates $M = 17$ patterns are present within the data and this takes account of the fact that there are no Malay Male non-smokers in this example. Adding smoking status to the previous model increases the number of regression coefficients in the fitted model to $k = 6$, hence $df = 17 - 6 = 11$. The corresponding test of the goodness-of-fit of the model gives $Pearson = 7.60$ and p-value $= 0.75$, and indicates that the model provides a good fit to these data.

CONDITIONAL LOGISTIC REGRESSION

A case-control study is an observational investigation in which persons with a disease (or relevant outcome) of interest are compared with a suitable control group of individuals without the condition in question. The relationship of a covariate to the condition in question is examined by comparing the change in its value between those with and without the condition. There are two distinct types of case-control study: one that is matched and one

(a) Predictions for E + G

table ihd ethnic gender

		gender and ethnicity				
		Male			Female	
ihd cases	chinese	malay	indian	chinese	malay	indian
no ihd	110	43	26	106	45	42
ihd	44	22	43	17	10	19

xi : logit ihd i.ethnic gender

Logistic regression   Number of obs = 527

ihd	Coef	SE	z	P>|z|	[95% CI]	
cons	-0.8827	0.1612				
Iethnic_2	0.2781	0.2580	1.08	0.28	-0.2275 to	0.7837
Iethnic_3	1.2624	0.2361	5.35	0.0001	0.7997 to	1.7252
gender	-1.0221	0.2122	-4.82	0.0001	-1.4380 to	-0.6062

estat gof, table

Logistic model for ihd, goodness-of-fit test

Group	Prob	Obs_1	Exp_1	Obs_0	Exp_0	Total
1	0.1296	17	15.9	106	107.1	123
2	0.1643	10	9.0	45	46.0	55
3	0.2926	44	45.1	110	108.9	154
4	0.3447	19	21.0	42	40.0	61
5	0.3533	22	23.0	43	42.0	65
6	0.5938	43	41.0	26	28.0	69

number of observations = 527
number of covariate patterns = 6
Pearson chi2 (2) = 0.85
Prob > chi2 = 0.65

(b) Model E + G + S

xi : logit ihd i.ethnic gender i.smoke

Log likelihood = -293.17547

ihd	Coef	SE	z	P > |z|	[95% CI]	
cons	-0.8920	0.1719				
Iethnic_2	0.2803	0.2589	1.08	0.28	-0.2271 to	0.7877
Iethnic_3	1.2642	0.2364	5.35	0.0001	0.8009 to	1.7275
gender	-1.0205	0.2124	-4.80	0.0001	-1.4368 to	-0.6042
Ismoke_2	-0.0288	0.6168	-0.05	0.96	-1.2377 to	1.1800
Ismoke_3	0.0501	0.2684	0.19	0.85	-0.4759 to	0.5761

estat gof
number of observations = 527
number of covariate patterns = 17
Pearson chi2 (11) = 7.60
Prob > chi2 = 0.75

Figure 4.17 Goodness-of-fit of the model including ethnicity, gender and smoking status on the probability of IHD (part data from the Singapore Cardiovascular Cohort Study 2)

```
list match anorexia Mage Parity gravwk bweight trauma
  +-----------------------------------------------------------------------+
  |      match   anorexia    Mage    Parity  Gravidity  Birthwght  Trauma |
  |----------------------------------------------------------------------|
  1.|      1       Control     30       1        39        3100       0    |
  2.|      1        Case       29       1        39        3250       0    |
  3.|      1       Control     25       2        40        3630       0    |
  4.|      1       Control     24       1        39        3360       0    |
  5.|      1       Control     22       1        40        3500       0    |
  6.|      1       Control     21       2        41        3720       0    |
    |----------------------------------------------------------------------|
  7.|      2        Case       33       2        38        3750       0    |
  8.|      2       Control     32       5        42        3320       0    |
  9.|      2       Control     27       3        42        3710       0    |
 10.|      2       Control     28       1        39        3210       0    |
 11.|      2       Control     27       1        42        3850       0    |
 12.|      2       Control     25       1        40        3680       0    |
  +-----------------------------------------------------------------------+
```

Figure 4.18   Listings of two 1:5 matched case-control sets, with the case having a diagnosis of anorexia nervosa – the variable 'match' defines those individuals that comprise the matched group (part data from Cnattingius, Hultman, Dahl and Sparén, 1999)

that is not. In the former, and this is the situation in Figure 4.18, a number of 'control' individuals are matched to a particular 'case'. The data listed form part of a case-control study conducted by Cnattingius, Hultman, Dahl and Sparén (1999), who wished to investigate whether factors at the time of birth contribute to the risk of an individual female developing anorexia later in life. Thus, the cases in this study are young women diagnosed with anorexia nervosa whereas the controls are other young women who do not have the condition. Each case was linked or matched to young women without a diagnosis of anorexia nervosa who were born in the same hospital and year. Using the birth records, mother's age (*Mage*), parity, gravidity, birth weight and experience of trauma at birth, were noted. The first case (match=1), whose data are in Row 2 of the database, is matched to 5 Controls, whose data are in rows, 1, 3, 4, 5, and 6. In contrast, an *unmatched* case-control study would be one in which a similar group (here young women) may be recruited to the study but the information recorded on the controls is not linked directly to a particular case. Then in the corresponding analysis, each group (controls and cases) is first summarized as a whole and then the two compared.

The data from each match-group can be summarized in a 2×2 table as those of Figure 4.19(a). In the first table of match-group 16, the anorexia case did not experience a trauma-at-birth, whereas, of the 5 controls, 1 did and 4 did not. In the second table of match-group 42, the case experienced a trauma, whereas the 5 controls did not. These tables, one for each match-group, form the units for analysis and thereby retain the essential linkage within each 6-subject group.

If the linking is ignored, then the 'broken-match' data would be summarized with respect to the risk posed from trauma-at-birth, as in Figure 4.19(b) from which $OR_{Trauma} = \dfrac{3787 \times 38}{743 \times 118} = 1.64.$

Alternatively, it can be calculated using (**logit anorexia trauma**) and which would also give the 95% CI as 1.13 to 2.39. However, the appropriate (matched) analysis can be conducted using *conditional* logistic regression. To fit the univariate model for trauma, *T*, the commands (**clogit anorexia trauma, group(match) vce(robust)**) which gives the estimated regression coefficients, and (**clogit anorexia trauma, group(match)**

(a) *Matched groups*	(b) *All data ignoring the matching*
tabulate anorexia trauma if match==16	tabulate anorexia trauma

(a) Matched groups

tabulate anorexia trauma if match==16

```
---------+------------------+--------
anorexia |      trauma      |
         |   No      Yes    |  Total
---------+------------------+--------
     No  |    4       1     |    5
     Yes |    1       0     |    1
---------+------------------+--------
  Total  |    5       1     |    6
---------+------------------+--------
```

tabulate anorexia trauma if match==42

```
---------+------------------+--------
anorexia |      trauma      |
         |   No      Yes    |  Total
---------+------------------+--------
     No  |    5       0     |    5
     Yes |    0       1     |    1
---------+------------------+--------
  Total  |    5       1     |    6
---------+------------------+--------
```

(b) All data ignoring the matching

tabulate anorexia trauma

```
---------+------------------------+--------
anorexia |         trauma         |
         |   No          Yes      |  Total
---------+------------------------+--------
     No  |  3,787        118      |  3,905
     Yes |    743         38      |    781
---------+------------------------+--------
  Total  |  4,530        156      |  4,686
---------+------------------------+--------
```

Figure 4.19 Examples of tabulations of anorexia nervosa status by presence or absence of trauma-at-birth for (a) two matched groups of size 6, and (b) a pooled summary from all subjects in the study ignoring the matching (data from Cnattingius, Hultman, Dahl and Sparén, 1999)

```
clogit anorexia trauma, group(match) vce(robust)

Conditional (fixed-effects) logistic regression          Number of obs = 4686
```

anorexia	Coef	SE	z	P>|z|	[95% CI]
trauma	0.5147	0.1910	2.70	0.0069	0.1405 to 0.8890

```
clogit anorexia trauma, group (match)  vce (robust) or
```

anorexia	OR	SE	z	P>|z|	[95% CI]
trauma	1.6732	0.3195	2.70	0.0069	1.1508 to 2.4327

Figure 4.20 Conditional logistic regression of a matched case-control study of risk factors associated with the development of anorexia nervosa (data from Cnattingius, Hultman, Dahl and Sparén, 1999)

vce(robust) or) which provides the corresponding OR, are used. These commands take note of the individual case-control groups and provide *robust* estimates of the standard errors (SE) of the regression coefficients. We explain in more detail the reason for use of the (so-called) robust estimates of the SEs in Chapter 5, *Over-dispersion and robust estimates*.

The output from these two commands is summarized in Figure 4.20. From this analysis the $OR_{Trauma} = 1.67$ with 95% CI 1.15 to 2.43, p-value=0.0069. In this example these values are very close to those obtained from the previous *suboptimal* calculations, although this will not always be the case. Indeed, the guiding principle of any analysis should be to follow that implied by the design.

(a) *Gravidity ignoring the matching*

tabulate gravwk anorexia

| | Anorexia | | |
gravvk	Control	Case	Total
26	0	1	1
27	2	0	2
28	3	0	3
29	0	0	0
30	8	4	12
31	7	3	10
32	3	6	9
33	18	3	21
34	15	9	24
35	44	7	51
36	73	13	86
37	144	34	178
38	359	66	425
39	746	154	900
40	1,100	219	1,319
41	811	154	965
42	396	78	474
43	105	22	127
44	49	6	55
45	2	0	2
Total	3,885	779	4,664

(b) *Gravidity in matched case-control groups*

tabulate gravwk anorexia if match==16

| | code | | |
gravwk	Control	Case	Total
39	2	0	2
40	1	0	1
41	1	1	2
42	1	0	1
Total	5	1	6
Mean	40.2	41.0	

Difference : Case − Control = 0.8 wks

tabulate gravwk anorexia if match==42

| | code | | |
gravwk	Control	Case	Total
37	1	0	1
38	1	0	1
40	1	1	2
41	2	0	2
Total	5	1	6
Mean	39.4	40.0	

Difference : Case − Control = 0.6 wks

Figure 4.21   Gravidity of cases and controls at birth from a study of risk factors for the development of anorexia nervosa (data from Cnattingius, Hultman, Dahl and Sparén, 1999)

In the situation where the covariate is continuous, or numerical as is gestational age at birth (*Gravwk* - gravidity assessed in weeks), the unmatched set of observations appears as in Figure 4.21(a) and examples of matched results in Figure 4.21(b). One summary obtained from each matched-group is the mean difference in gravidity between the average of the 5 controls and that of the case. In the matched-groups used for illustration, the gravidity of each case exceeds the mean of their controls. Thus, for match-set 16 the

---

(a) *Model Gr*

clogit anorexia gravwk, group(match) vce(robust) or

Conditional (fixed-effects) logistic regression   Number of obs = 4654

anorexia	OR	SE	z	P>|z|	[95% CI]
gravwk	0.9564	0.0192	−2.22	0.026	0.9196 to 0.9948

(b) *Model Tr + Gr*

clogit anorexia gravwk trauma, group(match) vce(robust) or

anorexia	OR	SE	z	P>|z|	[95% CI]
gravwk	0.9562	0.0191	−2.24	0.025	0.9195 to 0.9943
trauma	1.6665	0.3183	2.67	0.0076	1.1461 to 2.4231

Figure 4.22 Conditional logistic regression of gravidity and conditional multiple logistic regression of gravidity and trauma from a study of risk factors for the development of anorexia nervosa (data from Cnattingius, Hultman, Dahl and Sparén, 1999)

case has gravidity 41, and the controls, 39, 39, 40, 41, and 42 with mean 40.2 and so $d_{16}=41-40.2=0.8$ weeks. Similarly, $d_{42}=0.6$ weeks. Such differences form the units of analysis for these data, from which their mean, $\bar{d}$, and standard error would be calculated to form the basis of a paired t-test.

An alternative summary, is to estimate model **Gr** using the conditional logistic regression command (`clogit anorexia gravwk, group(match) vce(robust) or`) to determine the OR as illustrated in Figure 4.22(a). This suggests for every additional week of gravidity, the $OR=0.9564$ reduces the chance of anorexia.

The conditional regression commands can be extended to the multi-covariate situation as shown in Figure 4.22(b), where the model fitted involves both trauma and gravidity, that is, a linear model of the form: $Tr+Gr$. It is of note that the OR estimate for gravidity is little changed from the corresponding single-covariate model estimate of **Gr**.

ORDERED LOGISTIC REGRESSION

When describing the study of foetal loss in Example 1.3, we presented the ORs for those that were sampled using PUBS and by cardiocentesis compared with IHV as 1.85 and 13.85, respectively. In this calculation, the three types of fetal loss (at <2 weeks and >2 weeks following the procedure, and postnatal death) were merged into one group termed total fetal deaths to create a binary endpoint. The ORs just quoted were calculated on this basis and thereby took no account of the differing types of fetal loss. The Total column of Figure 4.23 indicates from 382 samples that 39 were lost in < 2 weeks, 18 at > 2 weeks, 30 were postnatal deaths, and the remaining were 295 live births. The proportion of live births is $p_1=295/382=0.7723$. If the live birth and postnatal death categories are merged, $P_2=(295+30)/382=0.8508$. Successively merging the other two categories in a similar way we obtain $P_3=(295+30+18)/382=0.8979$, and finally $P_4=(295+30+18+39)/382=1$. We have used the notation p_1, P_2, P_3 and P_4 to emphasize that the latter three are cumulative proportions. The corresponding cumulative

Foetal loss	IHV	PUBS	Cardio	Total	Unadjusted estimates Calculated from the Total column		Model estimates Taking account of puncture site	
< 2 weeks	21	7	11	39	$p_4 = 0.1021$ $P_4 = 1$		$Q_4 = 1$	$q_4 = 0.0690$
> 2 weeks	10	6	2	18	$p_3 = 0.0471$ $P_3 = 0.8979$		$Q_3 = 0.9310$	$q_3 = 0.0391$
Death	21	7	2	30	$p_2 = 0.0785$ $P_2 = 0.8508$		$Q_2 = 0.8919$	$q_2 = 0.0701$
Alive	240	50	5	295	$p_1 = 0.7723$ $p_1 = 0.7723$		$q_1 = 0.8218$	$q_1 = 0.8218$
Total	292	70	20	382				

Figure 4.23 Fetal loss following fetal blood sampling according to different puncture sites in both normal and abnormal fetuses (Source: Chinnaiya, Venkat, Chia, et al., 1998. Reproduced with permission of John Wiley & Sons Ltd.)

(a) *Assuming no influence of Puncture method*

olog Type

Ordered logistic regression   Number of obs = 382

```
---------------------------------
 Type  |   Coef      SE
--------+------------------------
 /cut1  |  1.2211    0.1220
 /cut2  |  1.7408    0.1436
 /cut3  |  2.1742    0.1690
---------------------------------
```

(b) *Taking account of Puncture method*

xi : olog Type i. Puncture, or

Ordered logistic regression   Number of obs = 382

```
------------------------------------------------------------------------
      Puncture |   OR       SE       z     P>|z|        [95% CI]
---------------+--------------------------------------------------------
 IHV           |   1
 PUBS          |   1.8170   0.5472   1.98   0.047    1.0070 to   3.2785
 Cardiocentesis|  15.6276   7.2903   5.89   0.0001   6.2633 to  38.9927
---------------+--------------------------------------------------------
        / cut 1 |   1.5286   0.1527
        / cut 2 |   2.1102   0.1776
        / cut 3 |   2.6020   0.2060
------------------------------------------------------------------------
```

Figure 4.24 Ordered logistic regression of fetal loss following fetal blood sampling according to different puncture sites (data from Chinnaiya, Venkat, Chia, et al., 1998)

logits are logit $p_1 = \log(295/[382 - 295]) = \log(295/87) = 1.2211$, logit $P_2 = \log([295 + 30]/[382 - 295 - 30]) = \log(325/57) = 1.7408$ and logit $P_3 = \log(343/39) = 2.1742$.

Ordered logistic regression takes note of the 4 categories (three different fetal loss types and live birth) rather than merges the fetal losses to create a binary outcome as was done in Example 1.3. If the analysis first focuses only on the Total column of Figure 4.23, and thereby ignores the design covariate *Puncture*, then the command (olog Type) of Figure 4.24(a) calculates the logit of the cumulative proportions of the preceding paragraph.

In contrast, the command (xi: olog Type i.Puncture) of Figure 4.24(b) takes account of the design covariate *Puncture* and also full note of the 4 categories of the outcome variable. This leads to *ORs* of 1.82 (95% CI 1.01 to 3.28) when comparing PUBS with IHV and

Fetal loss	IHV	PUBS
< 2 weeks	21	7
> 2 weeks	10	6
Death	21	7
Alive	240	50
Total	292	70

	IHV	PUBS
	31	13
52	20	
240	50	
$OR = 1.85$		

	IHV	PUBS
IHV	PUBS	21
31	13	271
261	57	
$OR = 1.92$		

	IHV	PUBS
21	7	
271	63	
$OR = 1.43$		

Figure 4.25 Cumulative ORs for fetal loss following fetal blood sampling according to IHV and PUBS puncture sites in both normal and abnormal fetuses (part data from Chinnaiya, Venkat, Chia et al., 1998)

15.63 (95% CI 6.26 to 38.99) when comparing cardiocentesis with IHV. In this example, although it will not always be the case, the ORs are very similar to the binary variable estimates of 1.85 and 13.85 of Example 1.3. However, the associated confidence intervals are narrower, indicating an increase in the precision of the estimated risks associated with the fetal sampling methods.

We note too that the logits associated with (/cut 1, /cut2, and /cut3) are modified somewhat from those given in Figure 4.24(a). Thus, we have $\text{logit}(q_1) = 1.5286$ as opposed to 1.2211, which leads to $q_1 = \dfrac{\exp(1.5286)}{1+\exp(1.5286)} = 0.8218$ rather than $p_1 = 0.7723$. Further, $Q_2 = 0.8919$, $Q_3 = 0.9310$ and $Q_4 = 1$. These lead by appropriate subtraction to $q_1 = 0.8218$ (as we have just calculated), $q_2 = 0.0701$, $q_3 = 0.0391$ and finally $q_4 = 0.0690$ as are shown in the last column of Figure 4.23.

In strict terms, the use of ordered logistic regression requires the assumption of proportional odds. This implies that wherever a cut is applied in dividing the ordered categorical variable into binary sections, the underlying odds ratio remains the same. To illustrate this point, the IHV and PUBs groups of Figure 4.23 are reproduced in Figure 4.25 and the 4 category ordered variable fetal loss is then dichotomized at three cut points to give three 2×2 tables. These provide the OR estimates of $(240 \times 20)/(52 \times 50) = 1.85$, 1.92 and 1.43. Proportional odds requires that these are all estimating the same underlying odds ratio, which may require some judgment on whether or not this is indeed the case. However, Whitehead (1993) suggests that proportional odds may reasonably be assumed if all the estimates indicate that the risk lies in the same direction such as in this example where each OR is greater than unity. Hence, it seems reasonable to take the $OR = 1.8170$ in Figure 4.24(b) as the 'averaged' estimate of the three ORs for comparing PUBs with IHV in terms of fetal loss. Similarly, we take $OR = 15.63$ when comparing the risk of sampling using cardiocentesis with IHV fetal sampling.

TECHNICAL DETAILS

Odds ratio (OR) and relative risk (RR)

From Figure 4.1, the proportion of infants developing asthma in those with no HRV experience in their first year of life is $p_{NoHRV} = \dfrac{c}{a+c} = \dfrac{50}{210} = 0.2381$, and for those with HRV it is $p_{YesHRV} = \dfrac{d}{b+d} = \dfrac{21}{45} = 0.4667$. Hence, the difference in proportions with asthma in the two groups is given by $d = p_{YesHRV} - p_{NoHRV} = 0.4667 - 0.2381 = 0.2286$ or 23%.

An alternative way of comparing the groups is to use the ratio of these proportions rather than their difference. Thus we define, in terms of the algebraic format of Figure 4.1, the relative risk (*RR*), as

$$RR = \frac{p_{YesHRV}}{p_{NoHRV}} = \frac{\dfrac{d}{b+d}}{\dfrac{c}{a+c}} = \frac{d(a+c)}{c(b+d)} \tag{4.15}$$

Using the corresponding data, this gives $RR=0.4667/0.2381=1.9601$ or approximately 2.

It is clear that equations (4.15) for the *RR* and (4.1) for the *OR* are not algebraically equivalent. However, when the probability of an event happening is rare, odds and probabilities become close. For example, if the probability $p=0.1$, then the odds are $0.1/0.9=0.11$, whereas if $p=0.01$, then the odds are $0.01/0.99=0.0101 \approx 0.01$. In the latter example, the probability and the odds are very similar. In terms of the cells of Figure 4.1, when the probabilities are small c will be much smaller than a and so $c/(a+c)$ is approximately c/a. Further, d will be much smaller than b and so $d/(b+d)$ is approximately d/b. In this case, the expression for the *RR* becomes that for the *OR*.

In our example, there appears no necessity for the odds ratio to be used given that we can calculate the relative risk directly from the 2×2 table. However, the *OR* has certain mathematical properties which render it attractive as an alternative to the *RR*.

One problem with using the *RR* as a summary is that there is no relationship between the relative risk defined as $RR_{Asthma} = \dfrac{p_{YesHRV}}{p_{NoHRV}}$ and $RR_{NoAsthma} = \dfrac{1-p_{YesHRV}}{1-p_{NoHRV}}$, except in the very exceptional single situation when $p_{YesHRV}=p_{NoHRV}=0.5$ in which case $RR=1$. In contrast,

$OR_{NoAsthma} = \dfrac{(1-p_{YesHRV})/p_{YesHRV}}{(1-p_{NoHRV})/p_{NoHRV}} = \dfrac{1.1427}{3.1999} = 0.3571 = 1/2.8003$ or $1/OR_{Asthma}$ and there is

therefore a direct relationship between the two.

Binomial distribution

Data that can take only a 0 or 1 response, such as treatment failure or treatment success, follow the *Binomial distribution* provided the underlying population response rate π does not change. The Binomial probabilities are calculated from

$$\text{Prob}(r) = \frac{n!}{r!(n-r)!}\pi^r(1-\pi)^{n-r} \tag{4.16}$$

for successive values of r from 0 through to n. In the above $n!$ is read as n factorial and $r!$ as r factorial. For $r=4$, $r!=4\times3\times2\times1=24$. Both 0! and 1! are taken as equal to unity. It should be noted that the mean or expected value for r, the number of successes yet to be observed if we treat n patients, is $n\pi$. The potential variation about this expectation is expressed by the corresponding standard deviation, $SD(r) = \sqrt{[n\pi(1-\pi)]}$. In the situation when π is very small, that is when it is close to 0, then $SD(r) \approx \sqrt{n\pi}$.

Maximum likelihood estimation (MLE)

Suppose we are estimating the probability of response to treatment in a group of n patients with a particular disease and the true or population value for this probability is π. Then an individual patient will respond with probability π and fail to respond with probability $(1 - \pi)$.

If, in our study, r of these patients respond and $(n - r)$ do not respond then, as can be seen from equation (4.16), the probability of this outcome is proportional to

$$\ell = \pi^r (1 - \pi)^{(n-r)} \tag{4.17}$$

Here ℓ is termed the likelihood. If we calculate $L = \log \ell$, then this is termed the log likelihood and we have

$$L = \log \ell = r \log \pi + (n - r) \log(1 - \pi) \tag{4.18}$$

It turns out that if we estimate π by $p = r/n$, then this corresponds to the value for π which maximizes the value of L and hence ℓ. We therefore state that $p = r/n$ is the maximum likelihood estimate (MLE) of π.

To obtain this estimate in a formal way, it is necessary to differentiate equation (4.18) with respect to π and equate the result to zero. The solution of this equation gives the estimate as $\pi = r/n$, which is hence the MLE estimate.

Likelihood ratio (LR) test

The likelihood ratio (LR) test calculates the likelihood under two different but nested hypotheses and compares these. For convenience, we term these the likelihood under the null hypothesis, ℓ_0, and the likelihood under the alternative hypothesis, ℓ_A. The likelihood ratio test is then

$$LR = -2 \log(\ell_0 / \ell_A) = -2(L_0 - L_A) \tag{4.19}$$

The quantities $-2L_0$ and $-2L_A$ are sometimes referred to as the deviances. If the null hypothesis was true, we would expect a small value of the LR, whereas a large value would indicate evidence against the null hypothesis. In the context of comparing models, the null hypothesis referred to here may correspond to a univariate model, say E and the alternative hypothesis to the model, $E+G$. So the test is to establish whether or not the regression parameters associated with the G component of the model can be regarded as essentially zero. If the null hypothesis is rejected, then the model becomes $E+G$, whereas if it is not, the model reverts to G.

In fact, it can be shown that the LR in equation (4.18) is approximately distributed as a χ^2 variable with the appropriate degrees of freedom, df. Irrespective of how many parameters are included in the null model, the degrees of freedom for comparing this with the alternative model with q additional parameters is also q. The value of the LR statistic is then referred to the χ^2 distribution, using $df = q$ to give the p-value.

The χ^2 distribution is tabulated in Table T5. However, in the case when $df = 1$, and only in this case, $z = \sqrt{\chi^2}$ so that Table T1 can then be used to obtain the p-value.

The empirical logit transformation

When calculating a proportion using the expression, $p=r/n$ results in the same value of $p=0$ when $r=0$ irrespective of the value of n. In a similar way, if $r=n$, then $p=1$ irrespective of the value n takes. However, it is intuitive that 0/100 contains more information than 0/10 and likewise for 100/100 compared with 10/10. Further, logit $0 = -\infty$ whereas logit $1 = +\infty$, and points with these extreme values cannot be used graphically. To overcome this difficulty, the logit transformation is sometimes modified to

$$\text{logit}(p) = \log\left[\frac{r+\dfrac{1}{2}}{n-\left(r-\dfrac{1}{2}\right)}\right] \qquad (4.20)$$

For the examples 0/10 and 0/100, equation (4.20) gives $\log(0.5/10.5)=\log(0.04762)=-3.04$ and $\log(0.5/100.5)=\log(0.004975)=-5.30$, respectively, whereas 10/10 and 100/100 give $\log(10.5/0.5)=\log(21.0)=+3.04$ and $\log(100.5/0.5)=\log(201)=+5.30$. This formulation enables plots similar to those of Figure 4.5 to have groups with 0% or 100% response rates represented.

5   Poisson Regression

SUMMARY

This chapter describes Poisson regression analysis, which may be utilized in situations where the event under study has a very small probability of occurrence and the group under study from which the events occur is large. In this situation the Poisson distribution is a special case of the Binomial distribution and so the regression methods utilized are a special case of logistic regression. Situations are described in which only the number of events is modeled, the individual group sizes concerned are incorporated, and when the exposure within each group is used as an indicator. Methods of dealing with over-dispersion are described, that is, when the observed variance is larger than would be anticipated from a Poisson distribution, using robust estimates for the estimated regression coefficients and their associated standard errors (SEs). Also included are details of zero-inflated models, which are designed to deal with situations where in some groups there are special reasons why excess counts of zero may be anticipated.

INTRODUCTION

In certain situations the number of events r occurring may be observed but it is difficult to establish the corresponding denominator, n, which is required if the estimated proportion is to be calculated. A typical example is the number of patients admitted to the Accident and Emergency Department of a specific hospital in a given period with serious injury following a road traffic accident. In such a situation, there are a large number of potential victims comprising all those using the roads during the time period of concern, and usually a very low chance of any one of these individuals being involved in an accident resulting in serious injury. Another example is that of Maheswaran, Pearson, Hoysal and Campbell (2010) discussed in *Example 1.4,* in which the impact of a health forecast alert service on admissions to hospital for chronic obstructive pulmonary disease (COPD) was evaluated. Each GP practice concerned consisted of a very large number of patients, so that among them a COPD represents a rare event. Another example is that of Wight, Jakubovic, Walters, *et al.* (2004) in which variations in cadaveric heart beating organ donor rates for kidney transplants between

Regression Methods for Medical Research, First Edition. Bee Choo Tai and David Machin.
© 2014 Bee Choo Tai and David Machin. Published 2014 by John Wiley & Sons, Ltd.

UK transplant centres was studied. Heart-beating donors are seriously ill patients who are placed on a ventilator in an intensive care unit (ICU). Here there is a very large population of potential donors living in the region of each of the 21 kidney retrieval areas (KRA), but each with a very low probability of being admitted to an ICU and thereby becoming a potential cadaveric donor. The authors estimated the UK-wide donor rate as 16.1 per million of the population per year and this ranged over the different KRA centers from 8.0 to 27.4. In addition, rates varied in relation to several factors including, for example, the proportion of ethnically non-white individuals living in each KRA.

In some circumstances, the extent of exposure (rather than population size) is used in the modeling process. Thus if the role of a potential carcinogen in inducing a particular form of cancer is to be determined in a group of industrial workers, the total work-time exposure of each worker to that factor will usually be accumulated.

POISSON OR BINOMIAL MODELS

To model the types of data of the preceding paragraph, the logistic model of the form of equation (4.4) is simplified by assuming the proportion being estimated is very small. In this case, the numerator on the right-hand side of the equation $\pi = \dfrac{\exp(\beta_0 + \beta_1 x_1)}{1 + \exp(\beta_0 + \beta_1 x_1)}$ will be very small and so the denominator will be approximately 1 (unity). Thus, the right-hand side effectively involves only the numerator. To distinguish this special situation, π is replaced by μ on the left-hand side. Hence, the Poisson regression model with a single covariate is

$$\mu = \exp(\beta_0 + \beta_1 x_1) \tag{5.1}$$

As the logarithm of this expression,

$$\log \mu = \beta_0 + \beta_1 x_1 \tag{5.2}$$

has a linear form the transformation is said to provide a 'log-link' function.

As we explain further in *Technical details*, the Poisson regression model, based on a count endpoint variable following a Poisson distribution, can be thought of as a special case of the logistic regression model based on a binary variable arising from a Binomial distribution. Once the model is fitted to the data the proportion of predicted events, q_j, for those with covariate value x_{1j} is given by

$$q_j = \exp(b_0 + b_1 x_{1j}) \tag{5.3}$$

An example in which a logistic regression model is appropriate is that of Viardot-Foucault, Prasath, Tai, *et al.* (2011) in which 606 women received intra-uterine insemination (IUI) and 118 (19.47%) of these achieved a successful pregnancy. Logistic regression on outcome (successful pregnancy) against age of the women at IUI makes use of both the number of those who and the number treated by the clinic. The command (`logit Preg Age`) gives estimates of the regression coefficients and (`logit Preg Age, or`) the estimated OR that are summarized in Figure 5.1(a). These indicate a reduced probability of successful pregnancy for every year of increased age since $b_{Age} = -0.0544$. If we take a woman exactly aged 35, then the chance of her successfully giving birth is

$$P_{35} = \frac{\exp[b_0 + (b_1 \times 35)]}{1 + \exp[b_0 + (b_1 \times 35)]} = \frac{\exp[0.3658 + (-0.0544 \times 35)]}{1 + \exp[0.3658 + (-0.0544 \times 35)]} = 0.1767.$$ A similar calcu-

lation for a woman exactly one year older gives $p_{36} = 0.1690$. This one extra year of age reduces

the possibility of a successful pregnancy by an $OR = \dfrac{0.1690/(1-0.1690)}{0.1767/(1-0.1767)} = \dfrac{0.2034}{0.2146} = 0.9478.$

This reduction is confirmed by the more accurately calculated output of Figure 5.1(a) as 0.9470.

On the other hand a Poisson regression model applied to these data ignores the total number treated and only utilizes whether or not a woman achieves a successful outcome. The necessary commands are (**poisson Preg Age**) and (**poisson Preg Age, irr**). In this case, $q_{35} = \exp[b_0 + (b_1 \times 35)] = \exp[-0.2034 + (-0.0438 \times 35)] = 0.1762$, while $q_{36} = 0.1686$ giving a ratio of $q_{36}/q_{35} = 0.1686/0.1762 = 0.9569$. This is verified by what is termed the incidence-rate

---

(a) Logistic regression

logit Preg Age
logit Preg Age, or

Number of obs = 606, LR chi2 (1) = 4.47, Prob > chi2 = 0.034

Log likelihood = −296.51715

Preg	Coef	SE	z	P>|z|	[95% CI]
b_0	0.3658	0.8554			
b_{Age}	−0.0544	0.0261	−2.09	0.037	−0.1056 to −0.0033

Preg	OR	SE	z	P>|z|	[95% CI]
Age	0.9470	0.0247	−2.09	0.037	0.8998 to 0.9967

(b) Poisson regression

poisson Preg Age
poisson Preg Age, irr

Number of obs = 606, LR chi2(1) = 3.61, Prob > chi2 = 0.058

Log likelihood = −309.26762

Preg	Coef	SE	z	P>|z|	[95% CI]
b_0	−0.2034	0.7596			
b_{Age}	−0.0438	0.0233	−1.88	0.060	−0.0894 to +0.0019

Preg	IRR	SE	z	P>|z|	[95% CI]
Age	0.9572	0.0223	−1.88	0.060	0.9144 to 1.0019

(c) Testing for Over-dispersion

estat gof, pearson
Goodness-of-fit chi2 = 485.2322, Prob > chi2(604) = 0.99.

Figure 5.1 Comparison of Logistic and Poisson regression analyses of successful pregnancies following intra-uterine insemination (IUI) (part data from Viardot-Foucault, Prasath, Tai, et al., 2011) ratio (*IRR*) of 0.9572 of Figure 5.1(b). Thus in this example q_{35}, q_{36} and *IRR* are very close to p_{35}, p_{36} and the *OR*. This close agreement illustrates the fact that the *IRR* from Poisson regression can be interpreted in much the same way as the *OR* of logistic regression. Specifically, if we were to compare women of ages 35 and 40, then the $IRR = 0.9572^{(40-35)} = 0.9572^5 = 0.8036$, indicating a much lower chance of achieving a pregnancy in the older women.

In this data set, there are $n_{35} = 5$ women who are recorded as 35.0 years of age, among whom 4 had successful pregnancies, and again $n_{36} = 5$ women who are recorded as 36.0 years of age among whom 0 pregnancies were recorded. As a consequence the corresponding predictions estimated from the Poisson model are $c_{35} = n_{35} \times p_{35} = 5 \times 0.1762 = 0.8810$ and $c_{36} = n_{36} \times p_{36} = 5 \times 0.1686 = 0.8430$ pregnancies. These are not very close to the observed values. However, the purpose of a model is to give a general description of the way in which the anticipated numbers of pregnancies changes, in this case in 606 women over the whole age range from 21.7 to 51.0 years, taking into account random fluctuations.

In general the number of predicted events is calculated by

$$c_j = E_j \times q_j = \exp(\log E_j + b_0 + b_1 x_{1j}) \tag{5.4}$$

where E_j is a measure of the *exposure* of group, *j*. In the above example, $E_{35} = n_{35}$ and represents the number of women in that particular group. However, in other examples, this may be a measure of time, for example, the total number of years of exposure to a particular carcinogen of a group of industrial workers. When, as in the next section, there is no measure of exposure, E_j is set equal to 1 in equation (5.4) and this gives the predicted counts $c_j = q_j$.

UNKNOWN POPULATION SIZE AT RISK

In the example of the women seeking help with conception, the number of women in the study is known and the chance of a pregnancy of 19.47% following IUI is quite high. Thus, logistic regression rather than Poisson regression is the appropriate method to use.

Figure 5.2 shows data for one year from a study conducted by Chia, Chia, Ng and Tai (2010), who investigated changing patterns and risk factors, including age and gender, for suicide in Singapore. This table shows, for example, that in the year concerned the number of suicides varied from 0 to 88 in the 10 gender by age groups. The distribution of the number of suicides in the 350 groups collated over 35 years varies considerably with very few suicides in the 5–9 year age groups of Figure 5.3(a) but ranging from 1 to 98 in the older groups of Figure 5.3(b). In view of this disparity, the youngest are excluded from the models that we present.

Gender	Age (years)					
	5–9	10–19	20–39	40–59	60+	Total
Male	0	10	88	75	59	232
Female	0	10	41	48	26	125
Total	0	20	129	123	85	357

Figure 5.2 Number of suicides in a particular year by age and gender (part data from Chia, Chia, Ng and Tai, 2010)

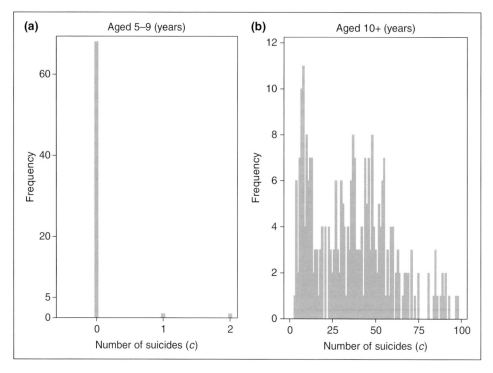

Figure 5.3 Histogram of the number of suicides committed in the (a) age 5–9 group, and (b) those groups 10 years and over (part data from Chia, Chia, Ng and Tai, 2010)

The simplest poisson model is when there are no covariates and equation (5.2) becomes the null model of $\log\mu = \beta_0$. Fitting this model using (**poisson Suicides**) to the data, excluding the 5–9 year group, gives the output summarized in Figure 5.4(a). From this, the average number of suicides is $c = \exp(3.5916) = 36.29$ with 95% CI $\exp(3.5722)$ to $\exp(3.6111)$ or 35.59 to 37.01. The second part of the output of Figure 5.4(a) provides this number and the confidence interval directly.

As with other regression model situations, if a continuous covariate, such as age, is to be included into the model it is important to verify if the assumptions made, for example the presumed linearity of the relationship, are reasonable. In this example, the age of the person who has committed suicide is categorized into the 5 age groups 5–9, 10–19, 20–39, 40–59, and 60+ years. These are coded from 1 to 5 in the database, and as such may be regarded as an ordered categorical variable. However, the band-width is not the same in all categories, so that it would not seem appropriate to assume equal divisions between categories. However, if we take the mid-category values, here essentially 7, 15, 30, 50 for the first four categories and (say) 70 years for the oldest, then on this scale we now have a numerical variable for age group, which we can use for model fitting purposes. However, as there are so few suicides in the 5–9 year groups, we have omitted these cases from the modeling, leaving 8 age by gender groups in each year.

The Poisson regression model including a single covariate of equation (5.2) can be extended to include two or more covariates. Thus, to investigate the influence of *Age* and *Gender* on the number of suicides, the corresponding command would be (**poisson Suicides Gender Age**). This calculation, using the mid-interval age of Figure 5.2 as a numerical variable, is summarized in Figure 5.4(c). An $IRR_{Gender} = 0.6852$ suggests that the females are less at risk of

---

(a) *Fitting the null (no covariate) model*

poisson Suicides,

Number of groups = 280

Suicides	Coef	SE	z	P>|z|	[95% CI]
cons	3.5916	0.009920	362.06	0.0001	3.5722 to 3.6111

poisson Suicides, irr

Suicides	IRR	SE	z	P>|z|	[95% CI]
cons	36.2929	0.3600	362.06	0.0001	35.5940 to 37.0054

(b) *Testing the null model for goodness-of-fit*

estat gof, pearson

Goodness-of-fit chi2 = 3998.25, Prob > chi2(279) = 0.0001

(c) *Assessing the influence of gender and age (using the mid-category value)*

poisson Suicides Gender Age
poisson Suicides Gender Age, irr

Suicides	Coef	SE	z	P>|z|	[95% CI]
cons	3.3445	0.0253			
Gender	−0.3780	0.0202	−18.72	0.0001	−0.4176 to −0.3384
Age	0.009655	0.0004788	20.16	0.0001	0.008716 to 0.01059

Suicides	IRR	SE	z	P>|z|	[95% CI]
Gender	0.6852	0.01384	−18.72	0.0001	0.6586 to 0.7129
Age	1.009702	0.0004835	20.16	0.0001	1.008754 to 1.010650

Figure 5.4 Poisson regression analysis of the number of suicides in eight age by gender groups collated over a 35-year period (part data from Chia, Chia, Ng and Tai, 2010)

committing suicide than the males. However, the $IRR_{Age}=1.0097$ per year suggests an increasing risk of suicide with increasing age. The fitted model is $c=\exp[3.3445-0.3780\,Gender + 0.009655\,Age]$, where $Gender=0$ for males and $Gender=1$ for females. From this, the expected number of suicides among females of age group (20–39), and hence with $Age=30$, is: $c=\exp[3.3445 - (0.3780\times1)+(0.009655 \times 30)]=25.95$. The actual mean suicide count for this group is 29.5 suggesting that the model describes the data relatively well.

OVER-DISPERSION AND ROBUST ESTIMATES

Over-dispersion

One basic requirement for count data to follow the Poisson distribution is that the mean and variance, *Var*, of such data should be equal and that both are described by the single parameter, μ. A similar requirement also relates to the Binomial distribution as the mean, $n\pi$, and the variance, $n\pi(1-\pi)$, are both connected through the value of the same parameter, π, where n is the number of subjects in the study. For both distributions, we assume successive observations are independent of each other. However, if there is a lack of independence between successive observations, for example following a road traffic accident several casualties from the same incident could arrive at the Accident and Emergency Department simultaneously, these relationships no longer hold. Thus, although the mean in the Binomial situation is still estimated by $n\pi$, the variance is increased to $Var = n\pi(1-\pi)\,[1+\rho\,(n-1)]$ where ρ is the correlation between the responses of any two subjects within the study. If observations are totally independent, $\rho = 0$, whereas if they are not ρ is likely to be greater than 0. In which case there is 'over-dispersion', that is, the variance is greater than we would expect under the Binomial distribution. In similar circumstances for the Poisson distribution, the variance increases from μ to $n\rho\mu$.

Other situations in which over-dispersion can arise are when one, or more, important (strongly influential) covariate is not considered within the model or if the model itself is incorrectly specified. A misspecified model is one that provides an unsatisfactory description of the data—perhaps by assuming a linear relationship that clearly does not hold. Although all models are misspecified to some extent in that they seldom if ever perfectly describe the data, there is particular concern here as highly inaccurate predictions can arise if the model chosen is not an appropriate one.

For both the Binomial and Poisson distributions, the link between the mean and *Var*, is often a rather severe restriction and so over-dispersion is quite a common phenomenon. This contrasts markedly with data having a Normal distribution where the value of the variance has no connection to the value of the corresponding mean. Hence, 'over-dispersion' is not a feature of continuous data.

If counts within n groups are made, for example the number of suicides in each of the age-gender-period groups in Singapore, with values, $c_1, c_2, \ldots, c_n$, then the corresponding test of over-dispersion is

$$Pearson = \sum\nolimits_{j=1}^{n} \frac{(c_j - \hat{c}_j)^2}{\hat{c}_j} \tag{5.5}$$

where c_j and $\hat{c}_j$ are the observed and predicted counts for group j, respectively. Under the null hypothesis of no over-dispersion *Pearson* follows the χ^2 distribution of Table T5, with $df = n - k$, where k is the number of parameters estimated in the model. This is essentially the same test as described by equation (4.14), but the expression for the calculation is simplified as we are now concerned with the Poisson rather than the Binomial distribution.

If the test is statistically significant, then this immediately suggests the presence of over-dispersion and, as the estimates of the SEs are being based on the assumption that the Poisson distribution holds, they will not be correctly estimated. Figure 5.4(b) uses the command (`estat gof, pearson`) to test the goodness-of-fit of the null model to the suicide data, and indicates quite clearly with *Pearson* = 3998.25, $df = 279$ and p-value = 0.0001 that over-dispersion is present. This implies that the estimated variance, calculated as the same value as the calculated mean, is likely to be seriously underestimated so that, for example, the confidence intervals quoted in Figures 5.4(a) and (c) should be wider than those given. In contrast to the over-dispersion present in the suicide data, when (`estat gof, pearson`) is applied to the pregnancy data in Figure 5.1(c) over-dispersion is not detected.

As we will discuss in the section *Zero-inflated models*, there are circumstances where a zero count among certain groups may be anticipated, for example very young children may not know how, nor have access to methods, nor the ability to commit suicide compared with older individuals and so excessive zeros might be anticipated among such population groups.

Robust procedures

As we have explained, the mean and variance of both the Binomial and Poisson distributions depend only on the value of a single parameter, and so over-dispersion is quite common in practice. Thus when over-dispersion occurs, the consequence of fitting a Poisson regression model is that the associated SEs of the regression coefficients are likely to be underestimated.

However, several (termed robust) methods of calculating SEs are available. In Stata the specific command is part of **vce(.)** (variance-covariance estimate), and among the possible options are (**robust**), (**jack**) and (**boot**), the latter being the most computer intensive. The terms 'jack' and 'boot' are abbreviations for 'jacknife' and 'bootstrap', respectively, whereas 'robust' is a more generic term that provides the 'sandwich' estimates of the SEs. The bootstrap involves the computer program taking many repeated samples with replacement from the observations actually obtained in a study. The sample size is that of the study itself, but sampling with replacement implies that each sample drawn is likely to contain repeats of some of the observations made and thereby excludes others. The parameter of interest is estimated for each of these samples and, from them all, the respective standard deviation is calculated. This standard deviation provides the estimate of the robust SE of the estimated regression coefficient of concern.

This parallels the situation shown in Figure 4.20, in which robust estimates of the SE were utilized when using conditional logistic regression. Boos and Stefanski (2010) give a non-technical description of bootstrapping.

The alternative robust estimators are compared in Figure 5.5 for the null model, that with no covariates and so $\beta_1 = 0$ in model (5.2), for which the number of suicides is $\exp(\beta_0)$. The first thing to note in this example is that $b_0 = 3.5916$ (the estimate of β_0) remains the same whether (or whichever) or not a robust method is utilized. However, the non-robust $SE(b_0) = 0.009920$ increases markedly to approximately 0.0375 (an almost fourfold increase) with only minor differences between the different robust approaches.

In Figure 5.6 the Poisson regression model of the number of suicide rates by gender and age conducted for Figure 5.4(c) is repeated, but using the bootstrap option. The SEs for the robust estimates over the non-robust estimates are all increased. For example, that for $SE(b_{Gender})$ increases from 0.02020 to 0.05935 and that for $SE(b_{Age})$ from 0.0004788 to 0.001558; each an approximately threefold increase. This consequently increases the width of the corresponding confidence intervals.

KNOWN POPULATION SIZE AT RISK

In actuality, as can be seen from Figure 5.7(a), for each gender by age group in the study by Chia, Chia, Ng and Tai (2010) the corresponding population size is known so that the respective suicide rates can be obtained. Thus, for the 20–39 year age group suicides of 88 males from 539,300 and 41 females from 553,000 were recorded. Suicide is clearly a rare event in all age-gender groups. In such circumstances, where populations are very large, rates are

```
poisson Suicides

Number of groups = 280

----------------------------------------------------------------------
  Suicides  |   Coef       SE        z       P>|z|        [95% CI]
------------+---------------------------------------------------------
      cons  |  3.5916    0.009920  362.06   0.0001    3.5722 to 3.6111
----------------------------------------------------------------------


poisson Suicides,vce(robust)

----------------------------------------------------------------------
            |             Robust
  Suicides  |   Coef       SE        z       P>|z|        [95% CI]
------------+---------------------------------------------------------
      cons  |  3.5916    0.03755    95.64   0.0001    3.5180 to 3.6650
----------------------------------------------------------------------


poisson Suicides, vce(jack)

----------------------------------------------------------------------
            |             Jackknife
  Suicides  |   Coef       SE        t       P>|t|        [95% CI]
------------+---------------------------------------------------------
      cons  |  3.5916    0.03757    95.59   0.0001    3.5177 to 3.6656
----------------------------------------------------------------------


poisson Suicides,vce(boot)

----------------------------------------------------------------------
            |             Bootstrap
  Suicides  |   Coef       SE        z       P>|z|        [95% CI]
------------+---------------------------------------------------------
      cons  |  3.5916    0.03743    95.96   0.0001    3.5183 to 3.6650
----------------------------------------------------------------------
```

Figure 5.5 Poisson regression analysis of the number of suicides in those of 10 years and older collated over a 35-year period using a non-robust and several robust methods of estimating the standard errors (part data from Chia, Chia, Ng and Tai, 2010)

```
poisson Suicides Gender Age, vce(boot)
poisson Suicides Gender Age, vce(boot) irr

Number of groups = 280, Wald chi2 (2) = 96.45

----------------------------------------------------------------------------
            |             Bootstrap
  Suicides  |   Coef       SE        z      P>|z|          [95% CI]
------------+---------------------------------------------------------------
      cons  |  3.3445     0.1428
    Gender  | -0.3780     0.05935   -6.37   0.0001    -0.4943   to -0.2617
       Age  |  0.009655   0.001558   6.20   0.0001     0.006601 to  0.01271
------------+---------------------------------------------------------------
            |             Bootstrap
  Suicides  |   IRR        SE        z      P>|z|          [95% CI]
------------+---------------------------------------------------------------
    Gender  |  0.6852     0.04727   -5.48   0.0001     0.5986 to 0.7845
       Age  |  1.0097     0.001743   5.59   0.0001     1.0063 to 1.0131
----------------------------------------------------------------------------
```

Figure 5.6 Poisson regression analysis of the variation in suicide rates by gender and age with bootstrap estimates of variance (part data from Chia, Chia, Ng and Tai, 2010)

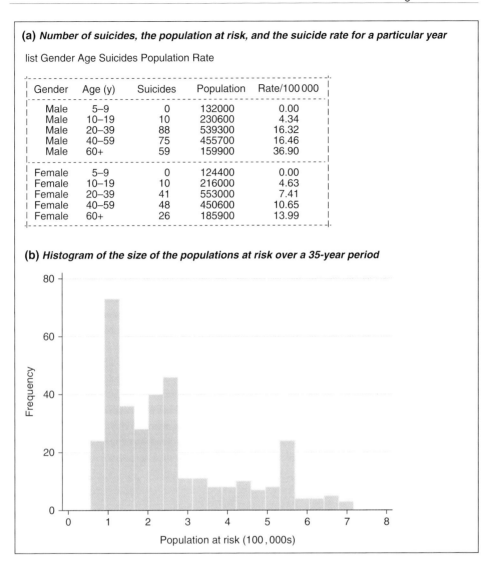

(a) *Number of suicides, the population at risk, and the suicide rate for a particular year*

list Gender Age Suicides Population Rate

Gender	Age (y)	Suicides	Population	Rate/100 000
Male	5–9	0	132000	0.00
Male	10–19	10	230600	4.34
Male	20–39	88	539300	16.32
Male	40–59	75	455700	16.46
Male	60+	59	159900	36.90
Female	5–9	0	124400	0.00
Female	10–19	10	216000	4.63
Female	20–39	41	553000	7.41
Female	40–59	48	450600	10.65
Female	60+	26	185900	13.99

(b) *Histogram of the size of the populations at risk over a 35-year period*

Figure 5.7 (a) Number of suicides in a particular year by age and gender with the corresponding populations at risk, and (b) frequency distribution of the populations at risk of the 350 age, gender by period groups (part data from Chia, Chia, Ng and Tai, 2010)

often quoted as per 100,000. These rates range from 0 to 36.90 per 100,000 in the 10 groups illustrated, with the zero rates among males and females aged 5–9 years and the maximum in males 60 or more years of age. The frequency distribution of the population sizes, excluding the 5–9 age groups, is shown in Figure 5.7(b) and ranges from 55,587 to 715,424 individuals.

Where the count, c, has an associated population size, P, we can then consider modeling $\log(\mu/P) = \beta_0 + \beta_1 x_1$. In which case equation (5.2) is modified to become

$$\log\mu = \log P + \beta_0 + \beta_1 x_1 \tag{5.6}$$

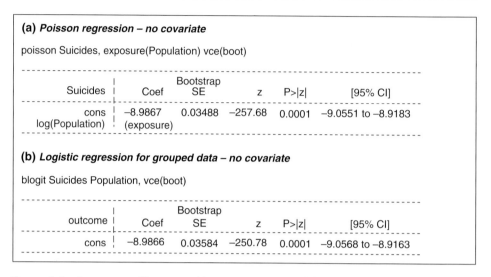

Figure 5.8 Comparison of Poisson and logistic regression models to estimate suicide rates when the corresponding population sizes are known (part data from Chia, Chia, Ng and Tai, 2010)

where the term $\log P$ is called the 'offset'. This model implies that

$$\mu = \exp\left[(1 \times \log P) + \beta_0 + \beta_1 x_1\right] \tag{5.7}$$

Equation (5.7) can be thought of as three-part linear model with parameters 1, β_0 and β_1. However, the first of these parameters is already known (and equal to unity) and so does not need to be estimated. If no covariate is involved, then (5.7) reduces to $\mu = \exp[(1 \times \log P) + \beta_0]$, and, when fitted to the suicide data using the command (**poisson Suicides, exposure(Population) vce(boot)**), this model gives the results of Figure 5.8(a). Applying this null hypothesis estimate $b_0 = -8.9867$ to a particular year, say 2000, when the total population was 2,791,000, gives $c = \exp[\log(2,791,000 - 8.9867)] = 349.05$, which is very similar to the 357 suicides actually recorded. A suicide rate is often expressed per 100,000 or in this case by $(349.05/2,791,000) \times 100,000 = 12.51$. In contrast, the null model of Figure 5.4(a), taking no account of population size, gave the anticipated number of suicides in each of the 8 gender by age groups concerned as 36.29 or only 290.34 in total, suggesting a lower rate of 10.40 per 100,000.

As the population of each age by gender group studied is known, the actual proportion of suicides can be calculated. This enables logistic regression methods to be used for analysis by means of the grouped data command (**blogit**) described in Chapter 4. Use of this command in Figure 5.8(b) gives an estimate $b_0 = -8.9866$, which is identical to that of Figure 5.8(a) except for a small rounding error in the calculations.

Taking note of the actual population sizes using the command (**poisson Suicides Gender Age, exposure (Population) vce (boot) irr**) of Figure 5.9 implements an extension of model (5.7) to two covariates. However, this model changes the $IRR = 0.6852$ of Figure 5.4(c) only marginally to $IRR = 0.6719$, but gives a wider 95% CI of 0.6089 to 0.7417 as the bootstrap method is used to obtain the SE.

```
poisson Suicides Gender Age, exposure (Population) vce(boot) irr
```

		Bootstrap				
Suicides	IRR	SE	z	P>|z|	[95%CI]	
Gender	0.6720	0.03383	−7.90	0.0001	0.6089 to 0.7417	
Age	1.0316	0.001410	22.78	0.0001	1.0289 to 1.0344	
log (Population)	(exposure)					

Figure 5.9 Poisson regression analysis of the variation in suicide rates by gender and age taking account of the size of the populations at risk (part data from Chia, Chia, Ng and Tai, 2010)

KNOWN CUMULATIVE EXPOSURE

In many epidemiological studies the actual exposure to a potential risk factor of interest is recorded. Thus, for example, if one is concerned with breast cancer risk in women using an oral contraceptive (OC), then each woman in the study will have their cumulative use of the OC recorded, which, when accumulated over all women to give T years of exposure, provides the denominator for the risk. Thus if n cancers are observed, the rate is then n/T per woman year. In this calculation the number of women recruited to the study, N, although likely to be much larger than n, plays no part in the calculation process. However, their 'exposure' can be used in the Poisson regression modeling process.

Figure 5.10 shows the cumulative survival time of three groups of psychiatric patients with tardive dyskinesia (*TarDy*), recorded as absent, mild or definitive, and the corresponding numbers of deaths recorded in each group. For all 608 patients, 72 deaths were recorded during a cumulative follow-up (their exposure) of 4509.005 years. This gives a rate of $72/4509.005 = 0.015968$ deaths per year. Such a result would be more often reported as 16.0 deaths per 1000 years.

This corresponds closely to the situation in which the population size, P, of equation (5.6) is known but is replaced here by the exposure, E, to give:

$$\log\mu = 1 \times \log E + \beta_0 + \beta_1 x_1 \tag{5.8}$$

Once again '1' is included in equation (5.8) to emphasize that there is an additional regression coefficient included but which is assumed to have value unity.

```
tabulate TarDy dead
```

	Living Status			Exposure (years)	
TarDy	Alive	Dead	Total	survy	Rate (/1000 y)
Absent	297	23	320	2392.8870	9.612
Mild	42	5	47	352.0767	14.201
Definitive	197	44	241	1764.0410	24.943
Total	536	72	608	4509.0050	15.968

Figure 5.10 Number of deaths and cumulative follow-up of psychiatric patients diagnosed with tardive dyskinesia as absent, mild or definitive (part data from Chong, Tay, Subramaniam, *et al.*, 2009)

We begin by ignoring the exposure, and applying the simple Poisson model to the extent of tardive dyskinesia of Figure 5.10 treated as an unordered categorical variable. This requires the creation of two dummy variables, which can be done automatically using the (**xi:**) function and including (**i.TarDy**) in the command. Alternatively, three dummy variables, one for each level of TD, denoted *TARD1, TARD2* and *TARD3,* can be created using the command (**tabulate TarDy, gen(TARD)**). This then enables the analyst to choose which two of these three are included in the regression command. Thus, the command (**poisson dead TARD2 TARD3, vce(boot)**) uses *TARD1* as the baseline group and compares *TARD2* and *TARD3* with that. If, inadvertently, the analyst makes the command (**poisson dead TARD1 TARD2 TARD3, vce(boot)**), then the program may recognize that one of these dummy variables is unnecessary and calculates the correct model in any event. The output of Figure 5.11(a) gives the fitted model $c = \exp[-2.6328 + (0 \times TARD1) + (0.3921 \times TARD2) + (0.9322 \times TARD3)]$. For emphasis, we have added the *TARD1* group here, and also in the corresponding edited output, although the associated coefficient of zero makes this unnecessary. For those without tardive dyskinesia, this model suggests $c = \exp(-2.6328) = 0.0719$ as $TARD2 = TARD3 = 0$. This corresponds to the actual proportion of deaths in this group, or 23/320.

However, taking exposure experienced, which is the cumulative survival from the initial census date of each *TarDy* category, into account, use of the command (**poisson dead TARD2 TARD3, exposure(survy) vce(boot)**) gives results as shown in Figure 5.11(b). The fitted model now becomes $c = \exp[\log(survy) -4.6448 + (0 \times TARD1) + (0.3904 \times TARD2) + (0.9536 \times TARD3)]$.

The estimate for those without TD have $TARD2 = TARD3 = 0$ and total exposure 2392.887 years, and so $c_{Absent} = \exp[\log(2392.8870) - 4.6448] = 22.9991$, which is essentially the actual number of deaths of 23. Thus, both models fitted reproduce the data summarized in Figure 5.10. However, a more parsimonous model for these data would be one in which the variable *TarDy* is used as an ordered categorical variable. The associated command is (**poisson dead TarDy, exposure(survy) vce(boot)**), and the output is summarized in Figure 5.11(c).

(a) *No account of exposure – unordered categorical variable*

tabulate TarDy, gen(TARD)

poisson dead TARD2 TARD3, vce(boot)
poisson dead TARD2 TARD3, vce(boot) irr

Number of obs = 608

dead	Coef	SE	z	P>|z|	[95% CI]
cons	−2.6328	0.1765			
TARD1	0				
TARD2	0.3921	0.4730	0.83	0.41	−0.5350 to 1.3192
TARD3	0.9322	0.2321	4.02	0.0001	0.4774 to 1.3871

dead	IRR	SE	z	P>|z|	[95% CI]
TARD1	1				
TARD2	1.4801	0.7303	0.79	0.43	0.5627 to 3.8932
TARD3	2.5401	0.6536	3.62	0.0003	1.5341 to 4.2061

Figure 5.11 Poisson regression analysis of the variation in death rates in psychiatric patients with tardive dyskinesia (part data from Chong, Tay, Subramaniam, *et al.*, 2009)

(b) *Accounting for exposure – unordered categorical variable*

poisson dead TARD2 TARD3, exposure(survy) vce(boot)
poisson dead TARD2 TARD3, exposure(survy) vce(boot) irr

Wald chi2 (2) = 14.44, Prob > chi2 = 0.0007, Log likelihood = −256.5431

dead	Coef	SE	z	P>|z|	[95% CI]
cons	−4.6448	0.2013			
TARD1	0				
TARD2	0.3904	3.3373	0.12	0.91	−6.1507 to 6.9314
TARD3	0.9536	0.2013	3.78	0.0002	−5.0393 to 4.2502
log(survy)	(exposure)				

dead	IRR	SE	z	P>|z|	[95% CI]
TARD1	1				
TARD2	1.4775	4.4008	0.13	0.90	0.0043 to 506.9
TARD3	2.5950	0.6823	3.63	0.0003	1.5500 to 4.3446
log(survy)	(exposure)				

estat ic

Model	Obs	ll (null)	ll(model)	df	AIC
.	608	−263.9058	−256.5431	3	519.0861

(c) *Accounting for exposure – ordered categorical variable*

poisson dead TarDy, exposure(survy) vce(boot)
poisson dead TarDy, exposure(survy) vce(boot) irr

Wald chi2 (1) = 10.23, Prob > chi2 = 0.0014, Loglikelihood = −256.5607

dead	Coef	SE	z	P>|z|	[95% CI]
cons	−4.6538	0.2336			
TarDy	0.4790	0.1498	3.20	0.0014	0.1854 to 0.7725
log(survy)	(exposure)				

dead	IRR	SE	z	P>|z|	[95% CI]
TarDy	1.6144	0.2403	3.22	0.0013	1.2059 to 2.1613
log(survy)	(exposure)				

estat ic

Model	Obs	ll(null)	ll(model)	df	AIC
.	608	−263.9058	−256.5607	2	517.1215

Figure 5.11 (Continued)

This model imposes equal steps when moving from Absent, to Mild to Definitive diagnoses of tardive dyskinesia. However, the unordered and ordered categorical models are not nested so how do we choose which to adopt? Introducing the command (**estat ic**) immediately after each model is fitted gives the Akaike criterion of equation (3.11) as 519.0861 and

517.1215 for the unordered and ordered categorical models, respectively. These estimates are similar in value but marginally give preference to the latter model, which, as it requires fewer parameters to estimate, is also the more parsimonious. Thus, we might conclude $c = \exp\left[\log(\text{survy}) - 4.6538 + (0.4790 \times TarDy)\right]$ where $TarDy$ takes the values 0, 1 and 2. Thus, for the absent, mild and definitive TD groups, we have $c_{Absent} = \exp[\log(2392.8870) - 4.6538] = 22.79$, $c_{Mild} = \exp[\log(352.0767) - 4.6538 + (0.4790 \times 1)] = 5.41$, and $c_{Definitive} = \exp[\log(1764.0410) - 4.6538 + (0.4790 \times 2)] = 43.80$. The corresponding $IRR = 1.6144$, hence the risk of death in those with mild dyskinesia is 1.6144 times that of those without signs, whereas for the definitive group it is $1.6144^2 = 2.6063$ or 2.6 times greater.

An alternative formulation $\log\mu = \log E + \beta_0 + \beta_1 x_1$ of equation (5.8) is to express the model as $\log\mu = E + \beta_0 + \beta_1 x_1$ in which case:

$$\mu = \exp(E + \beta_0 + \beta_1 x_1) \tag{5.9}$$

The corresponding command incorporating (**offset(logsurvy)**) produces the same output as using the command (**exposure(survy)**), provided the variable $E = \log(\text{survy})$ is calculated and added to the database.

ZERO-INFLATED MODELS

As we discussed earlier, there are situations where zero count may be more common than might be anticipated under the assumption that the counts follow a Poisson distribution. An example in which these occur is described by Böhning, Dietz, Schlattman, et al. (1999, Fig. 1) and Figure 5.12(a) illustrates the distribution of the Decayed Missing and Filled Teeth (DMFT) index amongst the 797 children concerned. Only the eight deciduous molars were considered in calculating the index, and so the index ranges from 0 to 8. The authors note: "There is a clear spike of extra zeros representing the caries-free children".

One way to model 'zero-inflation' is to create a model of two parts. One part concerns $c = 0$ and the other when $c > 0$. Both parts have a component described by the Poisson model, but that for $c = 0$ is a mixture of the Poisson component together with a proportion which describes those who are inflated. Thus, the combined model, the Zero-inflated Poisson (ZiP), is:

$$\text{ZiP}(c, \mu, \pi) = \begin{bmatrix} \pi + [(1-\pi) \times \exp(-\mu)\dfrac{\mu^0}{0!}] = \pi + [(1-\pi) \times \exp(-\mu)], & \text{if } c = 0 \\ (1-\pi) \times \exp(-\mu)\dfrac{\mu^c}{c!} & \text{if } c > 0 \end{bmatrix} \tag{5.10}$$

The model implies that the proportion, $1 - \pi$, of the individuals concerned follow the Poisson distribution with $c \geq 1$. For the remainder, π, do not and will have a corresponding count of zero. This model thus has two parameters, μ and π, that have to be estimated.

If we apply the usual Poisson model to all the DMFT data the commands and output are given in Figure 5.12(b). This implies the average count is estimated by $m = \exp(0.5922) = 1.81$ teeth. In order to fit model (5.10) to these data the command is (**zip DMFT, inflate(_cons)**) with the latter component (**_cons**) implying that the proportion π does not depend on any covariate. The results of Figure 5.12(c) identify 235 of 797 children (29.49%) that have zero count-inflation.

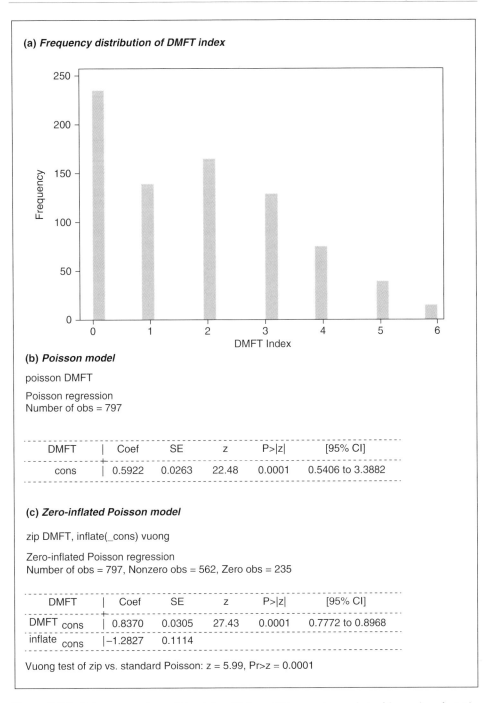

Figure 5.12 Poisson regression and Zero-inflated Poisson (ZiP) regression analysis of the number of suicides in 10 age by gender groups collated over a 35-year period (part data from Chia, Chia, Ng and Tai, 2010)

The command (**vuong**) implements the statistical test devised by Vuong (1989) which compares the ZiP and Poisson models. If the Vuong test is positive, as is the case here, then the test favours the ZiP model. In contrast, if the Vuong is negative the Poisson model is preferred.

The output also gives logit $p = -1.2827$ which confirms that π is estimated by $p = \exp(-1.2827)/[1+\exp(-1.2827)] = 0.2171$. Further, the estimate, m, is now increased to $\exp(0.8370) = 2.31$ teeth. This leads to ZiP(0, m, p) = $0.2171 +[(1 = 0.2171) \times \exp(-2.31)]$ = $0.2171 + (0.7829 \times 0.0993) = 0.2948$ and, provided $c > 0$, ZiP(c, m, p) = $0.7829 \times \exp(-2.31)\dfrac{2.31^c}{c!} = 0.0777 \times \dfrac{2.31^c}{c!}$. Thus, for example, when c = 5 are observed, then we would expect, $797 \times 0.0777 \times \dfrac{2.31^5}{5!} = 33.94$ DMFT from the model which is close to the 39 observed.

Where relevant, the ZiP model can be modified to take account of population sizes or the extent of exposure experienced by each group. It can also be extended to include one or more covariates in either or both of the component parts of equation (5.10). Thus going back to the earlier example on suicides, if we wish to investigate the role of *Gender* on suicide rates and take account of population size while acknowledging the possibility of zero-inflation which may be age dependent, then the command of Figure 5.13(a) would be appropriate.

The fitted model suggests that fewer suicides would be expected among females as the corresponding regression coefficient for *Gender* is negative, and is statistically significant as the p-value=0.0001. The Vuong test suggests that the ZiP regression analysis is appropriate, but that the inflation coefficient for *Age* is not statistically significant. Indeed the more parsimonious model (**zip Suicides Gender, exposure (Population) inflate(_cons)**) is more appropriate as this leaves the 'Suicides' section of Figure 5.13(a) unchanged, but gives the modified 'Inflate' section as in Figure 5.13(b). Once again, the Vuong test, with $z=8.14$, p-value=0.0001, suggests that the ZiP model is preferred.

RESIDUALS

As with other applications, residuals (see Figure 2.10) can be calculated following the fitting of a Poisson regression model. The command (**predict residTD**) is required to create the residuals of Figure 5.14(a), and thereby enables these to be plotted against the standard Normal distribution quantiles using the command (**qnorm residTD**). This plot zig-zags around the 45° line with mean values of residuals being -0.8307, -0.0568 and 1.1141 for the No, Mild and Definitive TD groups. These indicate that those with a definitive diagnosis of TD have the highest residuals although with wide variation from -1.73 to 1.41. The residual plot of Figure 5.14(b) obtained from the univariate model containing age alone indicates that there are some very large positive residuals indeed, with evidence of strong departure from linearity for the younger and older ages. This suggests that some transformation of *Age*, perhaps log(*Age*), would be more appropriate for modelling purposes. In this second example, the 45° line shown is distorted as the scales for the y- and x-axes are not the same.

We note that scores along the x-axis of these plots, refer to plotting the $z_{(i)}$ rather than the $Q_{(i)}$ of Chapter 2 and in which case these have to plotted against the standardized residuals or $e(i)/s_{Residual}$ where $s_{Residual}$ is obtained from the ANOVA for the corresponding fitted model.

(a) *Zero-inflation with no covariate*

zip Suicides Gender, exposure(Population) inflate(cons) vuong

Suicides	Coef	SE	z	P>|z|	[95%CI]
Suicides					
cons	−8.8247	0.0129			
Gender	−0.3651	0.0202	−18.08	0.0001	−0.4047 to −0.3255
ln(Population)	1	(exposure)			
inflate					
cons	−1.4224	0.1351			

Vuong test of zip vs.standard Poisson: z = 8.14, Pr>z = 0.0001

(b) *Zero-inflation adjusted for age*

zip Suicides Gender, exposure(Population) inflate(Age) vuong

Zero-inflated Poisson regression
Number of obs = 350, Nonzero obs = 282, Zero obs = 68

Suicides	Coef	SE	z	P>|z|	[95%CI]
Suicides					
cons	−8.8247	0.0129			
Gender	−0.3651	0.0202	−18.08	0.0001	−0.4047 to −0.3255
ln(Population)	1	(exposure)			
inflate					
cons	26.9554	2507.6			
Age	−23.4290	2507.6	−0.01	0.99	−4938.2 to 4891.3

Vuong test of zip vs. standard Poisson: z = 8.92, Pr>z = 0.0001

Figure 5.13 Zero-inflated Poisson (ZiP) regression analysis of the number of suicides collated over a 35-year period to compare the genders (a) with no covariate and (b) allowing the possibility for zero-inflation to depend on age (part data from Chia, Chia, Ng and Tai, 2010)

TECHNICAL DETAILS

Poisson distribution

We noted in Chapter 4, *Technical details*, equation (4.16), that the Binomial distribution takes the form $\text{Prob}(r) = \dfrac{n!}{r!(n-r)!}\pi^r(1-\pi)^{n-r}$, where r is the number of events observed among the n subjects concerned. We also noted that the mean number of events of this distribution is $n\pi$ and, in the circumstances when π is close to zero, the standard deviation of $\sqrt{n\pi(1-\pi)}$ is approximately $\sqrt{n\pi}$. Thus, in this latter situation the mean and variance, *Var* (the square of the standard deviation), are both equal to $n\pi$ and both depend on the value of the same single parameter, π.

Then if we set $\mu = n\pi$ and replace π by μ/n in equation (4.16) for the Binomial distribution, but use the notation c for counts, rather than r for events, the equation can be written as

$$\text{Prob}(c) = \frac{n!}{c!(n-c)!}\left(\frac{\mu}{n}\right)^c\left(1-\frac{\mu}{n}\right)^{n-c} \tag{5.11}$$

We now examine what happens to this expression as n gets larger and larger; alternatively stated as when $n \to \infty$. Thus, if we write $A = \dfrac{n!}{c!(n-c)!} = \dfrac{n \times (n-1) \times (n-2) \times \ldots \times (n-c+1)}{c!} =$

$\dfrac{n^c \times (1 - 1/n) \times (1 - 2/n) \times \ldots \times (1 - [c-1]/n)}{c!}$, so that when n is very large; $1 - 1/n \approx 1$,

$1 - 2/n \approx 1, \ldots, 1 - [c-1]/n \approx 1$, and $A \approx \dfrac{n^c}{c!}$.

(a) TardDy

```
poisson dead TarDy, exposure(survy) vce(boot)
predict residTD

table TarDy, contents (n residTD min residTD mean residTD max residTD) row
```

TarDy	N (residTD)	min (residD)	mean (residD)	max(residTD)
No TD	320	−1.9505	−0.8307	−0.7436
Mild TD	47	−1.3101	−0.0568	0.0758
Def TD	241	−1.7256	1.1141	1.4102
Total	608	−1.9505	0.0000	1.4102

```
qnorm residTD
```

Figure 5.14 Residual plots of Poisson regression analysis of the variation in death rates in psychiatric patients with respect to (a) diagnosis of TD and (b) age (part data from Chong, Tay, Subramaniam, *et al.*, 2009)

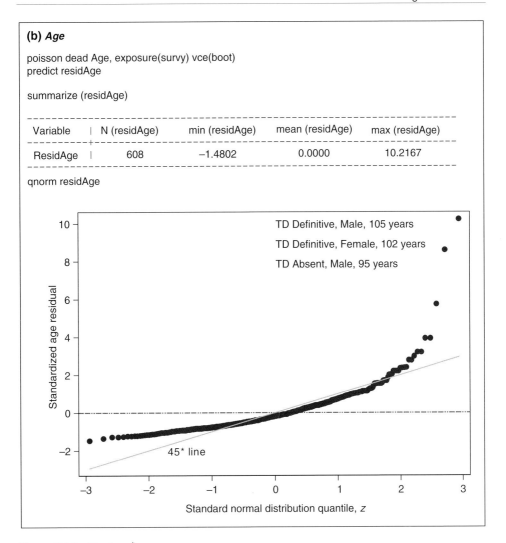

Figure 5.14 (Continued)

Also when n is very large and π very small but their product μ does not have an extreme value, $B = \left(1 - \dfrac{\mu}{n}\right)^{n-c} = \exp(-\mu)$. Substituting these parts into equation (5.11) results in

$$A \times \left(\dfrac{\mu}{n}\right)^c \times B = \dfrac{n^c}{c!} \times \left(\dfrac{\mu}{n}\right)^c \times \exp(-\mu) = \dfrac{\mu^c}{c!}\exp(-\mu) = \dfrac{\exp(-\mu)\mu^c}{c!}.$$ Here $\exp(-\mu)$ is a convenient way of writing the exponential constant e raised to the power of $-\mu$. The constant e being the base of natural logarithms which is 2.718281 ... as explained in Chapter 1, *Technical details*.

Thus, under these circumstances, the Binomial distribution of equation (5.11) becomes that of the Poisson distribution

$$\text{Poisson}(c) = \dfrac{\exp(-\mu)\mu^c}{c!} \qquad (5.12)$$

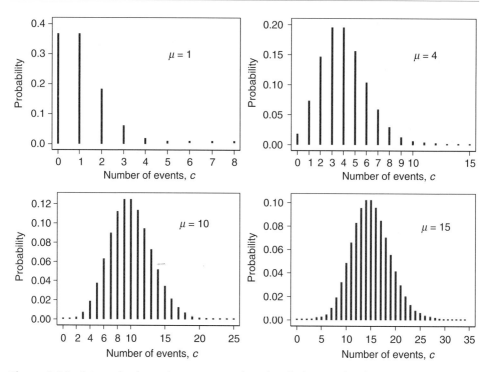

Figure 5.15 Poisson distribution for increasing values of μ. The horizontal scale in each diagram shows the value of c (adapted from Campbell, Machin and Walters, 2007, Figure 5.3)

where $c = 0, 1, 2, 3, \ldots$. The Poisson distribution has mean and variance both equal to μ.

The Poisson distribution is used to describe discrete quantitative data such as counts that occur independently and randomly in time at some average rate per unit of time, μ, as might be assumed for the number of cadaveric organs received by one Kidney Retrieval Area in a particular period as described by Wight, Jakubovic, Walters, et al. (2004).

Figure 5.15 shows the Poisson distribution for four different values of the mean, μ. For $\mu = 1$ the distribution is very skewed to the right, for $\mu = 4$ the skewness is much less and, as the mean increases to $\mu = 10$ or 15, the distribution becomes even more symmetric. Essentially, the distribution looks more like the Normal distribution shape as μ gets larger, although it is not concerned with a continuous variable.

Maximum Likelihood Estimation (MLE)

If in a study c subjects experience the event of interest, then the probability of this outcome, provided it follows the Poisson distribution of equation (5.12), is proportional to the likelihood:

$$\ell = \exp(-\mu)\mu^c \qquad (5.13)$$

The corresponding log likelihood is

$$L = \log \ell = -\mu + c \log \mu \qquad (5.14)$$

If we estimate μ by c, then $L = \log \ell = -c + c \log c$ corresponds to the largest value that L can take. We therefore state that c is the maximum likelihood estimate (MLE) of the parameter μ.

To obtain this estimate in a formal way, it is necessary to differentiate equation (5.14) with respect to μ and equate the result to zero. The solution of this equation gives the estimate as $\mu = c$, which is hence the MLE.

Relationship between Poisson and logit models

The relationship between the Poisson and logit models can be illustrated in the following way. If we first set $\pi = \mu/P$, where P is the population size, and note this is very large relative to the size of the associated count, μ. In this situation we have

$$\log\left[\frac{\pi}{1-\pi}\right] = \log\left[\frac{\mu/P}{1-\mu/P}\right] = \log\left[\frac{\mu}{P} \times \left(1 - \frac{\mu}{P}\right)^{-1}\right] \approx \log\left[\frac{\mu}{P} \times \left(1 + \frac{\mu}{P}\right)\right] \approx \log\left[\frac{\mu}{P}\right]$$

Thus from the logistic model, $\log\left[\frac{\pi}{1-\pi}\right] = \beta_0 + \beta_1 x_1 \approx \log\left[\frac{\mu}{P}\right]$. Consequently $\log\mu - \log P = \beta_0 + \beta_1 x_1$ or $\log\mu = \log P + \beta_0 + \beta_1 x_1$, which is the form of equation (5.6). If the population size is not known, $\log P$ and β_0 are merged into a single term, so the Poisson regression model becomes that of equation (5.2) or $\log\mu = \beta_0 + \beta_1 x_1$.

6   Time-to-Event Regression

SUMMARY

When the interval between two happenings, say date-of-birth to date-of-weaning of breast fed infants is recorded, the resulting 'time-to-event' data often require special regression techniques for their analysis, although time itself is measured on a continuous scale. In this chapter we describe how censored observations arise, essentially when the second happening or endpoint event has not occurred, although the initiation event has. It is these censored observations that cause the required technical changes to the statistical methods to be made. We describe the Kaplan-Meier method of summarizing in graphical form time-to-event data, which includes censored observations. The hazard ratio (HR) and the Cox regression model are introduced to enable comparison between two groups. The Cox model is then extended to allow for comparison of more groups, and also to take account of relevant covariates. Graphical and test-based methods for checking the proportional hazards (PH) assumption of the Cox model are described.

TIME-TO-EVENT DATA

In many clinical situations, a patient is diagnosed with a particular condition, receives appropriate treatment and, after a period, returns to full health. In this context, there are two critical events; the initial diagnosis and the final restoration of full health, each event with an associated date. The duration of time between these two dates is called the 'time-to-event'. However, in some circumstances, although the date-of-diagnosis is established, it is possible that the final 'event' does not occur or perhaps the time of that event may not be recorded. For example, in a clinical trial a participant may be recruited with a certain diagnosis, treated for their condition over a period of time, but then does not report back once their condition has resolved. From the investigators' perspective, the date-of-diagnosis is known, as is the last date-of-visit to the clinic. If they have also ascertained that the

Regression Methods for Medical Research, First Edition. Bee Choo Tai and David Machin.
© 2014 Bee Choo Tai and David Machin. Published 2014 by John Wiley & Sons, Ltd.

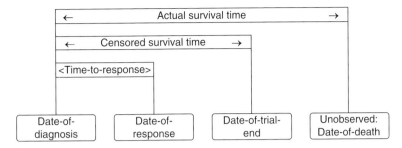

Figure 6.1 Critical events (Response and Death) and corresponding time-to-event relevant to a clinical trial

condition has not resolved by the latter date, then all the clinical team know for this individual is the duration of that interval and the fact that the condition has not yet been resolved. One presumes it will resolve some time later but the team will not know when. This interval (between diagnosis and last clinic visit) is still known as the 'time-to-event' but is now termed *censored* to acknowledge the fact that the critical event has not been observed. Thus, although time is measured on a continuous scale, special techniques have to be invoked for time-to-event data because censored observations often arise. The techniques employed with such data are conventionally termed 'survival analysis' methods.

One example of how censored observations arise is shown in Figure 6.1. There, a patient diagnosed with advanced cancer is recruited to an ongoing clinical trial. Initially, and relatively quickly, he or she responded to treatment and the date when this occurred is recorded. Subsequently, at a later date, the trial data collection ceases and as the patient is known to be alive, the censored survival time is noted and passed to the trial investigators. The patient clearly survives beyond that date until, hopefully much later, the date of their eventual demise.

Other examples of survival times include time from birth to onset of myopia (although many may never develop the condition), the time a broken bone takes to heal, the duration of an episode of influenza, how long an industrial worker has been exposed to a believed occupational hazard, or the time a transplanted kidney remains patent.

A key feature of many survival time studies is the distinction that needs to be made between calendar time, patient time-on-study, and ranked analysis time. Figure 6.2 shows a study including five patients who entered the study at different calendar times. This is typically the situation in any clinical trial in which the potential patients are those presenting at a particular clinic over a period of time, and not usually all on the same date. The progress of each patient recruited to the trial is then monitored for a period as is described in the appropriate trial protocol. Also, at some future date (calendar time), the trial will close and an analysis will be conducted. For a patient recruited late into the trial, this may imply that their endpoint observation (the event of concern) will not be made.

Thus, for patients B and D, in the example of Figure 6.2(a) both have *not* failed at the date of trial end, and so have censored 'time-to-fail' values. As D was recruited later, this is shorter than that for B. Patient C also has a censored 'time-to-fail', but this arises because of his or her loss to follow-up. In contrast, A and E both fail within the calendar time interval that the trial is open for recruitment, and therefore their actual 'time-to-fail' has been observed.

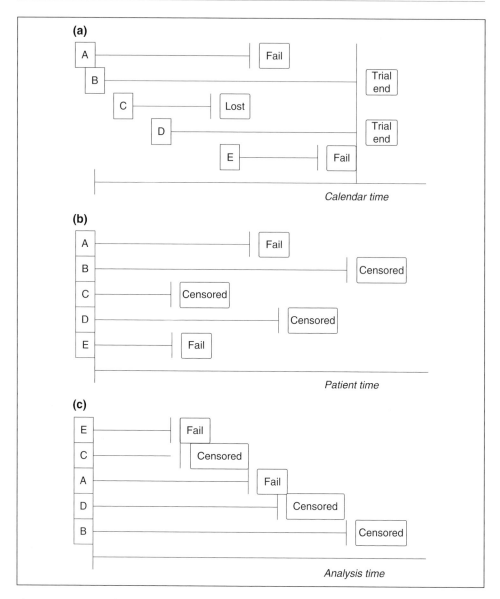

Figure 6.2   Time-to-fail endpoints for a clinical trial. (a) 'Calendar-time' when entering. (b) 'Patient-time' on the trial. (c) Rank-time for analysis purposes with censored patient C given a little (here exaggerated) extra survival over patient E who had failed with the same time-to-fail

At the close of the trial, the patients will now be viewed as in Figure 6.2(b). Here, time is measured for each patient from their date-of-entry to the trial. Thus, time is measured by patient (subsequent follow-up) time on trial, rather than in calendar time. Finally, for analysis purposes these times are ranked from smallest to largest as E, C, A, D, and B (Figure 6.2(c)). Although E and C both have the same time-to-fail, as C provides a censored observation it is presumed that whatever the eventual time-to-fail is (although we will never observe it), it will be larger than that recorded for individual E.

KAPLAN-MEIER SURVIVAL CURVE

Survival time is a continuous non-negative variable, but the corresponding distribution often has a long tail to the right and therefore, in most cases, is unlikely to have a Normal distribution shape. Nevertheless, it may be possible to find a transformation, such as taking its logarithm, which will make it appear so. Thus, it seems plausible that standard linear and multiple regression methods may be used for such transformed data. However, the reason for the use of special methods for survival data is not the shape of the distribution itself but rather the presence of 'censored' observations.

One method of summary of survival data is to specify in advance a fixed time-point, say 1-year, and then calculate the proportion of subjects whose survival times exceed this time period. However, this ignores the individual (and exact) survival times observed, and is therefore likely to be very wasteful of the available information. In particular, it does not utilize those observations censored at times less than 1-year from study entry. The Kaplan-Meier (K-M) method of calculation, and the associated survival curve, has been developed to deal with time-to-event data and make full use of all the individual survival times whether or not they are censored.

In the *unusual* situation where all subjects in a study experience the event of concern (say death) and so there are *no censored* observations, the K-M survival curve for n patients starts at time 0 with a value of 1 (or 100% survival) then continues horizontally until the time when the first death occurs, it then drops by $1/n$ at this point. The curve then proceeds horizontally once more until the time of the second death, when again it drops by $1/n$. This process continues until the time of the last death, when the survival curve drops by the final $1/n$ to take a value of 0 (0%). If two deaths happen to occur at the same time then the step down would be $2/n$.

The K-M estimate of the survival curve when there are censored observations mimics this process but essentially 'jumps' over the 'censored' observations, which then leads to steps down of varying magnitudes. The precise method of calculating the K-M survival curve is summarized in *Technical details*.

In the study of Sridhar, Gore, Boiangiu, *et al.* (2009) describing the post-diagnosis survival times of 35 patients with glioblastoma, 12 presented with very extensive disease, whereas in 23 the disease was less extensive. Figure 6.3(a) gives the survival times of the 12 patients with very extensive disease and, as all have died (Fail=1), there are no censored observations. In contrast, Figure 6.3(b) gives the survival times of the 23 patients with less extensive disease and in this latter group, 5 patients remain alive (Fail=0) at the time-of-analysis with censored survival times of 1.774, 1.823, 2.867, 2.897, and 3.422 years.

The command (`stset survy, fail(dead)`) first establishes that (`survy`) is a *time-to-event* variable and then identifies (`dead`) as that which provides the *censoring* mechanism. This illustrates that for survival time studies a pair of variables is required to define the event time. Thus, in the first row of the data of Figure 6.3(a), Time=0.0520 and Fail=1, whereas in the last row of Figure 6.3(b), Time=3.422+ and Fail=0. The latter Fail=0 indicates the patient is alive (not yet dead) at this time and so is a censored observation. In contrast, the former Fail=1 indicates that the patient died at this time and so the survival time is not censored. The second command (`sts list`) produces the K-M estimate of survival at every death time. The K-M curves for the Very and Less Extensive disease groups are shown in Figure 6.4. For those patients with very extensive disease the curve ends on the time-axis at the time of the longest survival time. In contrast, in those

(a) *No censored observation*				(b) *With some censored observations*			
stset survy, fail (dead) sts list				stset survy, fail (dead) sts list			
Time	Total	Fail	Survivor Function	Time	Total	Fail	Survivor Function
0.0520	12	1	0.9167	0.3641	23	1	0.9565
0.0575	11	1	0.8333	0.3943	22	1	0.9130
0.1150	10	1	0.7500	0.4736	21	1	0.8696
0.2272	9	1	0.6667	0.5941	20	1	0.8261
0.2820	8	1	0.5833	0.6297	19	1	0.7826
0.3149	7	1	0.5000	0.9418	18	1	0.7391
0.3751	6	1	0.4167	0.9610	17	1	0.6957
0.4298	5	1	0.3333	1.109	16	1	0.6522
0.6379	4	1	0.2500	1.136	15	1	0.6087
0.6790	3	1	0.1667	1.268	14	1	0.5652
0.7967	2	1	0.0833	1.415	13	1	0.5217
1.1500	1	1	0.0000	1.429	12	1	0.4783
				1.462	11	1	0.4348
				1.465	10	1	0.3913
				1.503	9	1	0.3478
				1.552	8	1	0.3043
				1.774+	7	0	0.3043
				1.823+	6	0	0.3043
				1.906	5	1	0.2435
				1.936	4	1	0.1826
				2.867+	3	0	0.1826
				2.897+	2	0	0.1826
				3.422+	1	0	0.1826

+Added to distinguish the censored
observations more clearly

Figure 6.3 Edited commands and output for calculating a Kaplan-Meier (K-M) survival curve for patients with glioblastoma (a) very extensive disease, no censored observations; (b) less extensive disease, some censored observation (data from Sridhar, Gore, Boiangiu et al., 2009)

with less extensive disease, the curve does not drop to the time-axis as the patient with the longest survival time remains alive at 3.422 years.

On the K-M survival curve of Figure 6.4(b), the small spikes correspond to the times of the censored observations. When there are a large number of patients and perhaps a large number of censored observations, the 'spikes' may clutter the K-M curve. In which case the numbers at risk, which are a selection of the Total columns of Figure 6.3, are tabulated at convenient intervals beneath the time-axis of the K-M curves. In our case, as there are so few patients, both spikes and numbers at risk are included.

When comparing two or more survival curves we usually assume that the mechanisms that result in censored observations do not depend on the group concerned, that is, the censoring is 'non-informative' in that it tells us nothing relevant to the comparison of the groups. For example, in a randomized clinical trial, it is assumed that patients are just as likely to be lost to follow-up in one treatment group as in another. If there are imbalances in such losses then this can lead to spurious differences in the apparent survival times of the groups concerned, leading perhaps to false conclusions being drawn from the analysis.

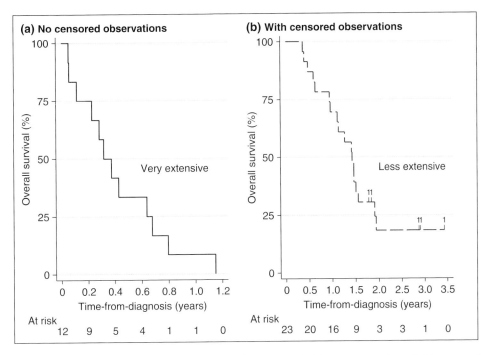

Figure 6.4 Examples of Kaplan-Meier survival curves with (a) no censored, and (b) censored observations from the glioblastoma cases of Figure 6.3 (data from Sridhar, Gore, Boiangiu, *et al.*, 2009)

THE HAZARD RATE AND HAZARD RATIO

Hazard rate

If we think of our own lives, we are continually exposed to the possibility of our demise. However, having lived until now, we can think of the chance of our demise in the next day, hour, or second as our hazard for the next interval be it, a second, hour or day. This can be thought of as our *instantaneous* death rate conditional on living until now. Clearly, the chance of our demise in the next very short interval of time will be small, but nevertheless the possibility remains. The hazard rate may be expressed as that of our particular age group, denoted $\lambda(Age)$, or more generally at a particular time t, denoted $\lambda(t)$. In general, we think of the hazard rate at a given value of t as the risk applying to what is just about to happen in the next (very short) period of time. It is mathematically defined in equation (6.11).

Our own hazard will fluctuate with time and will certainly increase for all of us as our age increases. Similarly, if we contract a life-threatening illness our hazard rate would unquestionably increase. In such a situation the aim of therapy would be to restore our elevated hazard to the former (lower) value, if possible. Individual hazards will differ, even in those of precisely the same age, and it may be that particular groups have (on average) higher values than others. Thus, the hazard of developing dental caries may be less in those who live in areas where fluoridation of the drinking water supply has occurred.

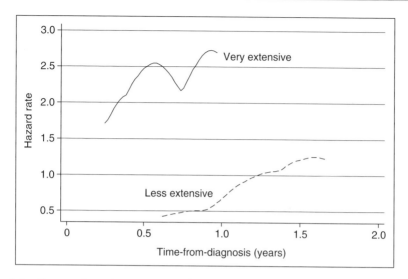

Figure 6.5 Changing hazard rates over time for glioblastoma patients with less and greater extent of disease at diagnosis (data from Sridhar, Gore, Boiangiu, *et al.*, 2009)

In investigating the patients with glioblastoma, it is clear from Figure 6.4 that those with very extensive disease at diagnosis have a worse prognosis than those with less extensive disease. Alternatively expressed, those with extensive disease have a greater hazard rate than those with less extensive disease. The corresponding hazard rates are shown in Figure 6.5, which clearly indicates generally increasing hazard rates with time-from-diagnosis which are higher (about five times greater) in those with very extensive disease.

Thus in general, we may wish to relate the hazard to various clinical characteristics among a particular group of individuals. In the case of two groups, we specify an underlying hazard function for those of one group (say those with very extensive disease) by $\lambda_0(t)$, which is often therefore termed the baseline hazard. We can then regard the hazard function for the less extensive disease group, $\lambda(t)$, in relation to this baseline as

$$\lambda(t) = h(t)\,\lambda_0(t) \tag{6.1}$$

Thus we describe the hazard function, $\lambda(t)$, of one group as a multiple, $h(t)$, of the other, $\lambda_0(t)$. In many situations the multiplier, $h(t)$, may not depend on time, and so could be expressed more simply as a constant, h. However, in most applications the value of h will depend on one or more covariates. For a single covariate, h is usually expressed in the form $h(x_1) = \exp(\beta_1 x_1)$, where the covariate is x_1 and has a corresponding multiplier (regression coefficient) β_1. If $\beta_1 = 0$, then $h(x_1) = \exp(0 \times x_1) = \exp(0) = 1$ and this implies that $\lambda(t) = \lambda_0(t)$. In view of this equation (6.1), for a single covariate, x_1, is usually expressed as

$$\lambda(t) = \lambda_0(t)\exp(\beta_1 x_1) \tag{6.2}$$

This equation can be extended to include more covariates as necessary.

Hazard ratio

When comparing two groups of individuals with respect to their survival times, the ratio of the two hazard functions is considered. Thus the hazard ratio, HR, for the situation of equation (6.2) where one group is designated by $x_1=0$, the other by $x_1=1$ is

$$HR = \frac{\lambda(t)}{\lambda_0(t)} = \frac{\lambda_0(t)\exp(\beta_1 x_1)}{\lambda_0(t)} = \exp(\beta_1 x_1) \tag{6.3}$$

This ratio does not depend on the changing baseline hazard, $\lambda_0(t)$, and neither does it change with time t. The situation is termed proportional hazards (PH). When the hazard functions of the two groups are identical the $HR=1$ and, in which case, the regression coefficient $\beta_1=0$.

An alternative format for equation (6.3) is

$$\log(HR) = \beta_1 x_1 \tag{6.4}$$

In equations (6.3) and (6.4) the value of the HR may depend on the value of the covariate, x_1, and so in this case it should be denoted more correctly $HR(x_1)$. However, for simplicity we will usually omit the associated covariates as the context usually makes it clear what they are.

THE COX REGRESSION MODEL

Single covariate

Equation (6.2) is the simplest form of the Cox proportional hazards regression model. The strength of the PH model developed by Cox (1972) is not only that it allows survival data arising from a changing hazard function to be modeled, but it does so without making any assumption about the underlying distribution of the hazards in the different groups concerned, except that these hazards remain proportional to each other over time.

As we have indicated, the null hypothesis of ultimate prognosis not being affected by membership of a particular group in this model is H_0: $\beta_1=0$. If this hypothesis is not rejected, then we infer that $HR=1$, which then implies that the risk of death in the two groups is the same.

Figure 6.6 gives the commands and output when the model of the form of (6.3) or (6.4) is fitted to the very extensive ($x_1=0$) and less extensive ($x_1=1$) disease groups of the glioblastoma patients. The associated commands are (**stcox Extent, nohr**), which estimates β_{Extent}, but when the HR is required, (**stcox Extent, hr**) is used. Here the (**hr**) component replaces (**nohr**) of the previous command, although it is often the default option and need not be stated explicitly. In this example, the null hypothesis H_0: $\beta_{Extent}=0$ is firmly rejected as the statistical test gives the p-value<0.0001. The estimated $b_{Extent}=-1.9821$. When the regression coefficient is negative, this indicates that the numerator group in equation (6.3) has a better outcome than the denominator or baseline group, and this implies that the corresponding estimated HR has a value less than 1 as here where $HR=0.1378$. Alternatively, had we coded very extensive ($x_1=1$) and less extensive ($x_1=0$), then the associated output would have given $b_{Extent}=+1.9821$ with $HR=7.2582=1/0.1378$. The associated K-M survival curves, generated by the command (**sts graph, by(Extent)**), provide a clear indication of a more favorable prognosis in those with less extensive disease as we noted previously in Figure 6.5.

The Cox regression model of equation (6.3), which involves a single binary covariate, can be adapted for ordered categorical, unordered categorical, numerical discrete and continuous

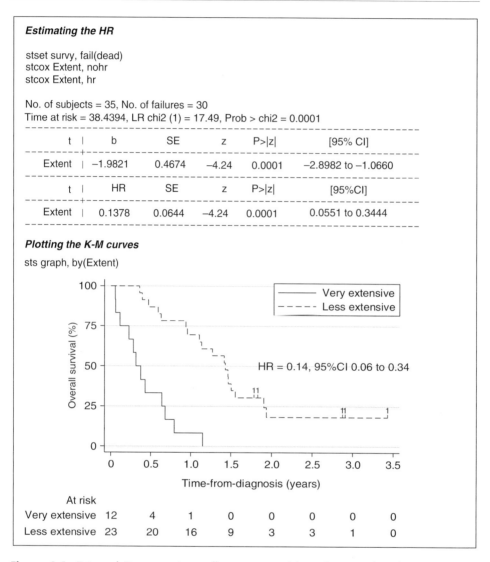

Figure 6.6 Estimated Cox regression coefficient, estimated hazard ratio and Kaplan-Meier survival curves for patients with glioblastoma by extent of disease at diagnosis (data from Sridhar, Gore, Boiangiu, et al., 2009)

covariates. Thus, Chong, Tay, Subramaniam, *et al.* (2009) assessed hospitalized patients with schizophrenia for evidence of tardive dyskinesia (TD) corresponding to a 3-level categorical variable, labeled *TarDy*, with categories of absent, mild and definitive TD. These patients were subsequently followed over an 8-year period and the dates of any deaths occurring noted. The cumulative death rate (CDR) plots (derived by subtracting the K-M estimate from 1) are obtained using the command (**st graph, failure by(TarDy)**)and are shown in Figure 6.7, from which it appears that those with definitive TD have the greatest CDR.

The corresponding model to describe their mortality experience is:

$$T: \log(HR) = \beta_{TarDy} TarDy \tag{6.5}$$

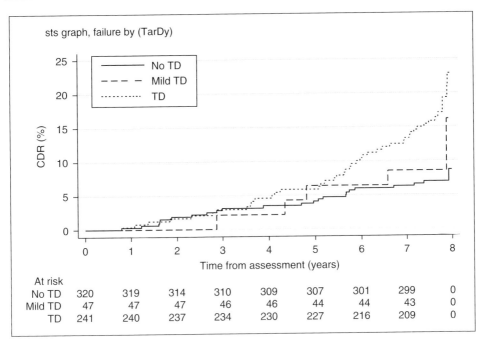

Figure 6.7 Estimated cumulative death rates (CDR) for patients with schizophrenia classified as having no, mild or definitive tardive dyskinesia (TD) (data from Chong, Tay, Subramaniam, *et al.*, 2009)

The 3-level covariate *TarDy* is clearly an ordered categorical variable taking values of (say) 0, 1 and 2, and can be used as such in a Cox regression model using the command (**stcox TarDy, nohr**) or the command (**stcox TarDy**): the latter giving the estimated HR.

The results of these analyses are given in Figure 6.8(a), which suggests that compared with those without TD, those with mild TD have a higher risk with $HR=1.6216$, and as the chosen divisions on the TD scale of severity are set as equal, the risk for those with definitive TD is $HR=1.6216^2=2.6296$.

The validity of the assumption of equal divisions on the TD scale can be verified by fitting the covariate *TarDy* as an unordered categorical variable, using the commands (**xi:stcox i.TarDy, nohr**) and (**xi:stcox i.TarDy**). Figure 6.8(b) gives estimates of the hazard ratios of mild and definitive as 1.4767 and 2.6177, which are very close to those estimated by the ordered categorical model and so justify the use of that scale. Consequently the first model is preferred as it is more parsimonious, being the simpler of the two.

Figure 6.9(a) shows, for example, that those with definitive TD are, on average, older at assessment than those without TD, and also indicates that the age-at-assessment ranges from 29 to 105 years: a difference between youngest and oldest of 76 years. Once again, no new principles are involved if there is only a single covariate, such as *Age*, which is continuous in nature. The Cox model for age-at-assessment is written

$$A: \log(HR) = \beta_{Age} Age \tag{6.6}$$

and this can be fitted to the data for patients with schizophrenia to examine how this influences their subsequent mortality.

(a) *Ordered categorical covariate*

stcox TarDy, nohr
stcox TarDy

No. of subjects = 608, No. of failures = 72
Time at risk = 4509.00, LR chi2(1) = 14.96, Prob > chi2 = 0.0001

t	Coef	SE	z	P>|z|	[95% CI]
TarDy	0.4834	0.1286	3.76	0.0002	0.2313 to 0.7356

t	HR	SE	z	P>|z|	[95% CI]
TarDy	1.6216	0.2086	3.76	0.0002	1.2602 to 2.0867

(b) *Unordered categorical covariate*

xi:stcox i.TarDy, nohr
xi:stcox i.TarDy

Time at risk = 4509.00, LR chi2(2) = 15.00, Prob > chi2 = 0.0006

t	Coef	SE	z	P>|z|	[95% CI]
TarDy_1	0				
TarDy_2	0.3898	0.4935	0.79	0.43	−0.5775 to 1.3571
TarDy_3	0.9623	0.2573	3.74	0.0002	0.4579 to 1.4667

t	HR	SE	z	P>|z|	[95% CI]
TarDy_1	1				
TarDy_2	1.4767	0.7288	0.79	0.43	0.5613 to 3.8847
TarDy_3	2.6177	0.6736	3.74	0.0002	1.5808 to 4.3347

Figure 6.8 Cox regression models for patients with schizophrenia assuming diagnosis of tardive dyskinesia (TD) as either an ordered or unordered categorical covariate (data from Chong, Tay, Subramaniam *et al.*, 2009)

However, as in other model-type situations, care has to be taken in using a sensible scale for the units of the covariate concerned. As age is a continuous variable, it could have been recorded in units ranging from seconds (more realistically days) to decades. Had it been assessed in months, the *HR* per month is given in Figure 6.9(b) as 1.0042, that for years as 1.0513 and that for decades as 1.6499. The investigator would choose the most appropriate for reporting purposes. We note that $1.0042^{12} = 1.0516$ and $1.0513^{10} = 1.6492$, and these indicate that whatever the scale chosen the interpretation remains the same. However, it is usually sensible in these circumstances to have no more than one '0' between the decimal point and the first non-zero digit in the reported estimate of the HR. Although a rather extreme situation when we span the full 76-year age range of this example, if we compare using the successive month, year and decade estimates of Figure 6.9(b) then $1.0042^{(76 \times 12)} = 45.71$, $1.0513^{76} = 44.79$ and $1.6499^{7.6} = 44.94$. The estimates for those who are 76 years older than the youngest patient at initial assessment are not numerically the same because of rounding errors, the latter being the most accurate in this case. Thus there is always a danger that a quoted estimate, here the *HR*, may be compromised by using an inappropriate choice of analysis scale.

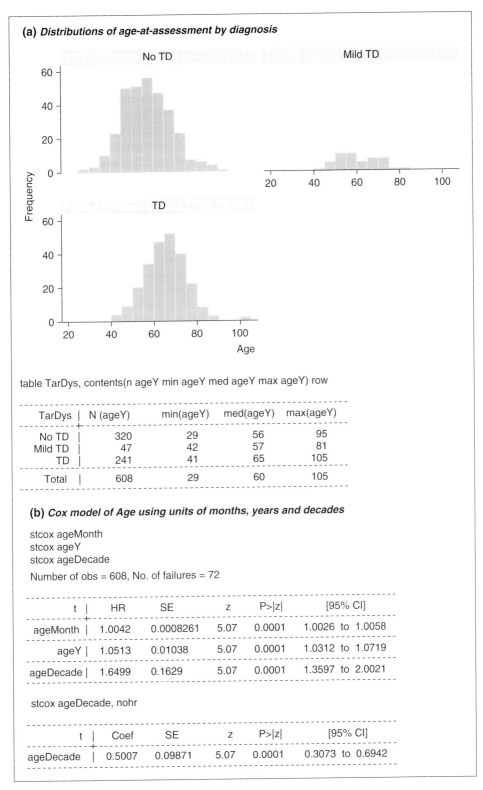

Figure 6.9 (a) Distribution of age at assessment, and (b) Cox regression models to investigate the influence of age on subsequent mortality in patients with schizophrenia classified as having no, mild or definitive tardive dyskinesia (TD) (data from Chong, Tay, Subramaniam, *et al.*, 2009)

In addition, such analyses assume a linear effect of age on the log*HR* scale and so it is usually prudent to verify if this is a reasonable assumption. This can be done either by adding a quadratic-in-age term or by creating a new variable with the covariate age represented as a categorical variable. The latter approach is usually more informative, although there is some subjectivity involved in selecting the location and number of cut-points to create the new variable. The optimum choice of the number of categories is likely to be very data-dependent, but a minimum of three and a maximum of seven categories are reasonable guidelines.

As an illustration, Figure 6.10(a) tabulates age-at-assessment in three groups 29–59, 60–69, and 70–105 years, to create the variable *AgeG3* and then fits the corresponding model using (**xi:stcox i.AgeG3, nohr**) and (**xi:stcox i.AgeG3**). The regression

---

(a) *Unordered categorical covariate*

tabulate AgeG3 TarDy

		TarDy		
age (Age)	No TD	Mild TD	TD	Total
29–59	195	26	67	288
60–69	89	13	106	208
70–105	36	8	68	112
Total	320	47	241	608

xi:stcox i.AgeG3, nohr
xi:stcox i.AgeG3

t	Coef	SE	z	P>|z|	[95% CI]
IAgeG3_1	0				
IAgeG3_2	0.7796	0.3022	2.58	0.010	0.1873 to 1.3720
IAgeG3_3	1.4526	0.3071	4.73	0.0001	0.8507 to 2.0545

t	HR	SE	z	P>|z|	[95% CI]
IAgeG3_1	1				
IAgeG3_2	2.1807	0.6590	2.58	0.010	1.2060 to 3.9431
IAgeG3_3	4.2742	1.3126	4.73	0.0001	2.3413 to 7.8027

(b) *Ordered categorical covariate*

stcox AgeG3, nohr
stcox AgeG3

t	Coef	SE	z	P>|z|	[95% CI]
AgeG3	0.7226	0.1510	4.78	0.0001	0.4266 to 1.0186

t	HR	SE	z	P>|z|	[95% CI]
AgeG3	2.0598	0.3111	4.78	0.0001	1.5321 to 2.7694

Figure 6.10 Cox regression model for subsequent mortality in patients with schizophrenia classified as having no, mild or definitive tardive dyskinesia (TD) on age at assessment regarded as a 3-level (a) unordered and (b) ordered categorical covariate (data from Chong, Tay, Subramaniam, et al., 2009)

coefficients of 0.7796 and 1.4526 represent approximately equal steps between the three categories as 0.7796 is relatively close to the mid-point $(0 + 1.4526)/2 = 0.7263$ of the other coefficients. This implies that the assumption of linearity may be reasonable, and further suggests that the variable *AgeG3* may be used as an ordered categorical covariate. This might then be modeled using (**stcox AgeG3, nohr**) and (**stcox AgeG3**). The results in Figure 6.10(b) give $HR = 2.0598$ for (AgeG3) category 60–69 compared with those 25–59. When the oldest group, 70–105, is compared with the youngest, the $HR = 2.0598^2 = 4.2428$. This is very close to the estimate of 4.2742 quoted in Figure 6.10(a).

Two covariates

As we have just seen, the age of the patients with schizophrenia at the study assessment point at which a diagnosis or otherwise of TD was made, has a considerable bearing on ultimate mortality. In the situation where more than one covariate may influence survival, here age as well as TD diagnosis, we can extend the Cox model to become:

$$\boldsymbol{T} + \boldsymbol{A}: \log HR\,(TarDy, AgeG3) = \beta_{TarDy} TarDy + \beta_{AgeG3} AgeG3 \tag{6.7}$$

In this situation if we take both *TarDy* and *AgeG3* as having the three ordered values of (say) 0, 1 and 2, then there are essentially nine patient groups. Thus, for those without TD who are aged 20–59 we have $(TarDy = 0, AgeG3 = 0)$, and so equation (6.7) becomes $\log HR(0, 0) = \beta_{TarDy} \times 0 + \beta_{AgeG3} \times 0 = 0$ or $HR(0, 0) = 1$. This implies that this particular group has the underlying hazard, $\lambda_0(t)$, and we therefore regard this as the baseline group against which we compare the other eight patient groups.

It is clear from Figure 6.11 that there is a higher CDR among those who were older when assessed for the purpose of this study, and there is a somewhat confusing pattern with respect to diagnosis essentially caused by the mild TD cases who are relatively few in number. However, the main focus of the analysis is whether or not a diagnosis of TD remains a risk factor for subsequent mortality after taking account of age-at-assessment. Thus, we have to compare model (6.7) including both *TarDy* and *AgeG3* with the simpler model (6.5) of *TarDy* alone.

The resulting calculations using (**stcox TarDy, nohr**) and (**stcox TarDy AgeG3, nohr**) are summarized in Figure 6.12(a). Comparisons of these two models are made using the likelihood ratio (LR) test which is described in more detail in Chapter 7, *Case study*. Thus, the models are tested by $LR = -2(L1 - L2) = -2[-440.42296 - (-433.20383)] = -2 \times -7.21913 = 14.44$. This is the same result as the difference of [**LR chi2 (2) – LR chi2 (1)**] $= 29.40 - 14.96 = 14.44$ from the same computer output. Under the null hypothesis, $H_0: \beta_{AgeG3} = 0$, the LR has a χ^2 distribution with $df = 1$ as the Cox model $(\boldsymbol{T} + \boldsymbol{A})$, including both *TarDy* and *AgeG3*, has two parameters; one more parameter than model $\boldsymbol{T}$ which is that for *TarDy* alone. Use of Table T5 with $df = 1$, implies a p-value < 0.001 as the calculated $LR = 14.44$ is greater than the tabulated $\chi^2 = 10.83$ under the column for $\alpha = 0.001$. This implies that the model $(\boldsymbol{T} + \boldsymbol{A})$ provides a better description of the situation. The corresponding estimated regression coefficient for *TarDy* has been reduced from $b_{TarDy} = 0.4834$ in model $\boldsymbol{T}$ to $b_{TarDy} = 0.3333$ in model $(\boldsymbol{T} + \boldsymbol{A})$: a reduction in value of $C = 0.3333/0.4834 = 0.69$ or 69%. This can be thought of as a major change and so the results from the extended model would be presented in any subsequent report.

The corresponding estimated hazard ratios are shown in Figure 6.12(b). Thus, for model $\boldsymbol{T}$, the estimate for *TarDy* is $HR = 1.62$ (95% CI 1.26 to 2.09, $p = 0.0002$), whereas that from

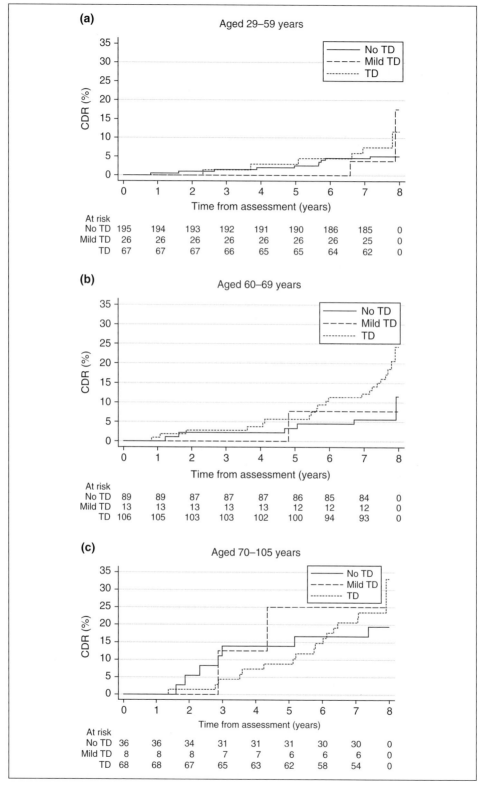

Figure 6.11 Cumulative death rates (CDR) for patients with schizophrenia classified as having no, mild or definitive tardive dyskinesia (TD) by age group at assessment (data from Chong, Tay, Subramaniam et al., 2009)

(a) *Comparing two models*

stcox TarDy, nohr

Subjects = 608, Failures = 72, **LR chi2(1) = 14.96**, Prob > chi2 = 0.0001

Log likelihood: **L1 = −440.42296**

t	Coef	SE	z	P>|z|	[95% CI]
TarDy	0.4834	0.1286	3.76	0.0002	0.2313 to 0.7356

stcox TarDy AgeG3, nohr

Subjects = 608, Failures = 72, **LR chi2(2) = 29.40**, Prob > chi2 = 0.0001

Log likelihood: **L2 = −433.20383**

t	Coef	SE	z	P>|z|	[95% CI]
TarDy	0.3333	0.1339	2.49	0.013	0.0709 to 0.5957
AgeG3	0.6052	0.1593	3.80	0.0001	0.2930 to 0.9175

(b) *HR estimates for TarDy from two models*

stcox TarDy

t	HR	SE	z	P>|z|	[95% CI]
TarDy	1.6216	0.2086	3.76	0.0002	1.2602 to 2.0867

stcox TarDy AgeG3

t	HR	SE	z	P>|z|	[95% CI]
TarDy	1.3955	0.1868	2.49	0.013	1.0734 to 1.8142
AgeG3	1.8317	0.2918	3.80	0.0001	1.3404 to 2.5030

Figure 6.12 Cox regression models for subsequent mortality on presence of tardive dyskinesia (TD) and age-at-assessment both regarded as ordered categorical covariates (data from Chong, Tay, Subramaniam, *et al.*, 2009)

model $T+A$ is reduced to $HR=1.40$ (95% CI 1.07 to 1.81, $p=0.013$). In broad terms, the conclusions of the simpler model are retained in that a diagnosis of TD is an adverse prognostic feature. However, the magnitude of this effect is reduced by taking account of the age-at-assessment of these patients with schizophrenia.

In general, despite a covariate being a strong predictor of outcome, adding this to the regression model may not substantially change the estimated value of the 'key' regression coefficient, which in the case just discussed is that of the TD group. Thus, the main concern here is the measure of the differences between the groups, and the role of the covariate age is to see if our view of this measure is modified or not by taking note of its presence. The aim of *this* study is not to establish or quantify the influence of the covariate itself.

More than two covariates

The Cox model can be extended to include more than two covariates. Thus, the influence of the binary covariate *Gender* could be added to the previous covariate model to give

$$T + A + G: \log(HR) = \beta_{TarDy}TarDy + \beta_{AgeG3}AgeG3 + \beta_{Gender}Gender \qquad (6.8)$$

The corresponding command takes the form (`stcox TarDy AgeG3 Gender`).

The number of variables that can be added to the Cox model is, in theory, without end. Thus, in general, by extending equation (6.4) we have the *k*-variable model

$$\log\left[HR(x_1, x_2, \cdots, x_k)\right] = \beta_1 x_1 + \beta_2 x_2 + \cdots, + \beta_k x_k \qquad (6.9)$$

Now, although the number of covariates we can add is without limit, there are practical constraints as estimates have to be obtained for the regression coefficients. Thus, for example, we cannot include more variables in a model than the number of events available for the analysis. Indeed the number of events should always exceed by far the number of parameters included in the model.

VERIFYING PROPORTIONAL HAZARDS

Complementary log-log plot

The complementary log-log plot used to verify PH is described in *Technical details*, and is obtained by using the command (`stphplot, by(TarDy)`). If the PH assumption is appropriate, the plots of each group concerned would all have a similar pattern, that is, they would change in 'parallel' with each other. If there were no real differences in prognosis between the groups concerned, then these 'parallel' patterns would lie over each other. However, if there is a difference in prognosis, then, although the patterns may be similar, some vertical shift between the plots of the different groups would be anticipated and they would not overlap.

Figure 6.13(a) shows the K-M survival curves for those patients with schizophrenia who do not have a diagnosis of TD and those with definitive TD. This is the same information (but excluding the mild TD cases) as provided in the cumulative plots of Figure 6.7. The corresponding complementary log-log plot is shown in Figure 6.13(b) and, as the profiles criss-cross, although approximately parallel, this provides some evidence of a departure from *PH* for these data.

Observed and predicted K-M plots

Another check for PH can be made by comparing the estimated K-M survival curves with those predicted after fitting a Cox model can be achieved by the command (`stcoxkm TarDy`). Thus, Figure 6.14 compares the estimated K-M curves of those with and without definitive TD with the curves predicted by the model. This suggests a departure from PH as the respective observed and predicted curves do not overlap for the majority of the years from the date-of-assessment. Indeed the predicted values appear above the K-M curve for patients of the No TD group and beneath the curve of the Definitive TD group.

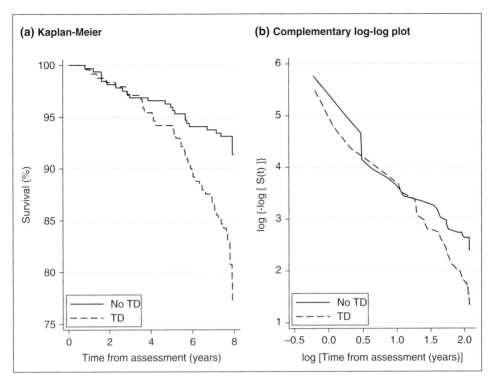

Figure 6.13 (a) Kaplan-Meier survival curves of patients with schizophrenia with or without a definitive diagnosis of tardive dyskinesia (TD), and (b) the corresponding complementary log-log plots (data from Chong, Tay, Subramaniam, *et al.*, 2009)

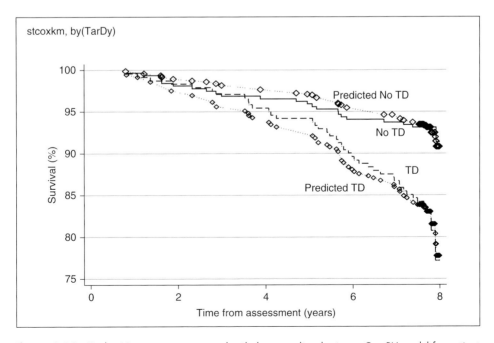

Figure 6.14 Kaplan-Meier curves compared with those predicted using a Cox PH model for patients with schizophrenia with or without a definitive diagnosis of tardive dyskinesia (TD) (data from Chong, Tay, Subramaniam *et al.*, 2009)

Schoenfeld residuals

Just as in the case of linear regression, residuals can be calculated and these used to help decide if the PH assumption is reasonable in a given situation. However, as is the case for logistic regression, the residuals for time-to-event studies are rather different in nature and are further complicated by the presence of censored observations as we explain in *Technical details*.

Suppose in the patients with schizophrenia we wish to evaluate the PH assumption for the Cox model when assessing *TarDy* alone, model *T*, and then again after adjustment for *AgeG3*, model *T+A*. As two covariates are to be included in the model, Schoenfeld residuals have to be calculated for each with the corresponding command (`stcox TarDy AgeG3, sch(ResidTD ResidAge)` (Figure 6.15a). In the situation of PH, Marubini and Valsecchi (1995) point out that a horizontal plot for each of the respective groups is to be anticipated. In our example, the residual plots of Figure 6.15(b) appear to gradually increase over time from the assessment suggesting a possible lack of proportionality. This is further supported by a global test of proportionality obtained from the command (`estat phtest`). The PH test assumes that under the null hypothesis, the regression coefficients $\beta_{TarDy}=\beta_{AgeG3}=0$. This is equivalent to testing that the log hazard ratio is constant over time. Thus, rejection of this null hypothesis indicates deviation from the assumption of PH. In this example, the test gives $\chi^2=6.76$ with $df=2$ as two parameters, one for *TarDy* and one for *AgeG3*, are estimated. The entry for $\alpha=0.03$ with $df=2$ in Table T5 is $\chi^2=7.01$ and suggests that the *p*-value ≈ 0.03. The more precise *p*-value$=0.034$ is given in Figure 6.15(c). This implies that the departure from PH is statistically significant. However, extending the test command to (`estat phtest, detail`) provides detail of the influence of the individual covariates in the model and suggests that the departures from PH are likely a result of *TarDy* as the corresponding $\chi^2=6.67$, $df=1$, *p*-value$=0.0098$. In contrast, the PH assumption with respect to *AgeG3* seems reasonable as $\chi^2=1.06$, $df=1$, *p*-value$=0.30$.

What if the proportional hazards assumption is wrong?

The violation of the PH assumption is not necessarily unacceptable, as to assume PH is essentially to estimate the effect of a covariate averaged over time and ignore the possibility that the effect of the covariate may vary over time. For example, females are known to have a longer life expectancy than males, although, when women become of child-bearing age, the risk difference between them and males of the same age group may lessen. However, in a study of gender differences in mortality which spans all age groups, a simple linear form for the age component of the regression model may be chosen. This model, based on the assumption of PH for the two genders, may be sufficient to conclude the presence of an important gender effect. In contrast, a more complex model, taking specific account of the child-bearing years, may suggest that the gender difference is diminished. However, unless this 'more correct' model identifies features of major clinical or scientific importance for the study findings, the simple but 'less correct' model may be adequate for the purpose of the study and therefore preferable in this instance.

Stratified Cox

One means of taking account of the lack of PH in a covariate is to make the 'major' comparisons of concern within the different levels of that covariate. Thus, if we use the randomized trial conducted by Pearson, Pinkerton, Lewis, *et al.* (2008) in children with

(a) *Cox model and estimating the residuals*

stcox TarDy AgeG3, sch(ResidTD ResidAge)

No. of subjects = 608, No. of failures = 72

```
    _t |     OR       SE       z     P>|z|        [95% CI]
-------+--------------------------------------------------------
TarDy (T) |  1.3805    0.1847   2.41   0.016    1.0620 to 1.7944
AgeG3 (A) |  1.8835    0.2956   4.03   0.0001   1.3847 to 2.5619
```

(b) *Residual plots*

scatter ResidTD survy
scatter ResidAge survy

(c) *Test of proportional hazards*

estat phtest

```
             |   chi2    df   Prob>chi2
-------------+-----------------------------
global test  |   6.76    2     0.034
```

estat phtest, detail

```
             |   chi2    df   Prob>chi2
-------------+-----------------------------
TarDy        |   6.67    1     0.0098
AgeG3        |   1.06    1     0.30
```

Figure 6.15 (a) Estimation of the Schoenfeld residuals, (b) scatter plot of the residuals against survival time, and (c) tests of proportional hazards after fitting a Cox model including diagnosis of tardive dyskinesia (TD) and age at initial assessment of patients with schizophrenia (data from Chong, Tay, Subramaniam, *et al.*, 2009)

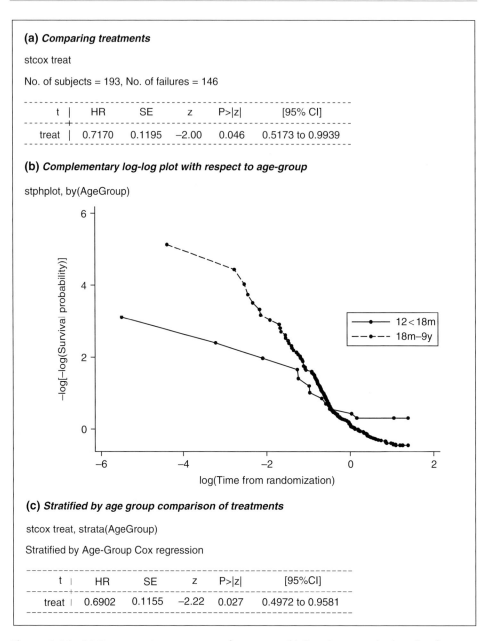

(a) *Comparing treatments*

stcox treat

No. of subjects = 193, No. of failures = 146

t	HR	SE	z	P>|z|	[95% CI]
treat	0.7170	0.1195	−2.00	0.046	0.5173 to 0.9939

(b) *Complementary log-log plot with respect to age-group*

stphplot, by(AgeGroup)

(c) *Stratified by age group comparison of treatments*

stcox treat, strata(AgeGroup)

Stratified by Age-Group Cox regression

t	HR	SE	z	P>|z|	[95%CI]
treat	0.6902	0.1155	−2.22	0.027	0.4972 to 0.9581

Figure 6.16 (a) Cox regression comparison of treatments, (b) Complementary log-log plot of two age groups, and (c) a Cox regression comparison of treatments stratified by age group, in children with neuroblastoma (part data from Pearson, Pinkerton, Lewis, *et al.*, 2008)

neuroblastoma (NB) as an illustration, then the main comparison of interest is the difference in effect of the randomized treatments: Standard and Rapid. When confined to children up to nine years of age, the command (**stcox treat**) gives in Figure 6.16(a) a $HR=0.7170$ in favour of Rapid.

However, Figure 6.16(b) suggests that when those of 12<18 months and 18 months–9 years are compared, the presence of non-proportional hazards is identified. In which case it might be important to examine the extent to which this lack of proportionality in the covariate age group affects the trial conclusions. Essentially such an analysis first compares the treatments given within each age group strata. It then combines these two to give an age group-adjusted hazard ratio. Such an analysis can be conducted using the command (**stcox treat, strata(AgeGroup)**) to give $HR_{Stratified}=0.6902$ of Figure 6.16(c). The corresponding p-value is now reduced from 0.046 to 0.027. Thus, in this illustration the stratified analysis suggests a greater difference between treatment groups and further suggests this is more statistically significant than initially concluded. However, the change in value of the estimate is $C=0.6902/0.7170=0.96$ or 4%, and may not be thought of as clinically important. In such circumstances the non-stratified estimate may be all that needs to be quoted in any report.

Further, in Chapter 10, *Time-varying covariates*, we introduce covariates which are termed time-varying or time-dependent and describe how they may be used in time-to-event regression models in situations where the hazards cannot be assumed to be proportional.

TECHNICAL DETAILS

Calculating a Kaplan-Meier survival curve

In what follows, we assume the event of concern is death.

(1) First order (rank) the survival times from smallest to largest. If a censored observation time and a time-to-death are equal, then the censored observation time is assumed to be a little after the death time in the ranking.

(2) Alongside the ranked times, record 1 if the time corresponds to a death and 0 if there is no associated death (to our knowledge the patient is still alive) and the time-to-event is therefore censored.

(3) Determine the number at risk, n_i, as the number of patients alive immediately before the death at time t_i.

(4) Calculate the probability of survival from t_{i-1} to t_i as $1 - d_i/n_i$.

(5) The cumulative survival probability, $S(t_i)$, is the probability of surviving from 0 up to t_i. It is calculated as

$$S(t_i) = (1 - d_i/n_i) \times (1 - d_{i-1}/n_{i-1}) \times \ldots \times (1 - d_1/n_1) \qquad (6.10)$$

This can be more briefly written as $S(t_i)=(1 - d_i/n_i) \times S(t_{i-1})$.
Note that we start at time zero with $t_0=0$ and $d_0=0$ and hence $S(0)=1 - d_0/n_0=1$.

(6) A censored observation at time t_i reduces the number at risk by one but does not change the cumulative survival probability at time t_i as $d_i=0$ and therefore $(1 - d_i/n_i)=1$.

(7) A plot of the cumulative survival probability $KM_i=S(t_i)$ against t_i, gives the K-M survival curve.

The calculations to obtain the K-M survival probability for the 23 patients with glioblastoma who have less extensive disease in the study of Sridhar, Gore, Boiangiu, *et al.* (2009) are shown in Figure 6.17. All those with survival times up to and including 1.552 years have died at the times indicated, and hence there are no censored observations among these. Up to this point the K-M estimate is therefore the simple proportion of the number remaining

Rank i	Ranked survival time (years) t_i	Total number at risk n_i	Number of deaths d_i	Probability of survival in interval t_{i-1} to t_i $1 - d_i/n_i$	KM$_i$ Cumulative survival probability $S(t)$
0	0	23	0	1	1
1	0.3641	23	1	0.9565	0.9565
2	0.3943	22	1	0.9545	0.9130
3	0.4736	21	1	0.9524	0.8696
4	0.5941	20	1	0.9500	0.8261
5	0.6297	19	1	0.9474	0.7826
6	0.9418	18	1	0.9444	0.7391
7	0.9610	17	1	0.9412	0.6957
8	1.109	16	1	0.9375	0.6522
9	1.136	15	1	0.9333	0.6087
10	1.268	14	1	0.9286	0.5652
11	1.415	13	1	0.9231	0.5217
12	1.429	12	1	0.9167	0.4783
13	1.462	11	1	0.9091	0.4348
14	1.465	10	1	0.9000	0.3913
15	1.503	9	1	0.8889	0.3478
16	**1.552**	**8**	**1**	**0.8750**	**0.3043**
17	1.774+	7	0	1	
18	1.823+	6	0	1	
19	1.906	5	1	0.8000	0.2435
20	1.936	4	1	0.7500	0.1826
21	2.867+	3	0	1	0.1826
22	2.897+	2	0	1	0.1826
23	3.422+	1	0	1	0.1826

+Indicates a censored survival time

Figure 6.17 Illustration of the calculations for the K-M survival curve for 23 patients with glioblastoma who have less extensive disease (data from Sridhar, Gore, Boiangiu et al., 2009)

alive (just) beyond this time-point, which is the simple proportion $(23-16)/23=7/23=0.3043$ indicated in bold type in Figure 6.17. Beyond that time the calculations must also take account of the censored observations, which are indicated by $+$.

The hazard function

The hazard function is the probability that an individual dies immediately after time t post diagnosis, conditional on having survived to that time. In formal terms this is defined by

$$\lambda(t) = \lim_{\delta t \to 0} \left[\frac{\text{Prob } (t \leq T < t + \delta t \mid T \geq t)}{\delta t} \right] \qquad (6.11)$$

Here Prob$(t \leq T < t + \delta t \mid T \geq t)$ is the probability that an individual's actual survival time, T, lies between t and a very short time after at $t + \delta t$, *provided* that they have already lived until t. This is termed a conditional probability. The hazard function $\lambda(t)$ is then the limiting value of this conditional probability divided by the small time interval δt, as the value of δt tends to zero, that is, gets smaller and smaller.

The complementary log-log transformation

As we have indicated, the PH assumption must hold for a valid interpretation of the regression coefficients obtained after fitting a Cox model. A graphical check on the proportionality is provided by a complementary log cumulative hazard plot.

If we represent the K-M estimate of survival of the baseline group by $S_0(t)$ then we are assuming this may change with time, t. We can then relate the survival of a comparison group, $S(t)$, to this by

$$S(t) = \left[S_0(t)\right]^{\exp(\beta x)} \tag{6.12}$$

If we then take the logarithm of both sides of the right-hand expression in (6.12), we obtain $\log[S(t)] = \exp(\beta x) \times \log[S_0(t)]$. The maximum value of $S(t)$ cannot exceed 1 (100% survival), and so $\log[S(t)]$ is negative as it cannot exceed $\log 1 = 0$ and this is also the case for $S_0(t)$. As a consequence it is necessary to negate both $\log[S(t)]$ and $\log[S_0(t)]$ before taking logarithms a second time to obtain

$$\log\left\{-\log[S(t)]\right\} = \log\left\{-\log[S_0(t)]\right\} + \beta x \tag{6.13}$$

The term $-\log[S(t)]$ in the above equation represents the cumulative hazard. As a consequence the complementary log-log plot, which is a plot of the left-hand side of equation (6.13), against $\log t$ will give separate curves depending on the number of distinct values of the covariate x. This is because the right-hand side of equation (6.13) has a part which varies with t, which is distinct from the part which varies with x. Any changes in the x term cause a step vertically up or down in the plot. The size of the step depends on the magnitude of the influence of the covariate on prognosis. In situations where the hazards are proportional, the shapes of the plots within each group of individuals with the same covariate value would follow the same general pattern as those with another covariate value apart from a possible constant (or zero) vertical shift.

Residuals

The situation with survival time studies is complicated by the censored observations and the fact that these observations have no 'event' associated with them.

Assuming a single covariate, x, the Schoenfeld residuals are calculated for the non-censored observations by

$$Sch_j = x_j - \frac{\sum x \exp(bx)}{\sum \exp(bx)}, \tag{6.14}$$

where j is the rank of each death time, t_j, among the n individuals in the study, and the summation, denoted Σ, is concerned with the subject whose rank is j and only those at risk at t_j beyond. As Marubini and Valsecchi (1995) point out, these residuals pertain only to time-points at which a death occurs. This contrasts with a residual for every individual, as is the case with the linear regression model of equation (1.5).

If we fit a Cox model with extent of disease (*Extent*) as the single covariate to the data from the 35 patients with glioblastoma using the command (**stcox Extent, nohr**), the corresponding output of Figure 6.18 gives the estimate of the regression coefficient β as $b = -1.9821$.

stcox Extent, nohr

No. of subjects = 35, No. of failures = 30, Time at risk = 38.4394

t	Coef	SE	z	P>|z|	[95% CI]
Extent	−1.9821	0.4674	−4.24	0.0001	−2.8982 to −1.0660

Rank	Patient	Extent	survy	status	exp(bx)	x*exp (bx)	Schoenfeld
1.	29	Very	0.0520	Dead	1	0	−0.2089
2.	32	Very	0.0575	Dead	1	0	−0.2236
3.	30	Very	0.1150	Dead	1	0	−0.2406
4.	31	Very	0.2272	Dead	1	0	−0.2604
5.	34	Very	0.2820	Dead	1	0	−0.2837
6.	35	Very	0.3149	Dead	1	0	−0.3116
7.	20	Less	0.3641	Dead	0.1378	0.1378	0.6544
8.	33	Very	0.3751	Dead	1	0	−0.3356
9.	7	Less	0.3943	Dead	0.1378	0.1378	0.6226
10.	27	Very	0.4298	Dead	1	0	−0.3666
11.	14	Less	0.4736	Dead	0.1378	0.1378	0.5803
12.	13	Less	0.5941	Dead	0.1378	0.1378	0.5921
13.	6	Less	0.6297	Dead	0.1378	0.1378	0.6044
14.	25	Very	0.6379	Dead	1	0	−0.3827
15.	26	Very	0.6790	Dead	1	0	−0.4526
16.	**24**	**Very**	**0.7967**	**Dead**	**1**	**0**	**−0.5536**
17.	**8**	**Less**	**0.9418**	**Dead**	0.1378	0.1378	0.2874
18.	1	Less	0.9610	Dead	0.1378	0.1378	0.2992
19.	21	Less	1.1088	Dead	0.1378	0.1378	0.3121
20.	3	Less	1.1362	Dead	0.1378	0.1378	0.3261
21.	28	Very	1.1499	Dead	1	0	−0.6586
22.	19	Less	1.2676	Dead	0.1378	0.1378	0
23.	10	Less	1.4155	Dead	0.1378	0.1378	0
24.	11	Less	1.4292	Dead	0.1378	0.1378	0
25.	15	Less	1.4620	Dead	0.1378	0.1378	0
26.	16	Less	1.4648	Dead	0.1378	0.1378	0
27.	12	Less	1.5031	Dead	0.1378	0.1378	0
28.	23	Less	1.5524	Dead	0.1378	0.1378	0
29.	22	Less	1.7741	Alive	0.1378	0.1378	.
30.	18	Less	1.8234	Alive	0.1378	0.1378	.
31.	4	Less	1.9055	Dead	0.1378	0.1378	0
32.	9	Less	1.9357	Dead	0.1378	0.1378	0
33.	5	Less	2.8665	Alive	0.1378	0.1378	.
34.	17	Less	2.8966	Alive	0.1378	0.1378	.
35.	2	Less	3.4223	Alive	0.1378	0.1378	.

Figure 6.18   The Schoenfeld residuals for patients with very and less extensive glioblastoma (data from Sridhar, Gore, Boiangiu, et al., 2009)

In order to calculate the Schoenfeld residuals, the survival time (survy) is ranked, and the survival status and extent group of each individual are required in the numerator and denominator components of equation (6.14). These are all given in the columns of Figure 6.18.

If we consider Patient 24, who has rank $j=16$, with very extensive disease (coded $x=0$) and who died at $t_{16}=0.7967$ years from diagnosis. As the covariate $x_{16}=0$, for this individual $x_{16} \times \exp(-1.9821 \times x_{16})=0 \times \exp(-1.9821 \times 0)=0 \times \exp(0)=0 \times 1=0$. In contrast Patient 8, who

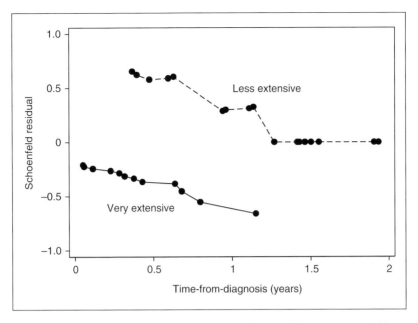

Figure 6.19   Plot of the Schoenfeld residuals for patients with very and less extensive glioblastoma (data from Sridhar, Gore, Boiangiu, *et al.*, 2009)

has rank $j=17$, with less extensive disease $(x_{17}=1)$ and who died at 0.9418, has $x_{17} \times \exp(-1.9821 \times x_{17})=1 \times \exp(-1.9821 \times 1)=1 \times 0.1378=0.1378$. To calculate the Schoenfeld residual for, for example, Patient 24, it is necessary to summate all values in the $\exp(bx)$ column for all ranks from $j=16$ to 35. Thus, $\Sigma\exp(bx)=1+(4 \times 0.1378)+1+(14 \times 0.1378)=2+(18 \times 0.1378)=4.4804$. Then it is necessary to calculate $\Sigma x^*\exp(bx)=0+(4 \times 0.1378)+0+(14 \times 0.1378)=18 \times 0.1378=2.4804$. Finally, $Sch_{16}=x_{16}-[\Sigma x^*\exp(bx)/\Sigma\exp(bx)]=0-[2.4804/4.4804] = -0.5536$.

It should be noted that Sch_j is negative for the very extensive disease patients who all have covariate $x=0$ and positive for the less extensive patients with $x=1$. However, once the last death occurs in one of the groups, here a death for Patient 28 with very extensive disease at $t_{21}=1.1499$ years, then either $Sch_j=0$ beyond this time or the residual is no longer defined for any patient who is alive. Thus, Patient 9 dies at $t_{32}=1.9357$ years with $Sch_{32}=0$, whereas Patient 5 is alive and therefore censored at $t_{33}=2.8665$ years with no defined Sch_{33}.

Judgment with respect to determining whether PH applies to these data is obtained by a scatter plot of Sch_j against t_j as in Figure 6.19. The plots for the extensive and less extensive disease groups appear approximately parallel justifying the PH assumption. However, if different or non-parallel patterns are displayed in the plot of the residuals against time, then this suggests that the PH assumption is violated.

The Schoenfeld (1982) residuals are only one of several alternative definitions of residuals in the time-to-event context. A fuller review is given by Marubini and Valsecchi (1995, pages 247–265), but their presentation is rather technical in nature.

7 Model Building

SUMMARY

This chapter describes some of the issues that need to be considered when building a parsimonious regression model. We stress that the purpose is to choose a modeling strategy that provides answers to the questions posed by the structure of the study design. In so doing it is important to identify the respective roles of the covariates concerned and to include them in, or omit them from, the final model in a constructive way. Statistical computer packages provide options that, following a basic set of chosen rules as determined by the analyst, select (usually) a subset of the possible covariates for the final model. Further, statistical packages may allow covariate selection procedures which can force certain pre-specified covariates to be mandatory components of the final model. Some of these options are described. We also caution against the indiscriminate use of automatic covariate selection procedures frequently involving numerous (unseen) multiple models being fitted within the program execution routines, and hence many tests of statistical significance of which the analyst may not be fully aware. We draw attention to difficulties in interpreting results following such procedures and suggest means by which some of these difficulties may be circumvented. An example of how a prognostic index is derived is also included.

INTRODUCTION

Purpose

We have given several examples of clinical studies in which the final analysis has been conducted using one form or another of a regression model. Some of these models have been very simple in structure such as that for comparing HDL levels in males and females shown in Figure 1.3. This model comprised a continuous explanatory variable, HDL and the single binary covariate, *Gender*. We also showed in Figure 3.3 that a parallel lines model, one for each gender, summarized the essential features of the influence of weight on HDL cholesterol values. In contrast, the multiple regression considered by Ng,

Regression Methods for Medical Research, First Edition. Bee Choo Tai and David Machin.
© 2014 Bee Choo Tai and David Machin. Published 2014 by John Wiley & Sons, Ltd.

Fukushima, Tai, *et al.* (2008) related log(ACR) in patients with type 2 diabetes to more than 20 potentially influencing covariates. We summarized in Figure 1.8 one of their reported models which included five of these covariates. In this model, the authors had made it clear that TNF-α score was the covariate of primary concern. In a similar way, Chong, Tay, Subramaniam, *et al.* (2009) of Figure 6.7 identified the diagnosis of absent, mild or definitive tardive dyskinesia (TD) as the primary covariate, although in this instance patient survival-time was the endpoint variable of concern. Thus, the primary purpose of the analysis is to identify a model that, once fitted, provides answers to the questions posed by the basic structure of the study design.

The dependent variable

Although the focus of this chapter is on the covariates, it must not be overlooked that the choice of dependent (y-variable) is crucial. In particular, it is important to retain the full information content of this variable. For example, if the continuous measurement values of ACR (g/kg) had been dichotomized by Ng, Fukushima, Tai, *et al.* (2008) into high and low values and logistic, rather than linear regression models used to assess the influence of the covariates then this would be wasteful of information and hence statistically inefficient. At worst, it could lead to misleading conclusions. In general, there is also a major concern as to how such a cut-point is determined. In most circumstances there are many options and one may imagine conclusions differing dependent on which is chosen. It would also be inefficient if Chong, Tay, Subramaniam, *et al.* (2009) were to ignore the individual survival times of the patients and merely record the proportion surviving at (say) 5-years post the census date at which the diagnosis of TD was determined. Perhaps, then using logistic regression rather than the more appropriate Cox regression to obtain a final model for their data. Equally for an ordered categorical variable, such as the 4-category foetal loss of the study conducted by Chinnaiya, Venkat, Chia, *et al.* (1998), it is better to preserve the categories of Figure 1.9 rather than choose one of the three possible cuts to create a binary endpoint.

We have also pointed out that when the endpoint variable is continuous then it is usually best to use it unchanged to develop the model, as this facilitates the final interpretation of the study results.

Despite these cautionary remarks, there will be occasions when, before analysis, converting a continuous to a binary endpoint or taking the logarithm of the endpoint will be entirely justified but the rationale for such decisions should be provided. For example, although the endpoint variable ACR itself might have led to an easier model to interpret, Ng, Fukushima, Tai, *et al.* (2008) noted that this had a skewed distribution and so, in order to normalize the data, chose to use log(ACR) as their endpoint for analysis instead.

TYPES OF COVARIATES

The covariates

Just as for the endpoint measures, care should be taken with the form that the covariates take before they are included into the model building process. Thus, if they take a continuous or ordered categorical form, then they should first be considered to have that same form in the prospective model. However, we have given an example in Figure 4.9 where the relationship of a covariate (age of the subject) to the endpoint of concern (presence or absence of IHD) may be non-linear, and, hence, if considered in the original continuous form, the corresponding model will be complex. In certain situations, this complexity may be avoided if, for example, some categories are merged, an ordered categorical covariate is regarded as unordered, or a continuous covariate is categorized. It is much better if there is 'external' evidence for such choices rather than them having been made on the basis of 'internal' examinations of the study data itself.

The situation for the covariates is additionally complicated by the possibility of adding a quadratic term (Figure 4.8) and/or an interaction with another covariate such as that between *HRV* and *Aero* (Figure 4.12) in the study by Jackson, Gangnon, Evans, *et al.* (2008) concerned with the possible development of childhood asthma following earlier wheezing rhinovirus illnesses. When there are several covariates to consider, and when linear assumptions do not appear to be supported, the potential complication of several interaction terms and/or trans-formations of the covariates needs to be contemplated.

Covariate role

The above considerations make it imperative to reflect carefully on which covariates to include (and in what form) in advance of commencing the model fitting. In this process, the main focus should be on the question(s) raised by the research design. Such a design should be developed taking note of pertinent research work done by others. This is very likely to help refine the research question, give clues as to the best endpoint to consider, and also provide some indication as to the role or otherwise of covariates.

In principle, a multivariable model of whatever kind can contain several covariates which can be broadly categorized into essentially three types: design (*D*); knowingly influential (*K*); and unknown, exploratory or query of uncertain influence (*Q*). A model for a particular situation can involve any of these types either singly or in any combination.

We can express the presence of the three types of explanatory variables in one model in an obvious format by:

$$y = \beta_0 + \beta_D D + \beta_k K + \beta_Q Q \tag{7.1}$$

Design covariates

Most studies are designed with a specific objective to estimate the effect of one or more key explanatory variables on the endpoint of concern. For example, in clinical trials, such a covariate is the intervention that is randomly allocated to patients. We call this a *D*-variable as it clearly plays a key role in the research design. In this case, one model, perhaps the only one of concern, must contain this covariate and so takes the form $y = \beta_0 + \beta_D D$. In the sim-plest of all situations $\beta_D = 0$, and so the intervention has no effect. In which case the 'null' model $y = \beta_0$ would describe the trial results, although in these circumstances it is usual to quote b_D (the estimate of β_D) with the *CI* (even though it will contain the null hypothesis value of 0) and the associated *p*-value.

In other situations the roles of the respective covariates may be less clear. Thus, in *Example 1.1* in which Busse, Lemanske Jr and Gern (2010) investigate how FEV_1

changes in relation to the recorded levels of interferon-λ (*Inter*, *I*), there are two groups of subjects (*Sub*, *Su*) concerned: asthma patients and healthy individuals. Clearly if there is no relationship between changes from baseline FEV$_1$ and interferon-λ, there is little point in comparing the subject groups. So the first model to examine would be of the main effect, *I*, alone, and if the associated regression coefficient is found to be statistically significant, the model *I + Su* is then considered. One then regards both *Inter* and *Sub* as *D*-covariates, although the first takes precedence over the second in the model building process.

Knowingly influential covariates

K variables are those known, or assumed to be, of major influence on the values taken by the endpoint variable, *y*, either from the researchers' own experience or from the published literature.

In the study reported by Sridhar, Gore, Boiangiu, *et al.* (2009), 35 patients with glioblastoma received temozolomide and radiation to treat their disease. The Kaplan-Meier estimate of their 1-year survival rate was 49%. However, it is well known that the prognosis for an individual with glioblastoma depends critically on the extent of disease at diagnosis. Thus, the covariate *Extent* (Very extensive or Less extensive) is a strong determinant of outcome with 1-year survivals of 8 and 70%, respectively, as shown in Figure 6.6. Thus, in any regression model that is constructed involving these patients, *Extent* (*E*) should be regarded as a *K*-covariate and therefore be a component of the final model. However, with so few subjects in this study, it is unlikely that the model would be extended further. In a sense, there is no *D*-covariate present as the objective is only to describe the outcome of a group of patients all receiving the same treatment.

Query covariates

Finally, the *Q*-covariates are those for which we do not know the magnitude of their influence on the endpoint and the objective of the study is to determine the extent, if any, of their influence. In certain situations, there may only be *Q*-covariates for the potential model and some automatic selection procedure may be invoked to help ascertain whether any of these are influential and, if there is more than one, assess their relative contribution in explaining the observed variation in the endpoint measure of concern. Thus, Jackson, Gangnon, Evans, *et al.* (2008, Table 2) include 13 covariates, involving estimates of 24 parameters, to establish risk factors for asthma at age 6 years (see Figure 4.1). After using a stepwise model selection procedure with backward elimination and Akaike's information criteria of equation (3.11), the final model included four variables: *Dog* in the household at birth (*p*-value=0.08); *Food* sensitization (1 year) (*p*-value=0.04); Other *Siblings* (*p*-value=0.03); and *Aeroallergen* sensitization (1 year) (*p*-value=0.02).

Transformations

Endpoint variable

When the endpoint is a continuous variable, it is quite useful to investigate the shape of the resulting distribution of all the cases in the study. Thus, for example, when examining the distribution of ACR in a sample from the study of Ng, Fukushima, Tai, *et al.* (2008) in this

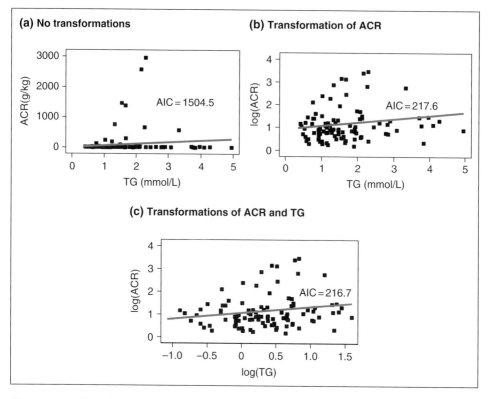

Figure 7.1 Effect of transforming the endpoint variable ACR (g/kg) and/or an associated covariate triacylglycerol (TG) (mmol/L) with the corresponding fitted linear regression lines indicated (part data from Ng, Fukushima, Tai, et al., 2008)

way, it is apparent that this has a very skew distribution. As is indicated in Figure 7.1(a), for the 100 subjects of the sample, the median was low at 8.4 g/kg, with a minimum of 1.5 but a high maximum of almost 3,000. Only eight patients have ACR > 250. Experience suggests that in this circumstance it may be better for modeling purposes to transform the scale and the logarithm is usually chosen. On this transformed scale the minimum, median and maximum of log(ACR) are 0.18, 0.93, and 3.47, and the distribution, indicated in Figure 7.1(b), is much less extreme in the upper tail.

Equally important to the above considerations, if other investigators have used log(ACR) in their reporting then (right or wrong; optimal or suboptimal) this provides a very cogent reason for modeling in the same way. However, if the current investigating team feel such a transformation is likely to be seriously misleading, they should say so, and explain why, in the subsequent publication of their own findings.

Of course, if the endpoint is binary we know that the logit transformation is necessary and this is applied by the statistical packages before the regression modeling begins. This too is the case for an ordered categorical variable such as the foetal loss following blood sampling as studied by Chinnaiya, Venkat, Chia, et al. (1998), which is then modeled using ordered logistic regression. However, in this latter case it is important to check if there are empty categories, which can be of particular concern if they are in a central position on the scale. Such gaps may cause difficulties at the analysis stage and it may be advisable to merge adjacent categories should they occur.

Covariates

Just as for an endpoint variable, if a covariate is continuous in form then it should be examined in a similar way to see if the modeling process is thereby improved. One can see from Figure 7.1(a) and (b) that triacylglyceride (TG) has a distribution with a long tail in the relatively few high values with a minimum, median, and maximum of 0.41, 1.40 and 4.95 mmol/L, respectively. After a logarithmic transformation, the distribution of log(TG) in Figure 7.1(c) is more symmetric in nature with a median of 0.33 and ranging from −0.89 to 1.60.

If a model is fitted to these data using the command (**regress logACR TG**) rather than (**regress ACR TG**), then the Akaike criterion, obtained by adding (**estat ic**) following each command, is reduced very substantially from 1504.5 to 217.6 and thereby very strongly supports the use of log(ACR) in the modeling. However, using the logarithmic transformation of the TG covariate via the command (**regress logACR logTG**) further reduces the Akaike criterion, but very marginally, from 217.6 to 216.7. On this basis, the linear model is best constructed on the log(ACR) scale but it is problematical as to whether the transformation of TG is necessary. Nevertheless, if such a transformation is standard practice then one should use it.

Derived covariates

In some situations there may be two, or possibly more, covariates that might be combined in a meaningful way before they are entered into the regression analysis. For example, Ng, Fukushima, Tai, *et al.* (2008) record the height (m) and weight (kg) of the individuals in their study from which they calculate the body mass index, BMI = weight/(height²). They also record the circumferences of both the waist (cm) and hip (cm), which they combine into the single covariate of the waist hip ratio, WHR = waist/hip. In either case, decisions on whether to use the BMI and WHR or their component covariates in the modeling process are probably best decided on the basis of published earlier work. If these are in common use in the research area then, even if the 'internal' evidence from the current study is not strong, it is probably advisable to use them. A clear advantage of using the derived variables, as Ng, Fukushima, Tai, *et al.* (2008) did, is that in each case one less parameter has to be estimated in the modeling process. In a different research area, Levitan, Yang, Wolk, *et al.* (2009) have suggested that both BMI and waist circumference (WC) are important predictors of hospitalization for heart failure among men but only WC for women.

CASE STUDY

One aspect of the Singapore Cardiovascular Cohort Study 2, which we have used extensively for illustration in earlier sections, investigated a variety of potential risk factors for IHD including the binary covariates gender (***G***), current smoking – yes/no (***S***) and drinking alcohol – yes/no (***D***), which are termed the 'main' effects. For these three variables of interest, the 8 possible logistic models are summarized in Figure 7.2. We use the shorthand

Model	Notation	Components of the model for logit (p)
Null		
–	(1)	β_0
One-variable		
Gender	**G**	$\beta_G x_G$
Smoke	**S**	$\beta_S x_S$
Drink	**D**	$\beta_D x_D$
Two-variable		
Gender and Smoke	**G+S**	$\beta_G x_G + \beta_S x_S$
Smoke and Drink	**S+D**	$\beta_S x_S + \beta_D x_D$
Drink and Gender	**D+G**	$\beta_D x_D + \beta_G x_G$
Three-variable		
Gender, Smoke and Drink	**G+S+D**	$\beta_G x_G + \beta_S x_S + \beta_D x_D$

Figure 7.2   All possible main effects logistic regression models for three binary covariates (gender, smoke and drink) for IHD (part data from the Singapore Cardiovascular Cohort Study 2)

description of these eight models among which (**1**) refers to the null or 'empty' model. Thus, model **G** includes gender, but no other variables, **G+S** gender and smoking, **D+G** drinking and gender, and **G+S+D** includes all three variables. In this context, the order we place **G**, **S** or **D** in any model with this notation is not important. The parameters, the different βs, within each model of Figure 7.2 are the regression coefficients to be estimated and the x's are the potential risk factors each taking values of 0 or 1.

To illustrate the model building process, the null model and the seven main effects logistic models have each been fitted to a sample of 300 subjects from the studies. These are summarized in Figure 7.3, where it should be noted that each model will also have an associated estimate for β_0 but to simplify the presentation only that for the null model is included.

A comparison between nested models is made by comparing the respective likelihoods. Two models are nested if all the covariates in the model with the fewer terms are included in the model containing more covariates. Thus, for example, model **G** is nested within model **G+S+D**, but it is not nested within model **S+D**.

Thus, to compare the fit of model **G** with that of the null model (**1**) of Figure 7.3, the likelihood ratio (LR) of $LR_{G,(1)} = 2[L_G - L_{(1)}]$ is calculated. Using the corresponding values from Figure 7.3 gives $LR_{G,(1)} = 2[-168.1400 - (-170.8624)] = 2 \times 2.7224 = 5.4448$ as shown in Figure 7.4 (column 2). As the models are nested, the corresponding number of *df* is the difference in the number of parameters in the two models. Model **G** has $v_G = 2$ parameters, β_0 and β_{Gender}, whereas the null model, (**1**), has $v_{(1)} = 1$ as only β_0 is estimated. Hence, $LR_{G,(1)}$ has $df = v_G - v_{(1)} = 2 - 1 = 1$. Under the null hypothesis that fitting the model **G** does not explain significantly more of the variation in the data than the null model, $LR_{G,(1)}$ has a χ^2 distribution with $df = 1$. The corresponding p-value can then be obtained from Table T5. The entry in Table T5 that is closest to that of $LR_{G,(1)} = 5.44$ is $\chi^2 = 5.41$. This is found in the row for $df = 1$ and the column with $\alpha = 0.02$. Thus, the p-value obtained is approximately 0.02.

The LR statistics for the differences between all possible main effects models and the null model, together with comparisons between nested models (obtained from the difference of their respective LRs when compared with the null model) are summarized in Figure 7.4. For example, the comparison of the model **D+G** with the nested model **D** gives $LR = 7.48 - 0.47 = 7.01$ while comparing it with the null model (**1**) the $LR = 7.48$.

Model	b	SE(b)	OR	p-value	L = logℓ
Null or Empty					
(1)	$b_0 = -1.0634$	0.1322	–	–	-170.8624
One-variable					
G	-0.6465	0.2831	0.52	0.022	-168.1400
S	-0.1015	0.3365	0.90	0.763	-170.8174
D	-0.2104	0.3083	0.81	0.495	-170.6250
Two-variable					
G+S					-168.1007
Gender	-0.6459	0.2831	0.52	0.023	
Smoke	-0.0957	0.3396	0.91	0.778	
S+D					-170.5818
Smoke	-0.0995	0.3368	0.91	0.768	
Drink	-0.2097	0.3084	0.81	0.497	
D+G					-167.1232
Drink	-0.4525	0.3229	0.64	0.161	
Gender	-0.7637	0.2950	0.47	0.010	
Three-variable					
G+S+D					-167.0881
Gender	-0.7630	0.2950	0.47	0.010	
Smoke	-0.0906	0.3409	0.91	0.790	
Drink	-0.4516	0.3230	0.64	0.162	

Figure 7.3 Logistic regression models, for IHD using the three binary covariates: gender (G), smoking (S) and drinking alcohol (D) fitted to data from 300 subjects (part data from the Singapore Cardiovascular Cohort Study 2)

	Contrasting with the null model (1)			LR for comparing nested models			
				Two-variables			Three-variables
Model	LR	df	p-value	G+S	S+D	D+G	G+S+D
(1)	–		–	–	–	–	–
G	5.44	1	0.0196	0.08	–	2.04	2.11
S	0.09	1	0.7640	5.43	0.47	–	7.46
D	0.47	1	0.4908	–	0.09	7.01	7.08
G+S	5.52	2	0.0632	–	–	–	2.03
S+D	0.56	2	0.7553	–	–	–	6.99
D+G	7.48	2	0.0238	–	–	–	0.07
G+S+D	7.55	3	0.0563	–	–	–	–

Figure 7.4 Likelihood ratio (LR) statistics and degrees of freedom (df) for main effects logistic models for IHD including gender, smoking and drinking alcohol (part data from the Singapore Cardiovascular Cohort Study 2)

SELECTION PROCEDURES

At the design stage of a clinical investigation there may appear to be several covariates that might contribute to explaining the variability in the values of the endpoint of concern. In such situations it is tempting for investigators to record a relatively large number of covariates, which they will then need to deal with at the analysis stage. We stress that considerable thought should be focused on whether or not a particular covariate should be studied.

However, for the majority of purposes of this section, we assume that the investigators have several Q-covariates to consider and wish to identify which, if any of these, has an important influence on the endpoint concerned. In these circumstances most computer packages provide covariate selection procedures to assist the analyst with their choice.

In broad terms, the methods of deciding on which of (usually) several covariates should be included in the final model describing the results of the study, can be categorized as: user controlled, semi-automatic or automatic, although the possibility of using all approaches in developing one model is not excluded. Also, within each of the three general approaches there are options available and therefore choices to make. Some options, together with details of how they are activated, are summarized in Figure 7.5.

Selection Type	Selection criteria for the available covariates
User controlled	
1. Forced	No selection – chosen covariate(s) always in the final model.
2. Lock	Enables the first covariate in the model to be retained and not subjected to any selection criteria. This would usually be a *D*-covariate.
3. Changes in estimates	*C* or 1/*C* – suggested *C*=1.1 (10%). A possible criterion that indicates that any covariate influencing a *D*-covariate to this extent or more should be retained in the final model (Rothman, 2002).
4. Retaining	If a covariate requires indicator variables, then these can be included (or not) together. Similarly if two or more covariates have to be assessed simultaneously then these can be only included (or not) together.
Semi-automatic	
5. Hierarchical	*p*-value after examination of each sequence of tested covariates.
Forward selection	Rank the order of the covariates with the primary for consideration in the model ranked first. Stipulate probability of entry, pe. Fit "empty" model. While the last covariate added remains "significant", add the next and re-estimate.
Backward selection	Stipulate probability of removal, pr. Rank the order of the covariates with the least important for consideration in the model ranked last. Fit full model on all covariates. While the last covariate added is " not significant", remove it and re-estimate.
Automatic	
6. Consider all possible models	Choose the final model as that with the smallest *p*-value.
7. Selection	
Forward	Stipulate pe. Fit "empty" model. While the most-significant excluded covariate is "significant", add it and re-estimate.
Backward	Stipulate pr. Fit the full model on all covariates. While the least-significant covariate is "not significant", remove it and re-estimate.

Figure 7.5 Some model building options for identifying influential covariates for the final model with associated computer search logic utilized as appropriate (partially based on StataCorp, 2007c, Reference Q-Z, p. 343)

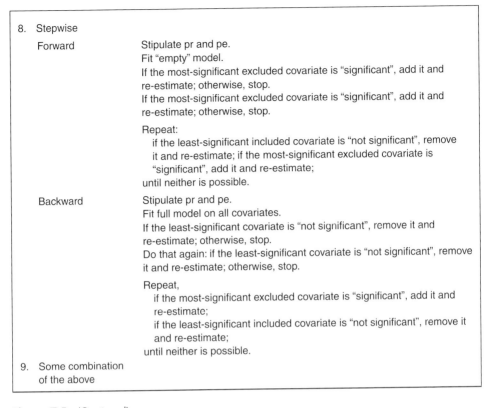

8. Stepwise

    Forward
    Stipulate pr and pe.
    Fit "empty" model.
    If the most-significant excluded covariate is "significant", add it and re-estimate; otherwise, stop.
    If the most-significant excluded covariate is "significant", add it and re-estimate; otherwise, stop.

    Repeat:
    if the least-significant included covariate is "not significant", remove it and re-estimate; if the most-significant excluded covariate is "significant", add it and re-estimate;
    until neither is possible.

    Backward
    Stipulate pr and pe.
    Fit full model on all covariates.
    If the least-significant covariate is "not significant", remove it and re-estimate; otherwise, stop.
    Do that again: if the least-significant covariate is "not significant", remove it and re-estimate; otherwise, stop.

    Repeat,
    if the most-significant excluded covariate is "significant", add it and re-estimate;
    if the least-significant included covariate is "not significant", remove it and re-estimate;
    until neither is possible.

9. Some combination of the above

Figure 7.5   (Continued)

Forced

By 'forced' one means that a particular covariate must be present in the final model. One example would be the variable *TarDy* describing the diagnosis of tardive dyskinesia in patients with schizophrenia in the study of Chong, Tay, Subramaniam, *et al.* (2009). Whereas in the context of the models summarized in Figure 7.3, one may envisage that the investigating team may learn from external sources that *Gender* is known to be an important risk factor for IHD and so insist that only models *G*, *G+S*, *G+D*, and *G+S+D* should be considered. With this constraint they may then choose one of the other selection options in Figure 7.5 to decide which of these four models should be the final one. In this case, the corresponding forward selection command (**stepwise, pe(0.05) lockterm1 : logit IHD Gender Smoke Drink**) of Figure 7.6(a) will select a model. However, (**lockterm1:**) ensures *Gender* is always in the model whereas other covariates remain only if they are statistically significant at the 5% level. The latter is the requirement set by the (**pe(0.05)**) term in the command. In this case, neither *Drink* nor *Smoke* are added to *Gender*, as the corresponding *p*-values are greater than 0.05, so the (single-covariate) model chosen is *G*. In contrast, if *Smoke* is locked into the model as in Figure 7.6(b), then *Gender*, but not *Drink*, is added so model *S+G* is chosen. Similarly, if *Drink* is locked into the model, then *Gender*, but not *Smoke*, is included and so the model *D+G* is chosen as in Figure 7.6(c). The term (stepwise) in the preceding commands is a generic instruction that features in many of the examples of this section.

Forward selection with the first term locked into the model

(a) *Selection chooses G*

stepwise, pe(0.05) lockterm1 : logit IHD Gender Smoke Drink

Begin with term 1 model

p >= 0.05 for Drink and Smoke

LR chi2(1) = 5.44, Prob > chi2 = 0.020

IHD	Coef	SE	z	P>|z|	[95% CI]
cons	−0.8232	0.1632			
Gender	−0.6465	0.2831	−2.28	0.022	−1.2013 to −0.0917

(b) *Selection chooses S + G*

stepwise, pe(0.05) lockterm1: logit IHD Smoke Drink Gender

Begin with term 1 model

p = 0.0225 < 0.05 adding Gender

LR chi2(2) = 5.52, Prob > chi2 = 0.063

IHD	Coef	SE	z	P>|z|	[95% CI]
cons	−0.7456	0.3193			
Smoke	−0.0957	0.3396	−0.28	0.78	−0.7613 to 0.5700
Gender	−0.6459	0.2831	−2.28	0.023	−1.2008 to −0.0910

(c) *Selection chooses D + G*

stepwise, pe(0.05) lockterm1: logit IHD Drink Gender Smoke

Begin with term 1 model

p = 0.0096 < 0.05 adding Gender

LR chi2(2) = 7.48, Prob > chi2 = 0.024

IHD	Coef	SE	z	P>|z|	[95% CI]
cons	−0.6641	0.1956			
Drink	−0.4525	0.3229	−1.40	0.16	−1.0853 to 0.1804
Gender	−0.7637	0.2950	−2.59	0.010	−1.3419 to −0.1855

Figure 7.6 Alternative logistic models for IHD using forward selection but depending on which of gender, drinking or smoking is first forced into the model (part data from the Singapore Cardiovascular Cohort Study 2)

Change in estimates

One way of determining whether a covariate (*New*) is important or not when added to an existing model is to examine the resulting changes to the regression coefficients for the covariates of the initial model (say Model 1) when compared with the model with the new covariate added (Model 2). If the change is large, then one may conclude that *New* is influential and should therefore be retained in the model. Thus, one is not examining the statistical significance of *New* itself but rather assessing the strength of its influence on (say) the estimated regression coefficient of the design covariate. Thus, in Figure 7.3, if we presume *Drink* is the design variable and *Gender* a *K*-covariate, the models to compare are D and $D+G$. This presumes that the main objective of the study is to determine the influence of alcohol consumption (*Drink*) on IHD. The first model established $b_{Drink1} = -0.2014$, the second $b_{Drink2} = -0.4525$. The relative change from one to the other is calculated as $C = b_{Drink2}/b_{Drink1} = -0.4525/-0.2014 = 2.25$ and this is a substantial change! This suggests that the model $D + G$ is necessary to provide the answer to the alcohol consumption question posed. The quantity C reflects the researchers' judgment of what constitutes the level of influence, termed confounding, that must therefore be adjusted for. The choice of either C or $1/C = 1.1$ is suggested (see Figure 7.5) as a practical guide as to whether or not *New* needs to be added to the model. Thus, if the main concern of the study had been smoking (*Smoke*), then we would compare models S and $S + G$ in which case $C = b_{Smoke2}/b_{Smoke1} = -0.0957/-0.1015 = 0.94$. On the above criterion for C, this is not regarded as a big change and so the chosen model to report is S.

Hierarchical selection

When we have defined a main effects model such as $G+S+D$, we have stated that this is the same model as, for example $S+D+G$, and equally for any other order of the three components. However, knowledge of what design type a component covariate is, may provide a natural ordering of their relative importance. So let us presume *Drink* is the *D*-covariate, *Gender* a *K*-covariate, and *Smoke* is a *Q*-covariate. In this case it would be natural to write the corresponding model to consider in the order $D+G+S$. If the order is regarded as important, then the model is termed hierarchical.

Hierarchical backward

The backward hierarchical approach proceeds by first fitting the full model $D+G+S$, then checks whether or not the last term, here S, can be removed from the model without significant loss. If removal incurs statistically 'significant loss', then the *final* model chosen is the first model examined, $D+G+S$. However, if there is no 'significant loss' the reduced model $D+G$ is then checked to see if G has or has not to be retained in the model. If G is retained, then no test of the component D alone will be made. On the other hand, should G be removed, then a test of whether or not D should be retained in the model would be made. In this way, but only if appropriate, the removal process can continue until only the null model is retained.

   To implement the procedure, the analyst has to specify the value of the *significance* level (pr) to be used for the test of the null hypothesis that the regression parameter associated with the covariate for the first step (*Smoke* in our example) equals zero and should therefore be *removed* from the model. If the calculated *p*-value is greater than (pr), then that covariate will be removed from the model. In the event, as Figure 7.7(a) shows, for *Smoke* the *p*-value$=0.79$, which is greater than the 0.1 set by the analyst, so S is removed from the model. In contrast, when *Gender* is subsequently tested, the *p*-value$=0.0096$, which is less than 0.1 and therefore this covariate is retained. Because of the hierarchical nature of the model, the selection process then stops with the final model chosen as $D+G$.

(a) *Hierarchical backward – hierarchy: Drink, Gender, Smoke*

stepwise, pr(0.1) hierarchical: logit IHD Drink Gender Smoke

Begin with full model

p = 0.79 >= 0.1 removing Smoke

p = 0.0096 < 0.1 keeping Gender

LR chi2(2) = 7.48, Prob > chi2 = 0.024

IHD	Coef	SE	z	p-value	[95% CI]
cons	−0.6641	0.1956			
Drink	−0.4525	0.3229	−1.40	0.16	−1.0853 to 0.1804
Gender	−0.7637	0.2950	−2.59	0.010	−1.3419 to −0.1855

(b) *Hierarchical forward – hierarchy: Drink, Gender, Smoke*

stepwise, pe(0.05) hierarchical: logit IHD Drink Gender Smoke

Begin with empty model

p = 0.49 >= 0.05 testing Drink

p >= 0.05 for all terms in model

LR chi2(0) = 0.00, Prob > chi2 = 1

IHD	Coef	SE	z	p-value	[95% CI]
cons	−1.0634	0.1322	−8.04	0.0001	−1.3224 to −0.8043

(c) *Hierarchical forward – hierarchy: Gender, Drink, Smoke*

stepwise, pe(0.05) hierarchical: logit IHD Gender Drink Smoke

Begin with empty model

p = 0.022 < 0.05 adding Gender

p = 0.16 >= 0.05 testing Drink

LR chi2(1) = 5.44, Prob > chi2 = 0.0196

IHD	Coef	SE	z	p-value	[95% CI]
cons	−0.8232	0.1632			
Gender	−0.6465	0.2831	−2.28	0.022	−1.2013 to −0.0917

Figure 7.7 Hierarchical selection methods for logistic models for IHD potentially including gender, smoking and drinking alcohol (part data from the Singapore Cardiovascular Cohort Study 2)

Hierarchical forward

In contrast to the backward hierarchical approach, forward hierarchical selection starts with the null or empty model and attempts to build on this. Consequently, the probability of entry (pe) to the model has to be specified. In Figure 7.7(b) this is set as 0.05 and the first covariate to be examined is *Drink*. The corresponding *p*-value=0.49, which is much greater than 0.05 and so *D* is not included in the model. However, because of the hierarchical structure no other covariates will then be considered. Hence, the chosen model is the empty model (**1**).

In contrast, forward selection of the hierarchical model *G*+*D*+*S* in Figure 7.7(c) first allows *G* into the model as the *p*-value=0.022. It then tests if the covariate *Drink* should be added. The *p*-value=0.16, which is greater than 0.05, and so *D*, and consequentially *S*, are not added. In general, the final model chosen will depend on the analyst's choice of hierarchy for the covariates concerned and also on the values set for (pe) and (pr).

Grouping terms

In some circumstances the analyst may require particular covariates (say two) to either both be in the final model or both out. In which case the covariates are grouped together as in the following command: (**logit IHD (Smoke Drink) Gender**). Here the covariates *Smoke* and *Drink* are either both to be in the final model or both out. Such circumstances may arise if the primary purpose of the study is to quantify the magnitude of the influence of both smoking and alcohol consumption, and to check if these are modified in any way by other covariates; only *Gender* in this example. When the forward hierarchical selection of Figure 7.8(a) is made,

---

(a) *Hierarchical Forward – linked covariates: (Drink, Smoke)*

stepwise, pe(0.05) hierarchical: logit IHD (Drink Smoke) Gender

Begin with empty model

p = 0.76 >= 0.05 testing Smoke Drink
p >= 0.05 for all terms in model

LR chi2(0) = 0.00, Prob > chi2 = 1

IHD	Coef	SE
cons	−1.0634	0.1322

(b) *Hierarchical Backward – linked covariates: (Drink, Smoke)*

stepwise, pr (0.1) hierarchical: logit IHD (Drink Smoke) Gender

Begin with full model

p = 0.0097 < 0.1 keeping Gender

LR chi2 (3) = 7.55, Prob > chi2 = 0.056

IHD	Coef	SE	z	p-value	[95% CI]	
cons	−0.5909	0.3371				
Drink	−0.4516	0.3230	−1.40	0.16	−1.0846 to	0.1814
Smoke	−0.0906	0.3409	−0.27	0.79	−0.7587 to	0.5775
Gender	−0.7630	0.2950	−2.59	0.010	−1.3413 to	−0.1847

Figure 7.8 Logistic models for IHD with linked covariates smoking and drinking as either both in or both out of the final model using (a) hierarchical forward, and (b) hierarchical backward selection (part data from the Singapore Cardiovascular Cohort Study 2)

the output excludes both *Smoke* and *Drink*, and thereby also excludes *Gender*. In contrast Figure 7.8(b) uses a backward hierarchical approach and now keeps them both in the chosen model as well as also adding *Gender*, In this latter case, the overall test with $df=3$ has a p-value$=0.056$, which is less than 0.1.

The grouping terms option, here in the form (`Smoke Drink`), is useful if one of the potential covariates to be included in a model is a categorical variable of more than two groups. Thus, the command of (`regress v1 v2`) of Figure 2.5(b) would be better formatted as (`regress (v1 v2)`). This would ensure that both of the two dummy variables created to describe the three ethnic groups, Chinese, Malay, and Indian, would always be retained (or removed) were they to be part of a selective regression analysis possibly including other covariates.

All possible combinations

By its very name this implies that every one of the seven different models associated with the covariates concerned first need to be fitted to the data. The *LR* statistic is then calculated against the empty model for each of these, and the associated p-values determined. For all the models of Figure 7.4 (column 2), the LR statistics when contrasting each model with the null model range from 0.09 to 7.55. Among these, the three that have a $LR<3.84$ have a p-value>0.05. This is because in order for the LR with $df=1$ to be statistically significant at the significance level of $\alpha=0.05$, its value must be greater than 3.84. Any LR with $df=2$ or more will require an value even larger than 3.84 to be significant. This can be seen from Table T5 where, for example, to be significant with $df=2$ and $\alpha=0.05$, the value of χ^2 must exceed 5.99, and for $df=3$ it must exceed 7.81 and so on. Consequently, all we have to examine are the *LR*s with the following values 5.44 ($df=1$) and 7.48 (2). As given in Figure 7.4 (column 4), these have respective p-values of 0.0196 and 0.0238 of which that for model *G* is the smallest and so this is selected as the final model.

Selection and stepwise

The precise details of how the selection and stepwise methods (both Forward and Backward) are implemented are described in Figure 7.5 and the corresponding associated commands are listed in Figure 7.9. Essentially, forward selection specifies (`pe`) and begins with the empty model and backward selection specifies (`pr`) and begins with the full 3-covariate model. In contrast, stepwise specifies both (`pe`) and (`pr`) whether implemented by the forward or backward option. However, for our example, each of these four options identifies the same final model as *G*, although the details of this model are not reproduced in Figure 7.9.

Choosing the best approach

In choosing the selection method it is important to first identify the respective design roles of the covariates concerned and eventually to include them in, or omit them from, the final model in a constructive way. As we have shown in, for example, Figure 7.7, quite different models (with the same data) can arise depending on the 'design' specification, which is set *before* the study data are collected.

In general terms, there is no single 'best' option for selecting which of several covariates should be included in the final model unless there is strong *prior* knowledge with respect to how some of these are likely to influence the outcome of concern.

The choice is even more uncertain in situations where the research purpose is to 'explore' or 'identify' associations. As we have already indicated, the different options can result in

---

(a) *Forward selection*

stepwise, pe(0.05) : logit IHD Drink Gender Smoke

Begin with empty model

p = 0.022 < 0.05 adding Gender

Chooses **G**

(b) *Backward selection*

stepwise, pr(0.1): logit IHD Drink Gender Smoke

LR test begin with full model

p = 0.79 >= 0.1 removing Smoke
p = 0.16 >= 0.1 removing Drink

Chooses **G**

(c) *Forward stepwise*

stepwise, pr(0.1) pe(0.05) forward: logit IHD Drink Gender Smoke

Begin with empty model

p = 0.022 < 0.05 adding Gender

Chooses **G**

(d) *Backward stepwise*

stepwise, pr (0.1) pe(0.05): logit IHD Drink Gender Smoke

Begin with full model

p = 0.79 >= 0.1 removing Smoke
p = 0.16 >= 0.1 removing Drink

Chooses **G**

Figure 7.9 Selection and stepwise methods from models for IHD including gender, smoking and drinking alcohol (part data from the Singapore Cardiovascular Cohort Study 2)

quite different final models so the analyst needs to be aware of this possibility when choosing the selection method. One option is to choose several approaches, and, should each of these indicate the same 'final' model, this will provide some reassurance that the conclusions drawn from the study may be robust. On the other hand, if the different approaches select different covariates, then the investigators should report this and perhaps conclude that no reliable indication as to their relative importance can be drawn from the current study.

DERIVING A PROGNOSTIC INDEX

Once the format of the endpoint variable and those of the covariates are chosen, the selection process is used to derive the final model. This model will form the basis from which the conclusions of the study are drawn. However, in many instances the regression model fitted to data arising from a clinical study will be used to predict the outcome for future subjects

		FFR75			Poor prognosis FFR75=1 (%)
		< 75%	≥ 75%		
Covariate		1	0	Total	
PB	0	1	38	39	2.5
	1	32	14	46	69.6
MLA	0	32	18	50	64.0
	1	1	34	35	2.9
LL	0	5	30	35	14.3
	1	28	22	50	56.0

Figure 7.10 Association between fractional flow reserve (FFR) and potential prognostic factors for outcome (part data from Lee, Tai, Soon, et al., 2010)

with particular values of the covariates that are included in the model. For example, Tan, Law, Ng and Machin (2003) found that Zubrod score, presence or absence of ascites and alpha-fetoprotein (AFP) levels at diagnosis were indicators of subsequent survival outcome in patients with hepatocellular carcinoma. These were combined into a Cox regression model from which a prognostic index (PI) for outcome was developed for use in future patients.

Although not the approach used by Lee, Tai, Soon, et al. (2010) to investigate criteria for defining functionally significant stenoses in small coronary arteries, we use a subset of their data to illustrate how a PI may be derived from a logistic regression model fitted to their data. The outcome variable is whether or not the fractional flow reserve (FFR) is less than 75% indicating an arterial blockage which is severe enough to obstruct blood flow. Thus, the binary endpoint is FFR75=1 if FFR <75% else FFR75=0 and the covariates are plaque burden (%), minimum lumen area (mm^2) and lesion length (mm), respectively. For our purpose we dichotomize these at 79%, 2.25 mm^2 and 12.55 mm, respectively, and label the corresponding binary covariates PB, MLA and LL with 0 for the lower and 1 for the higher levels of the covariates. The data are summarized in Figure 7.10, and suggest that values of PB=LL=1 are indicative of poor prognosis, whereas MLA=1 indicates a good prognosis.

The logistic regression analysis of FFR75 based on 85 subjects with all three covariates included and using the command (**logit FFR75 PB MLA LL**) results in the model of Figure 7.11(a), in which each of the covariates concerned is highly statistically significant. Choosing one particular subject group, from the set of the $2^3 = 8$ covariate combinations, (say) PB=MLA=LL=1 (Figure 7.11(b), Column (ii), Group 3), gives a score of logit(FFR 75)=−5.3789+5.3491−4.5479+3.3870=−1.1907. From which, by use of equation (4.4), the corresponding estimated FFR75 rate is p_{FFR75}=exp(−1.1907)/[1+exp(−1.1907)]=0.2331 or approximately 23%. The score calculation, and those for the other seven covariate combinations, is listed in Figure 7.11(b), Column (v), which shows that logit(FFR75) ranges from −9.93 to +3.36 and the anticipated proportion with poor prognosis ranges from 0.00% to 96.63% (Column (vi)) with 15 patients in the former and 27 in the latter group (Column (iii)). However, the regression model provides non-zero predictions for those of Groups 5, 6, and 7 despite zero counts of FFR75=1 in these.

In developing a PI one may wish to form a collection of groups (each comprising groups with a similar prognosis) and also facilitate the calculations for determining the eventual

(a) *Logistic regression*

logit FFR75 PB MLA LL

FFR75	Coef	SE	z	p-value
cons	−5.3789	1.5494		
PB	5.3491	1.4437	3.71	0.00021
MLA	−4.5479	1.4678	−3.10	0.0019
LL	3.3870	1.1724	2.89	0.0039

(b) *Potential risk groups defined by combinations of the three covariates*

Group	PB, MLA, LL	n	Observed FFR75=1 (%)	Regression Score	Regression Predicted FFR75=1 (%)	PI Score	PI Predicted FFR75=1 (%)
(i)	(ii)	(iii)	(iv)	(v)	(vi)	(vii)	(viii)
1	(1, 0, 1)	27	96.3	+3.36	96.63	12	96.3
2	(1, 0, 0)	10	50.0	−0.03	49.25	9	50.0
3	(1, 1, 1)	4	25.0	−1.19	23.31	8	25.0
4	(0, 0, 1)	8	12.5	−1.99	12.01	7	12.5
5	(1, 1, 0)	5	0.0	−4.58	1.02	5	0.0
6	(0, 0, 0)	5	0.0	−5.38	0.46	4	0.0
7	(0, 1, 1)	11	0.0	−6.54	0.14	3	0.0
8	(0, 1, 0)	15	0.0	−9.93	0.00	0	0.0

(c) *Simplifying the estimated regression coefficients of a fitted model*

	Development steps	PI
0	From logistic regression	$-5.3789 + 5.3491 PB - 4.5479 MLA + 3.3870 LL$
1	Drop constant term	$5.3491 PB - 4.5479 MLA + 3.3870 LL$
2	Divide by each regression coefficient by 4.5479	$1.1762 PB - MLA + 0.7447 LL$
3	Simplify the coefficients	$1.25 PB - MLA + 0.75 LL$
4	Multiply coefficients by 4 to make integers	$5 PB - 4 MLA + 3 LL$
5	Add 4 to avoid negative integers	$4 + 5 PB - 4 MLA + 3 LL$

Figure 7.11   Logistic regression of FFR75 on the potential prognostic factors for outcome (part data from Lee, Tai, Soon, *et al.*, 2010)

risk score. Figure 7.11(c) outlines the steps that might be taken in simplifying the regression model to enable a PI to be derived. The aim here is to arrive at a PI which can be easily utilized within a clinical setting.

Once the (simple) PI is derived then it can be calculated for all the subjects from whom the initial regression model was obtained. The results of the calculation using PI=4+5PB − 4 MLA+3LL are tabulated in Figure 7.11(b), Column (viii) indicates that none of those with a PI of 5 or less have FFR75=1, whereas almost all of those with PI=12 do.

As is now evident, in this example, the simplification of the regression coefficients of the fitted model to those of the PI makes no difference to the actual numbers of patients falling into the eight groups. This is caused both by having only eight combinations possible as a consequence of the binary nature of three covariates plus the fact that they each appear to have a strong prognostic impact. In general, this will not be the case and the ability to distinguish groups is likely to diminish as the rounding procedure of Figure 7.11(c) evolves.

It is well recognized in such studies that PI models that appear to be quite satisfactory when used with the data from which they are generated turn out to be of little value for prospective use. In view of this, it is usually recommended that, before prospective use, any derived PI should be validated in some way. One approach is to repeat the initial study (perhaps by an independent group of researchers) and to test the PI on this new data – if it is satisfactory for these new subjects, then this would provide reassurance for its possible use in routine clinical practice. If it is not satisfactory, then further use (without refinement) would not be anticipated. An alternative strategy is to divide the initial data set randomly into (say) two equal parts, derive the PI in one of these and then validate with the other. A difficulty here, as would be the case in the above example, is that the formative data set will now include only half as many patients so that the associated regression coefficients of the fitted model will be less reliably estimated. Consequently, the resulting PI may not reflect the true situation particularly well. More details of such cross-validation (CV) techniques are given in Chapter 9, *Practical considerations*.

Altman and Royston (2000) describe in careful detail how a prognostic model should be validated. Further, Altman, Lausen, Sauerbrei and Schumacher (1994) point out the dangers of using binary cut-points of essentially continuous covariates in the evaluation of prognostic factors.

PRACTICAL CONSIDERATIONS

A multivariable regression model can include many covariates in a single model. However, the final model is subject to the practical constraints imposed by the type and quantity of data available for analysis. Furthermore, inclusion of unnecessary variables in a model reduces statistical efficiency, as reflected in larger *SE*s, wider *CI*s, and larger *p*-values. In general, a 'parsimonious' model is preferred, but this is only so if it serves the specific research purposes to a sufficient degree. We emphasize too that the model building often involves some subjectivity so that it is important that as much of the intended process is documented in the study protocol, that any deviations from the procedures anticipated are also documented, and wherever possible the consequence of 'subjective' decisions are checked for their robustness.

The primary purpose of the analysis is to identify, and then once fitted, a model that provides answers to the questions posed by the basic structure of the study design. In clinical trials, the ICH E9 Expert Working Group (1999) insists that a trial protocol includes sections identifying the research question(s), the choice of appropriate design to answer these questions, together with details of the proposed statistical procedures to be implemented at the analysis stage. These essential recommendations have been adopted internationally as requirements by many Ethical and Regulatory Authorities responsible for approving and overseeing such trials. Following similar guidelines should be a key requirement for investigators planning any type of study.

Study size

A first consideration when planning a study of whatever type is the detailed discussion of the intended design. Once this is determined, a key next step is to determine the necessary study size to answer the question(s) posed by the design. Too many subjects are wasteful of resources, whereas too few may be insufficient for the study purpose as equivocal results may be the consequence.

Further, although the number of covariates we can add to a regression model is theoretically without limit, there are practical constraints as estimates have to be obtained for the regression coefficients. Thus, for example, we cannot include more variables in a model than the number of events available for the analysis.

Much has been written on how to determine study size which, in the context of regression models, hinges on how reliably we wish to estimate the 'key' regression parameters anticipated for the final model. If D-covariates are involved, then, for example, the anticipated magnitude of the difference between two interventions may represent a clinically meaningful benefit and one may wish to establish this with the planned randomized trial.

On the other hand, if only Q-covariates are concerned then some degree of judgment is required as, by their very nature, little is known of their respective influences. However, a 'rule-of-thumb' suggests that for every Q-covariate added, or more precisely for every additional parameter investigated (each categorical covariate involves $G - 1$ parameters), 20 more subjects should be recruited. One rationale here is that if y is a continuous variable and x a continuous covariate, then a scatter plot, with associated linear regression line fitted, is unlikely to be very informative unless 20 or more observations are included. The motivation is that if there is only one Q-covariate involved, one should include such a plot when reporting the study. For example, in Figure 2.11 in which there are only eight subjects concerned, we showed that by removing one point (admittedly carefully selected by us) from the scatter plot the subsequent fitted linear regression of change in FEV_1 against interferon-λ levels brought a substantial change in the estimated slope of the relationship. Had numbers in the plot been larger (20 or more), then such a marked disturbance is clearly less likely by the removal of a single point—hence, the larger study is more 'robust'.

The above is also based on the suggestion by Altman and Royston (2000) that the number of *Events Per* candidate co*Variate* (*EPV*) is calculated for which a minimum value of 10 (or the safer 20) is advocated. The multivariable analysis of Jackson, Gangnon, Evans, *et al.* (2008, TABLE 2) in which from 259 subjects, $E=107$ events (asthma at six years of age) were observed, the number of covariates, $v=13$, so that $EPV=E/v=107/13=8.2$, which fails the above criteria. However, this calculation implies that a single parameter is estimated per covariate, but among the covariates concerned is *BirthMonth*, which one may presume is regarded as an unordered categorical variable of 12 levels, so rather than a single parameter for this variable, there will be 11 parameters to estimate. Thus, $EPV=107/24=4.5$, which is far fewer than recommended.

A more formal approach to the calculation of study size may take the following form. Suppose again we are investigating the relationship between a continuous endpoint y and a continuous covariate x, and that they are thought to be linearly related through the simple linear regression model $y=\beta_0+\beta_{Covariate}x$. Then suppose we know something of the range of the possible values of x for the intended study, and this is from approximately x_{Low} to x_{High}. The values of y at these two extreme x values will be, $y_1=\beta_0+\beta_{Covariate}x_{Low}$ and

$y_2 = \beta_0 + \beta_{Covariate} x_{High}$. Thus, the difference between these two quantities is: $\delta = y_2 - y_1 = (\beta_0 + \beta_{Covariate} x_{High}) - (\beta_0 + \beta_{Covariate} x_{Low}) = \beta_{Covariate}(x_{High} - x_{Low})$.

Cohen (1988) relates the difference, δ, to the standard deviation of the y-variable, termed σ_y, and thereby defines the standardized difference or effect size as:

$$\Delta = \frac{\delta}{\sigma_y} = \frac{\beta_{Covariate}(x_{High} - x_{Low})}{\sigma_y} \tag{7.2}$$

with Δ pre-specified by the investigating team.

In terms of the eventual statistical test, the null hypothesis (H_0) is that $\beta_{Covariate} = 0$, which is equivalently expressed as $\Delta = 0$. The alternative hypothesis (H_A) is that: $\Delta = \Delta_{Plan}$, where the latter is the investigator's judgment of the ultimate (post-study) size of equation (7.2) while still at the design (pre-data) stage of the trial.

If the probability of falsely rejecting H_0 when it is true (termed the Type 1 error) is set to α, and the probability of falsely rejecting H_A when it is true (Type 2 error) is set to β, the number of subjects required for the study is:

$$N = \frac{4(z_{1-\alpha/2} + z_{1-\beta})^2}{\Delta_{Plan}^2} \tag{7.3}$$

where $z_{(1-\alpha/2)}$ and $z_{(1-\beta)}$ are obtained from Table T1 of the standard Normal distribution. The usual value for $\alpha = 0.05$, whereas for β it is often 0.2 but is preferably smaller at 0.1. When $\alpha = 0.05$, $z_{(1-\alpha/2)} = z_{0.975} = 1.96$ from Table T1, whereas for $\beta = 0.2$, $z_{(1-\beta)} = z_{0.8} = 0.8416$ and for $\beta = 0.1$, $z_{0.9} = 1.2816$. These values are more directly obtained from Table T3.

Cohen (1988) then goes on to argue that in many practical situations at the design stage of a study, one is more likely to have a feel for an appropriate value for Δ_{Plan} rather than the individual values of $\beta_{Covariate}$ and σ_y. Further, he suggests a realistic range for Δ_{Plan} is from 0.1 to 1.0, and defines a 'small' effect, that is a stringent criterion, as $\Delta_{Plan} = 0.2$, a 'moderate' effect $\Delta_{Plan} = 0.5$ and a 'large' effect, that is a liberal criterion, $\Delta_{Plan} = 0.8$.

So the key debate when planning a study of whatever type is: Do we anticipate a small, moderate, or large effect of the covariate under discussion?

Table T7 indicates how the sample size calculated from equation (7.3) changes as Δ_{Plan} increases from the 'small' Cohen effect size of 0.2 until a very 'large' effect' of 1.0. For the Type 1 error $\beta = 0.2$, study sizes would range from as few as 34 to as many as 788, whereas for a Type 2 error of $\beta = 0.1$, they increase from 44 to 1054. On this basis our suggestion of 20 subjects, for a study examining a single Q-variable, is widely optimistic as the size of effect associated with this, $\Delta_{Plan} = 1.35$, is much larger than Cohen's anticipated range of values. He is effectively implying, that whatever the study, it is very unlikely that the observed effect size will exceed $\Delta = 1$. Thus, our presumption of very large $\Delta_{Plan} = 1.35$ would appear to be unrealistic. In fact, Table T7 suggests any study with less than 44 subjects is unlikely to be sensible.

Suppose investigators have access to information on a sample of 100, of the 320, patients selected from the study of ACR and its relation to triacylglycerol (TG). Further, suppose they wished to replicate the findings of Ng, Fukushima, Tai, et al. (2008) then: How big a study should they conduct?

The sample log(TG) values range from −0.9 to +1.60, although the investigators recognize that there are very few observations close to the maximum. So, in planning a new study, they anticipate $x=\log(TG)$ to vary from -0.8 to 1.40. Further, this study has shown that $y=\log(ACR)$ ranges from 0.18 to 3.47 and this includes relatively few very high values. They know from experience that were $\log(ACR)$ to follow an approximately Normal distribution, then the range of the data would not exceed approximately 4 standard deviations, that is, be equal to approximately $2 \times 1.96 \times \sigma_y$. If they assume the range is essentially from 0.2 to 2.8 (ignoring some of the lowest and highest values), this provides them with an estimate of $\sigma_{y.Plan}=(2.8-0.2)/(2 \times 1.96) \approx 0.65$.

The components of equation (7.2) are now in place with $\Delta = \beta_{TG} \times [1.40 - (-0.8)]$ $/0.65 = 3.38\,\beta_{TG}$. If the planners are anticipating a medium effect size, that is $\Delta_{Plan}=0.5$, then this is equivalent to specifying $\beta_{TG}=0.5/3.38=0.15$ $\log(ACR)$ units per unit change in $\log(TG)$. By coincidence, this corresponds to the value given by Ng, Fukushima, Tai, *et al.* (2008, Table 2) for their multivariable Model 1.

From Table T7 the study size contemplated with $\Delta_{Plan}=0.5$ would be 128 or 172 depending on the Type 2 error chosen. However, as the sample sizes obtained are based on assumptions made by the investigators, some caution is required so that these numbers would be rounded upwards to 130 and 180, respectively. With these in mind, the investigators might then argue that 150 subjects is a feasible compromise and opt for that number for their study. So in the final study design they would plan to recruit 150 subjects in whom $\log(ACR)$ and $\log(TG)$ values would be recorded. Of course, the rule-of-thumb can then be implemented to add 20 further subjects for every additional covariate to be studied.

Different sample size calculation methods are necessary depending on the endpoint of concern, whether continuous, binary, ordered categorical, numeric or survival time based and are also governed by specific features of the study design. Further details are provided by Machin, Campbell, Tan and Tan (2009).

It is important to be aware that if a logistic model is anticipated, then the balance of the number of events (coded 1) and non-events (coded 0) is important. Thus, if the proportion of either one of these is very high (and consequently the other is very low) then this tends to imply that more subjects would be needed than for a situation where the events and non-events are more evenly balanced. Also when the study involves the Cox proportional hazards model it is not the actual number of subjects recruited, N, that determines the precision of the parameter estimates but rather the number of events, E, observed. As time-to-event models incorporate censored observations, E, is often substantially smaller than N.

Data acquisition

Volume, complexity and nature

The desired volume, complexity and nature of data to be collected will vary from study to study. The temptation to collect more data than is strictly necessary for the purpose at hand should be resisted as this often leads to a disproportionate amount of missing data and a loss of focus on the important research questions posed.

Checking

Much of the data in medical studies is captured in paper-based form, although there is an increasing trend for electronic data capture. The advantage of electronic forms is that range and cross-checks (checking the consistency of the new data with itself and with that already in the database) and value checks can be instantly applied. In addition, missing values can be immediately queried and irrelevant questions, such as asking a non-smoker for details of cigarette consumption can be skipped. However, paper forms are often used for convenience.

In spite of all precautions that may be taken in the study protocol to ensure that measurements are made according to carefully documented procedures, mistakes do occur in the recording of such values. Some of these errors may be detected by a quick check of the form on which the result has been recorded, whereas others may be missed and passed to the data file. At this stage range and cross-checks, easy programming of which needs to be an integral feature of the database, may help to identify such problems. If problems are found, these can be checked against case-records for correction of any erroneous values identified. In some cases, this will provide confirmation that the 'apparent error' is not an 'error' at all. Also, some 'outlier' values may not necessarily be identified by range checks alone, but by previous or subsequent data collected on the same subject or by comparison with data from other subjects in the total data set.

Missing data

A major cause for concern is if data items go unrecorded. Such items of *missing* data may result in bias (see *Technical details*) and, if large in number, this may cause the apparent results of a pre-clinical, clinical or epidemiological study not to reflect the true situation.

If the dependent variable y is missing from the database, then no modeling can be conducted including those subjects for which this is the case. Thus, it is clearly vital that the endpoint measures are recorded for all concerned. In certain circumstances, even if y is missing, the covariates for that individual may be available, in which case once the selected model is determined and the regression coefficients estimated, Y_{Miss} could be predicted. The value obtained for Y_{Miss} may then provide a clue as to why y_{Miss} may be missing in the first place. For example, suppose the model predicts the individual to have a very low value, then this low value may indicate the reason he or she had not been assessed at the clinic. On the other hand, if $Y_{Miss} \approx \bar{y}$, then one might assume the observation may be missing at random and hence any bias resulting from the observation missing from the dataset is likely to be small.

In general, however, it is the covariates that are likely to be missing. The number of missing items within (say) a questionnaire may relate to how easy it is to complete, its length or the nature of the questions concerned. Thoughts with respect to all these details need to be discussed by the project development team. It is important that the proportion of data items that are missing or unknown in the data set is minimal. Experience suggests that as the number of variables requested by the research teams increases, the proportion of 'missing' data also increases.

One simple approach to 'avoid' missing data at the analytical stage is to delete all patients from the analysis who have any missing data in the covariates of interest. This makes all the analytical procedures such as the statistical tests and the associated p-values comparable at every stage in the variable selection process. However, exclusion of patients on this basis may be very wasteful of information as this leads to, for example, excluding a patient with only a single missing value in a covariate that turns out to be of little explanatory value. So in practice one may start by excluding all patients with missing values at the early stages of the selection process but bring them back into the process as it becomes clear which of the covariates are likely to be in the final model. Some subjectivity will be required in making this judgment.

A useful approach, at least for categorical variables, is to create a distinct category for those covariates with missing data. If the data are missing at random, then this category should behave in a central manner as it will comprise a (random) mixture of the other category levels. Were the missing category to correspond to (say) the highest risk category, then this may indicate that 'missing' is a sign of poor prognosis. Perhaps it is then 'missing' as the patient was too ill for the measure to be recorded. For example, when a patient is an emergency admission, time for less routine assessments may not be available and so they may go unrecorded. In which case the absence of these values may be indicative of a poor condition and hence the fact that the data are 'missing' is prognostic for outcome.

Although there are no formal rules attached to an acceptable level of missing data, if more than 15% are missing for a particular variable then serious consideration should be given to excluding it entirely from the modeling process. If the missing data comprise less than 5%, then the bias introduced may be regarded as small. These are only pragmatic suggestions, however, and may have to be varied with circumstance. No useful model can result if a vital piece of information cannot be easily collected. Also, no strategy to compensate for missing data is any substitute for 'real' data values. Further serious concern must be raised about the potential practicability of any variable for which there is a large proportion of missing data.

Multiple tests

In the relatively straightforward example of Figure 7.3, there are eight models including the empty model concerned, and among these there are 19 nested comparisons that can be made between them. These comparisons do not include models that allow for the presence of possible interaction terms. The conventional test of the null hypothesis of any regression parameter, $\beta_{Covariate}=0$, at say the $\alpha=0.05$ level, anticipates that even if the null hypothesis is true it will be rejected five times in every 100 independent tests of the hypothesis. Thus, the test has a 5% false-positive rate (Type I error). This implies that if we conduct a large number of significance tests then it is likely that there will be a surfeit of false positive outcomes from these significance tests. In other words, we will include terms in our final model that perhaps should not be there.

One suggestion to circumvent this problem is to reduce the significance level of the multiple tests using the Bonferroni correction, which takes account of the number of tests contemplated, k. The practical way of implementing this change in reporting the results of multiple comparisons is to multiply each p-value actually obtained by k, and judge statistical significance or otherwise on the basis of this modified value.

However, in selective regression techniques if $\alpha=0.05$, but there are $k=19$ possible models to be compared, then the probability of entry (pe) into the model would be reduced to α/k or $0.05/19=0.0026$. If we applied this rule to the three binary covariate models for the 300 subjects of Figure 7.3 using the selection command (**stepwise, pe(0.0026): logit IHD Drink Gender Smoke**), then only the empty model would have been selected.

Although the above is only an illustrative example, multiple testing frequently occurs in practice. Thus, there are 45 different p-values included in the tables, and there are others within the text (hence at least 45 tests of statistical significance have been conducted) presented by Jackson, Gangnon, Evans, *et al.* (2008). In which case, Bonferroni suggests considering $\alpha/k=0.05/45=0.0011$ rather than 0.05 to judge statistical significance. Nevertheless, the authors have provided careful detail of the selection processes they have used so that the reader can judge what impact the multiple testing may have had on the study conclusions.

The difficulty here is that the Bonferroni correction assumes that all the statistical tests are independent of each other, which is not the case when we are fitting all the different (sometimes nested) models to the same (or at least overlapping) data. Hence, Bonferroni is likely to over compensate but, as far as we are aware, there is no simple answer as to the extent of this.

We advise testing all D-variables at the conventional $\alpha=0.05$, applying no significance tests to any K-variables, initially allowing all Q-variables into the model at $\alpha=0.05/k$, where k corresponds to the number of β_D and β_K parameters, plus β_0, that are already included in the model so far. Any Q-covariate then subsequently added to the model, should be checked for the magnitude of its influence on the regression coefficient(s) of the primary D-covariate. If the influence is small, then this should be reported, although the final model would not include that variable. In contrast, if the influence is large it should be retained in the final model.

Multiple modeling

In the example, taken from Jackson, Gangnon, Evans, *et al.* (2008), we referred to the fact that the results of 45 or more statistical tests were included their report. However, 17 of this number relate to the two multivariable models presented. One model contains all 13 of the potential risk factors, whereas the second contains only four of these following the use of a stepwise selection with backward elimination based on Akaike's information criterion. In this type of situation, Young and Karr (2011) make an important distinction between multiple testing and multiple modeling as they point out that the selection process can involve (computer algorithm) looking at many models but only the final one is presented. What is more, precise features of the selection processes involved are not necessarily fully revealed, the consequence is that the reader of the report (and even the analyst responsible) may have little idea of the number of multiple tests involved.

Young and Karr (2011) raised major concerns with respect to how observational studies are analyzed, their findings reported, and how they are subsequently interpreted. In our context, their concerns arise from studies in which there are a large number of potential covariates and therefore a very large number of models from which the 'final' model is selected. However, we have suggested that indiscriminant use of selection methods can be avoided by giving careful consideration at the design (pre-data) stage of a study and setting out clearly what is intended. In any research context, the indiscriminant use of any statistical procedure may lead to false conclusions but the application of selective methods (given the wide choice of alternative strategies) is particularly prone. Nevertheless, concern should not be entirely focused on large observational studies, there is also a concern at the extent of false conclusions arising from basic scientific research where studies are not large but are insufficiently replicated. In contrast, Ince (2011) highlights the major problems of (so-called) data mining experiments in which computer-based searches are made to establish 'interesting' associations.

Confirmatory studies

As we have indicated when discussing the development of a PI, in many instances once a study has been conducted and reported a second study to verify the same findings will not be undertaken, although there are sometimes cogent reasons why it should be. Thus, when deriving a prognostic model for hepatocellular carcinoma in developing countries the paper by Tan, Law, Ng and Machin (2003) was initially rejected (and rightly so) by the reviewers concerned with a rider, from the editor, that if a confirmatory data set could be identified, and the model subsequently validated, then the journal would review the paper again sympathetically. Fortunately, data from a randomized trial became available, the proposed model was validated, and the revised paper subsequently published. This might be regarded as a type of cross-validation by use of a 'split-sample' analysis advocated by Young and Karr (2011) to help avoid some of the problems associated with interpreting observational studies.

Stratification

One particular feature of randomized controlled trials is the recognition that patients with a particular disease or condition may present at diagnosis with good or poor diagnostic features, which will have an important influence on the ultimate outcome. Thus, for example, it is known that nodal status in patients with nasopharyngeal cancer acts in this way. In the randomized trial of Wee, Tan, Tai, *et al.* (2005) described in *Example 1.5* two groups were formed according to the nodal status (*Node*, *N*) of the patient (Group 1: N0, N1, or N2; Group 2: N3) at diagnosis. In these circumstances the binary covariate *Node* would be thought of as a *K*-covariate, whereas the treatment allocated (*Treat*, *T*), of either RT or CRT, is the *D*-covariate.

At the design stage of the trial, in view of the fact that those of nodal Group 2 were antic-ipated to have a much worse survival, the investigators were concerned that despite a pro-posed 1:1 randomization to RT or CRT, there could ultimately be a severe imbalance between the treatment arms with respect to nodal status when recruitment was completed. To deal with this possibility, two options were contemplated.

The first was merely to record the nodal status at diagnosis and then verify in the eventual analysis, by comparing model $T+N$ with T, if the estimated hazard ratios (HR) for com-paring treatments were materially different when determined by the two models. The second option, and the one implemented, was to stratify the randomization within the nodal groups. That is, before randomization, the nodal status of the patients was to be determined and, once determined, randomization to *Treat* was made within that *Node* group on a 1:1 basis. In this situation, the *K*-variable *Node*, becomes a second (and secondary) design variable *D*, and as such must be dealt with appropriately in the analysis.

In this second case, although not necessarily apparent from the associated computer output, the analytical process has several stages. First, the comparison between RT and CRT is made within the node Group 1 (*Node*=0), and this is repeated for Group 2 (*Node*=1). These calculations provide two estimates of the HR which are then combined, taking account of the different patient numbers in the two *Node* groups, to produce a stratified HR and the associated confidence interval. This process follows the same lines that we described in Chapter 6, *Verifying proportional hazards*, when describing an example in which a strat-ified Cox model was used to take account of non-proportional hazards.

It is important to stress, that only if the first option is taken (and so the randomization is not stratified) is the regression model comparison of T with $T+N$ valid. Equally, only if the sec-ond option is taken (and the randomization is stratified) is the stratified model approach valid.

Figure 7.12(a) gives the number of patients with nasopharyngeal cancer randomized within the two nodal groups and their assignment to each treatment group. As was planned, the numbers in each treatment group are broadly equal within each nodal group. The unadjusted analysis following the command (**stcox Treat**) gives a *HR*=0.5697 (95%

(a) Allocation to treatment following a randomization stratified by nodal status

tabulate Node Treat

```
------------+-------------------+---------
            |    Treatment      |
     Node   |   RT      CRT     |   Total
        +                       +
 N0, N1, N2 |   77       82      |   159
        N3  |   33       29      |   62
            +-------------------+---------
     Total  |  110      111      |   221
------------+-------------------+---------
```

No. of subjects = 221, No. of failures = 88
stcox Treat

```
-----------------------------------------------------------
   t  |   HR       SE       z     P>|z|        [95% CI]
------+----------------------------------------------------
Treat | 0.5697    0.1248   -2.57   0.010    0.3708 to 0.8753
-----------------------------------------------------------
```

(b) Incorrect analysis: Treatment adjusted for nodal status

stcox Treat Node

```
-----------------------------------------------------------
   t  |   HR       SE       z     P>|z|        [95% CI]
------+----------------------------------------------------
Treat | 0.5958    0.1310   -2.36   0.018    0.3872 to 0.9166
Node  | 1.8192
-----------------------------------------------------------
```

(c) Correct analysis: Treatment stratified by nodal status

stcox Treat, strata (Node)

```
-----------------------------------------------------------
   t  |   HR       SE       z     P>|z|        [95% CI]
------+----------------------------------------------------
Treat | 0.5826    0.1282   -2.45   0.014    0.3784 to 0.8969
-----------------------------------------------------------
```

Figure 7.12 Comparison of results following (a) an unadjusted analysis, (b) an adjusted analysis and (c) a stratified analysis, with the latter two analyses taking account of the nodal status at diagnosis of patients with nasopharyngeal cancer (part data from Wee, Tan, Tai, et al., 2005)

CI 0.3708 to 0.8753, p-value=0.010) suggesting a benefit of CRT over RT in terms of event-free survival (EFS).

The inappropriate adjusted analysis of Figure 7.12(b) using (`stcox Treat Node`), gives HR=0.5958 suggesting a marginally reduced benefit to CRT than previously indicated with an increased p-value=0.018. The stratified, and now correct, analysis of Figure 7.12(c) using (`stcox Treat, strata(Node)`), gives an intermediate HR=0.5826 with p-value=0.014. In both instances, the analyses taking account of nodal status had little impact on the magnitude of the estimated treatment effect, although this will not always be the case. However, it is important that the analysis conducted, and reported, is that which reflects the underlying design.

Subgroup analysis

In some situations, once a study is completed a comparison (although not planned at the design stage) of, for example, the effect of treatment in a randomized trial within a subgroup of patients is made in order to reveal 'interesting' groups who may do especially well (or especially badly) with the test treatment concerned. Such unplanned comparisons may result in spurious findings partially as a result of multiple modeling and multiple testing, but more importantly as a result of the reduced sample sizes that are involved.

To use the example of the trial of Pearson, Pinkerton, Lewis, *et al.* (2008) involving patients with neuroblastoma (NB), suppose we wish to see if the *HR* was materially different within those of different ages who have been categorized into the four groups, *AgeG4*, of Figure 7.13(a). The first thing to note is that the patient numbers in the youngest group and the two categories of older patients are rather small.

(a) *Allocated treatment within four age-groups*

tabulate AgeG44 Treat

```
--------+--------------------+--------
        |        Treat       |
AgeG4 | Standard       Rapid | Total
--------+--------------------+--------
12<18m |     13           10 |    23
18m–9y |     84           86 |   170
10–15y |      2            3 |     5
16–20y |      2            0 |     2
--------+--------------------+--------
 Total |    101           99 |   200
--------+--------------------+--------
```

(b) *Treatment comparison within Age-groups*

12<18m *months*

stcox Treat if AgeG4 == 1

No. of subjects = 23, No. of failures = 12

t	HR	SE	z	P>|z|	[95% CI]
Treat	1.0164	0.5970	0.03	0.98	0.3215 to 3.2138

18 *months – 9 years*

stcox Treat if AgeG4 == 2

No. of subjects = 170, No. of failures = 134

t	HR	SE	z	P>|z|	[95% CI]
Treat	0.6681	0.1163	–2.32	0.020	0.4750 to 0.9397

10–20 *years*

stcox Treat if AgeG4 > 2

No. of subjects = 7, No. of failures = 6

t	HR	SE	z	P>|z|	[95% CI]
Treat	2.8527	2.6291	1.14	0.26	0.4686 to 17.3677

Figure 7.13 Subgroup comparison of treatment outcome for three age groups of young patients with neuroblastoma (part data from Pearson, Pinkerton, Lewis, *et al.*, 2008)

The relevant command in Figure 7.13(b) for those aged 12-18 months is (`stcox Treat if AgeG4==1`). In this case, only 12 failures are observed from the 23 patients concerned, and this leaves very low precision (wide confidence intervals) for the estimated $HR=1.02$ (very close to the null) in favor of *Standard* over *Rapid*. The small numbers in the older age groups suggest that these groups might best be merged, although this larger group of those aged 10-20 years and comprising seven patients and six failures remains very small. However, the command (`stcox Treat if AgeG4 >2`) estimates a $HR=2.85$ (a very large effect) for these patients which again favors *Standard*. However, the lower limits of the corresponding confidence intervals of 0.3215 and 0.4686 from these two analyses are both consistent with *considerable* benefit for patients receiving the *Rapid* treatment approach.

In contrast, those aged 18 months to 9 years comprise a large group of 170 patients with 134 failures. The corresponding command (`stcox Treat if AgeG4==2`) gives an estimated $HR=0.67$ indicating a strong benefit for those receiving *Rapid* which is statistically significant, p-value$=0.020$. However, even this alleged benefit has an associated confidence interval which is very wide—consistent both with a dramatic effect (less than 0.5) and one not too distant from the null hypothesis, H_0: $HR=1$, value of no effect. Further, as there is multiple (triple) testing, following the Bonferroni suggestion the associated p-value is likely to be closer to $3 \times 0.020=0.06$, which is no longer statistically significant. Thus, at best, these analyses can only give an indication of the situation that exists with respect to age.

Although this is clearly an extreme example, it would not be correct to infer *Standard* is best for the Youngest and Oldest patients, whereas *Rapid* is best for those of Intermediate age. However, similar dangers are likely to be encountered whenever a subgroup analysis is conducted.

If subgroup analyses are to be made, then they should be stated in the study protocol itself and, at that stage, the design team should decide whether or not they are warranted. It is very tempting for those who get a null result for the basic question(s) they pose with their choice of design to look for tempting 'tit-bits' for those to whom the actual study report is targeted.

TECHNICAL DETAILS

Bias

There are two types of measures of concern, those that relate to the endpoint(s) and those which relate to the corresponding covariates. Care has to be taken whichever of these, possibly many variables, has to be measured or assessed. Clearly some will be easily determined, such as the intervention allocated in a randomized trial, or the gender of the subjects concerned, whereas others may need detailed (and possibly repeated) assessments before they can be established. It is important that these assessments are made in a manner to minimize the possibility of bias.

Just as equation (1.7) summarizes the linear regression model associating the endpoint to a key covariate, we can describe aspects of the measurement process in a model framework in the following way

$$v = V + \varepsilon \tag{7.4}$$

Here V is the true value of the reading that we are about to take on an experimental unit. After we have made the measurement, we record the values of V value as v. We know, with most measures we take, that we will not record the true value but one that we hope is close enough to this for our purpose thereby implying the errors (or residuals), $\varepsilon = V - v$ of equation (7.4), will be small. We also hope, over the series of measurements we take (one for each experimental unit), that the individual ε will not be too large and that their mean, $\bar{\varepsilon}$, will be close to zero. In which case, any errors we make will have little impact on the final conclusions.

However, if there is something systematically wrong with what we are doing (possibly being quite unaware of this), then the model we are concerned with is now

$$v = B + V + \varepsilon \tag{7.5}$$

This second model implies that even if we average out ε to be close to zero over the course of the study, we are left with a consistent difference, B, between the true value V and that we actually record, v. This is termed the bias. Thus, the measurements should be taken to try to ensure that $B = 0$ from the onset.

8   Repeated Measures

SUMMARY

This chapter describes studies that involve repeated measures of the same endpoint variable taken on individual subjects over time in a longitudinal manner. In essence, the measure repeated on the same subject implies that the successive observations are not likely to be independent of each other. This association is termed auto-correlation and needs to be accounted for in fitting an appropriate regression model. The types of model described include those that assume all subjects follow a single model with fixed parameters which are to be estimated. Such models are termed population-averaged. These are compared with random-effects models, which allow each subject followed longitudinally to have individual values for their own parameters, although the model structure remains common across all subjects in the study. A mixed model is one in which some of the parameters are fixed and others are random. These approaches are illustrated using endpoints of a continuous and binary nature. We point out that some care is needed in defining the layout (wide or long) of the associated database and how the variables included may be named.

LONGITUDINAL STUDIES

We introduced in Figure 1.12 the longitudinal study (longitudinal as the patients concerned are followed over time) described by Poon, Goh, Kim, *et al.* (2006) where repeated measures of a visual analogue scale (VAS) of self-reported pain levels experienced by patients arising from their oral lichen planus (OLP) were summarized. However, the plots within each of the panels in this longitudinal randomized trial do not distinguish the individual profiles of, for example, the 71 patients who were allocated to receive steroid treatment. Nevertheless, the fact that successive measurements from a patient are linked to each other needs to be accounted for in any model fitting process. Further, the profiles within each treatment group do not appear linear over time. This non-linearity makes the appropriate model difficult to determine and thereby further complicates the situation.

Regression Methods for Medical Research, First Edition. Bee Choo Tai and David Machin.
© 2014 Bee Choo Tai and David Machin. Published 2014 by John Wiley & Sons, Ltd.

Medical time series

In contrast to the rather complex example of the trial in patients with OLP, Figure 8.1(a) gives the weight of one individual determined from time-to-time over a period of approximately three months. These 16 observations have mean 76.71 kg and standard deviation (SD) of 0.4703 kg. The corresponding scatter plot of the changing weight over time, comprising the data points of Figure 8.1(b), might reasonably be described by a simple linear model, although the amount of variation appears somewhat exaggerated in this instance by the choice of scale for the y-axis. However, successive readings are likely to be correlated so that any model fitted to describe the relationship has to take into account the associated auto-correlation pattern and magnitude. Nevertheless, the corresponding linear model for the single subject assessed at different times, t

$$y_t = \beta_0 + \beta_1 t + \eta_t \qquad (8.1)$$

looks very similar to that of equation (1.7), except that y_t replaces y_i and the covariate x_i is replaced by t. Further, η_t replaces the residual ε_i. The reason for this latter change is to emphasize that the residuals are no longer independent as the model is describing changes over time in one individual. The subscript 't' indicates that y and η may vary with time for the *individual* of concern whereas, in equation (1.7), 'i' takes a value from 1 to n depending on which of the n individuals is concerned. We can express the lack of independence by anticipating that the correlation between the residual at (say) t_1 and that at any other time (say) t_2, will not be zero, that is, $\rho(\eta_{t_1}, \eta_{t_2}) \neq 0$.

The command (**regress Weight Day**) of Figure 8.1(c) provides the estimates of the regression coefficients as $b_0 = 77.0674$ and $b_{Day} = -0.008205$ to establish this line. Further, the residual standard deviation $s_{Residual} = 0.4575$ (denoted Root Mean Square Error, MSE) is not very different from $SD = 0.4703$ quoted earlier (which can also be obtained from the ANOVA table by $s_{Total} = \sqrt{[3.3175/15]}$). The close similarity of the two values ($s_{Residual}$ and s_{Total}) suggests that the linear model explains little of the variation in body-weight over time.

As this model takes no account of the auto-correlation between successive measures, it may be misleading. Nevertheless, the regression coefficients are likely to be approximately correct, although $s_{Residual}$ is less reliable and may be under- or overestimated by assuming that the successive observations are independent. In fact there are several ways in which the auto-correlation can be accounted for but all require one or more assumptions to be made. The assumptions can often be verified as appropriate or not by looking for patterns in the residuals. However, the 'correct' residuals can only be obtained once the 'correct' model is fitted. Hence there is some circularity in the verification process.

One approach to estimating equation (8.1) is to fit a 'time-series' model using the command (**prais Weight Day, rhotype(tscorr)**) where (**prais**) refers to the Prais-Watson method, which takes account of the fact that the residuals, η_t, are auto-correlated in a particular way. To implement this command it has to be preceded by (**tsset Day, daily**), which establishes that the variable *Day* (our time covariate) is measured in days. The command then anticipates daily data and further takes note that, in this example, the observations made are not equally spaced in time. The fitted model is summarized in Figure 8.1(d) and provides $b_0 = 77.0707$ and $b_{Day} = -0.008347$ as the corresponding estimates. These are very close to those obtained when assuming the observations were independent. The standard error of $SE(b_{Day}) = 0.006059$ has now marginally increased over the OLS value, $SE(b_{Day}) = 0.006028$. This regression model (hatched line) is added to Figure 8.1(b) and this overlaps almost entirely with the ordinary least squares (OLS) regression line obtained using (**lfit Weight Day**).

Database format

In the weight change example, we were modeling the behavior of a single individual over time. Diggle (1990) gives more details of such 'medical time-series'. However, we are more concerned with modeling situations for a group of individuals such as those patients receiving treatment for their OLP which we summarized in Figure 1.12. In which case, it is

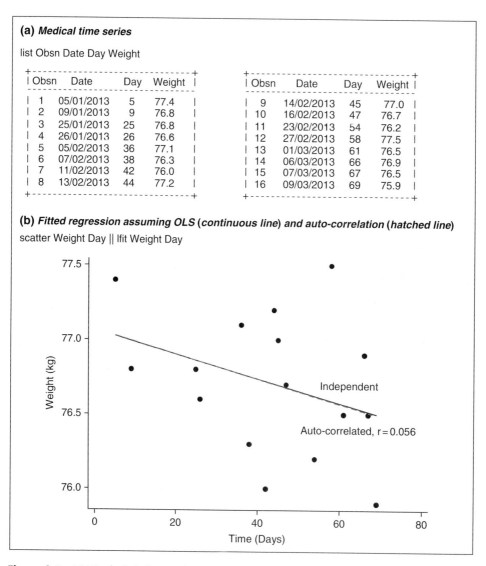

(a) *Medical time series*

list Obsn Date Day Weight

Obsn	Date	Day	Weight
1	05/01/2013	5	77.4
2	09/01/2013	9	76.8
3	25/01/2013	25	76.8
4	26/01/2013	26	76.6
5	05/02/2013	36	77.1
6	07/02/2013	38	76.3
7	11/02/2013	42	76.0
8	13/02/2013	44	77.2

Obsn	Date	Day	Weight
9	14/02/2013	45	77.0
10	16/02/2013	47	76.7
11	23/02/2013	54	76.2
12	27/02/2013	58	77.5
13	01/03/2013	61	76.5
14	06/03/2013	66	76.9
15	07/03/2013	67	76.5
16	09/03/2013	69	75.9

(b) *Fitted regression assuming OLS (continuous line) and auto-correlation (hatched line)*

scatter Weight Day || lfit Weight Day

Figure 8.1 (a) Weight (kg) of one individual taken on 16 occasions over a three-month period, and (b) almost identical estimated regression lines, one assuming independent observations using ordinary least squares (OLS), and the other taking accounting of auto-correlation

(c) *Assuming independence*

regress Weight Day

Number of obs = 16, F(1, 14) = 1.85, Prob > F = 0.20

Source	SS	df	MS	F	p-value
Model	0.3877	1	0.3877	$1.85 = (-1.36^2)$	0.20
Residual	2.9298	14	0.2093	**Root MSE = 0.4575**	
Total	3.3175	15			

Weight	Coef	SE	t	p-value	[95% CI]
b_0	77.0674				
b_{Day}	−0.008**205**	0.006028	−1.36	0.20	−0.02113 to 0.00472

(d) *Assuming auto-correlation present*

tsset Day, daily

prais Weight Day, rhotype(tscorr)

Prais-Winsten AR(1) regression -- iterated estimates

Weight	Coef	SE	t	p-value	[95% CI]
b_0	77.0707				
b_{Day}	−0.008**347**	0.006059	−1.38	0.19	−0.02134 to 0.00465
ρ	0.0556				

Figure 8.1 (Continued)

very likely that the variation between individuals will be greater than that observed within a single individual.

Figure 8.2(a) gives part of the data from a study conducted by Nejadnik, Hui, Choong, *et al.* (2010) involving changes in the self-assessed Physical Component Summary (PCS) score of the SF-36 quality-of-life instrument in patients undergoing cartilage repair. The clinical trial protocol specified that patients were to be self-assessed prior to surgery (Day 0), and then post-surgery at 3, 6, 9, 12, 18, and 24 months. The variables listed include a baseline assessment, `PCS0`, and up to six subsequent measures, `PCS3, PCS6, PCS9, PCS12, PCS18, and PCS24`, recorded at the times `t0, t3, t6, t9, t12, t18, and t24` respectively. Using the command (`twoway connected PCS and t`), Figure 8.2(b) gives a connected line plot of the data from these 15 patients and illustrates very different patient profiles over time. This contrasts with the example of Figure 1.12, which does not identify individual patients so distinct profiles cannot be distinguished. For the current example, patient (`id`=7) has the lowest `PCS0`=22.7, which then falls post-surgery to `PCS3`=16.5 and eventually rises to `PCS24`=45.0. In contrast, patient (`id`=11) has `PCS0`=51.1 but does not recover to this value over the study period of assessments as `PCS24`=39.1. Overall, PCS scores declined over baseline values (`PSC0`) following surgery but subsequently gradually improved over time.

However, as shown in Figure 8.2(c), the number of patients with PCS assessments (variable *FUPCS*) declined with follow-up time with, for example, only 21 of 71 were assessed

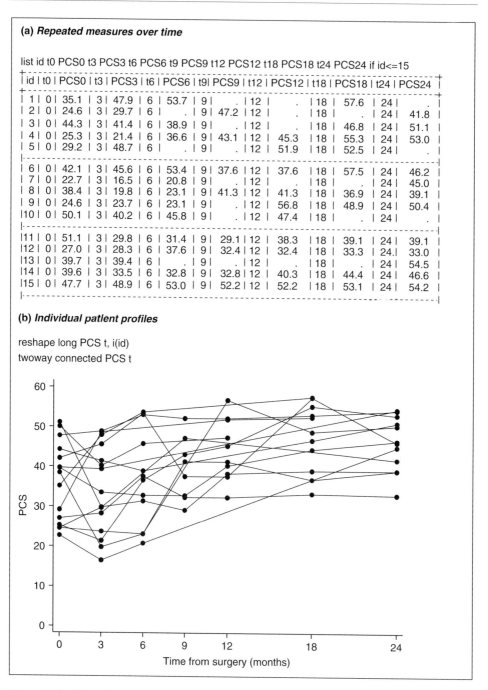

(a) *Repeated measures over time*

```
list id t0 PCS0 t3 PCS3 t6 PCS6 t9 PCS9 t12 PCS12 t18 PCS18 t24 PCS24 if id<=15
+-----------------------------------------------------------------------------+
| id | t0 | PCS0 | t3 | PCS3 | t6 | PCS6 | t9| PCS9 | t12 | PCS12 | t18 | PCS18 | t24 | PCS24 |
+-----------------------------------------------------------------------------+
|  1 | 0 | 35.1 | 3 | 47.9 | 6 | 53.7 | 9 |   . | 12 |    . | 18 | 57.6 | 24 |    . |
|  2 | 0 | 24.6 | 3 | 29.7 | 6 |   . | 9 | 47.2 | 12 |    . | 18 |    . | 24 | 41.8 |
|  3 | 0 | 44.3 | 3 | 41.4 | 6 | 38.9 | 9 |   . | 12 |    . | 18 | 46.8 | 24 | 51.1 |
|  4 | 0 | 25.3 | 3 | 21.4 | 6 | 36.6 | 9 | 43.1 | 12 | 45.3 | 18 | 55.3 | 24 | 53.0 |
|  5 | 0 | 29.2 | 3 | 48.7 | 6 |   . | 9 |   . | 12 | 51.9 | 18 | 52.5 | 24 |    . |
|-----------------------------------------------------------------------------|
|  6 | 0 | 42.1 | 3 | 45.6 | 6 | 53.4 | 9 | 37.6 | 12 | 37.6 | 18 | 57.5 | 24 | 46.2 |
|  7 | 0 | 22.7 | 3 | 16.5 | 6 | 20.8 | 9 |   . | 12 |    . | 18 |    . | 24 | 45.0 |
|  8 | 0 | 38.4 | 3 | 19.8 | 6 | 23.1 | 9 | 41.3 | 12 | 41.3 | 18 | 36.9 | 24 | 39.1 |
|  9 | 0 | 24.6 | 3 | 23.7 | 6 | 23.1 | 9 |   . | 12 | 56.8 | 18 | 48.9 | 24 | 50.4 |
| 10 | 0 | 50.1 | 3 | 40.2 | 6 | 45.8 | 9 |   . | 12 | 47.4 | 18 |    . | 24 |    . |
|-----------------------------------------------------------------------------|
| 11 | 0 | 51.1 | 3 | 29.8 | 6 | 31.4 | 9 | 29.1 | 12 | 38.3 | 18 | 39.1 | 24 | 39.1 |
| 12 | 0 | 27.0 | 3 | 28.3 | 6 | 37.6 | 9 | 32.4 | 12 | 32.4 | 18 | 33.3 | 24.| 33.0 |
| 13 | 0 | 39.7 | 3 | 39.4 | 6 |   . | 9 |   . | 12 |    . | 18 |    . | 24 | 54.5 |
| 14 | 0 | 39.6 | 3 | 33.5 | 6 | 32.8 | 9 | 32.8 | 12 | 40.3 | 18 | 44.4 | 24 | 46.6 |
| 15 | 0 | 47.7 | 3 | 48.9 | 6 | 53.0 | 9 | 52.2 | 12 | 52.2 | 18 | 53.1 | 24 | 54.2 |
|-----------------------------------------------------------------------------|
```

(b) *Individual patient profiles*

```
reshape long PCS t, i(id)
twoway connected PCS t
```

Figure 8.2 Physical Component Summary (PCS) scores using the SF-36 obtained from patients undergoing cartilage repair (part data from Nejadnik, Hui, Choong, *et al.*, 2010)

(c) *Details of the number of assessments made*

tabulate FUPCS

FUPCS	Freq.	Percent
1	3	4.2
2	9	12.7
3	8	11.3
4	14	19.7
5	16	22.5
6	21	29.6
Total	71	100.0

Figure 8.2 (Continued)

at baseline and also at all the six succeeding time points. Consequently, for many patients the PCS information is incomplete. Such *gaps* in the data can complicate the analytical processes and curtail the choice of model that can be fitted. There are also three patients for whom only a single post-surgery PCS assessment was made (as **PCS0** may be regarded as a covariate rather than an endpoint measure) and so there are no *repeated* measures for these. They are therefore omitted from the repeated measures modeling process. Figure 8.2(a) also illustrates that there are also many *gaps* in the data, for example, patient (**id**=13) has **PCS0**=39.7, **PCS3**=39.4 then no further assessments until **PCS24**=54.5.

It is customary when creating a database for a study to include all the data from an individual in one (perhaps very wide) row. Thus, the database corresponding to the data of Figure 8.2(a) would contain in the first column a unique patient identifier, say **id**, for each row. Then along a row for a specified **id** the subsequent variables recorded on that individual. For example, for the fifth individual (**id**=5), the row would comprise: 5: 0, 29.2; 3, 48.7; 6, . ; 9, . ; 12, 51.9; 18, 52.5; 24, . . This format can be compared with that of Figure 8.1(a), which contains the information on a single individual. In that case, the rows have an identifier (**Obsn**) tracking the different weighing occasions but, in contrast to Figure 8.2(a), the information on the changing (**Day**) and (**Weight**) of the individual is contained in two columns. Here the information is contained in a so-called *long* file format of 16 rows and (ignoring **Obsn** which is merely the row number and the date) two columns for the variables (**Day, Weight**). Had this been in the *wide* file format of Figure 8.2(a), then the database for this one individual would comprise a single row containing 32 variables and take the form: 5, 77.4, 9, 76.8, … , 66, 76.5, 68, 75.9. Were the data in this wide format, then sensible names for the variables would be: **day0, weight0, day1, weight1, … , day15, weight15.** This variable name structure then reflects that of Figure 8.2(a), which is: **id, t0, PCS0, t3, PCS3, … , t24, PCS24,** although (**id**) has to be added here as there are 15 patients each with their own row in the database.

As will be the case in most studies including several subjects, in repeated measures studies the data are usually held in the *wide* format. However, for analysis purposes the data often have to be rearranged into the *long* format. Indeed the database has to be reshaped in

```
list id _j Age Gender Implant t PCS if id<4

+-----------------------------------------------------+
| id    _j    Age    Gender    Implant    t      PCS  |
|-----------------------------------------------------|
| 1     0     41     Male      ACC        0      35.1 |
| 1     1     41     Male      ACC        3      47.9 |
| 1     2     41     Male      ACC        6      53.7 |
| 1     3     41     Male      ACC        9        .  |
| 1     4     41     Male      ACC        12       .  |
|-----------------------------------------------------|
| 1     5     41     Male      ACC        18     57.6 |
| 1     6     41     Male      ACC        24       .  |
| 2     0     64     Female    BMSC       0      24.6 |
| 2     1     64     Female    BMSC       3      29.7 |
| 2     2     64     Female    BMSC       6        .  |
|-----------------------------------------------------|
| 2     3     64     Female    BMSC       9      47.2 |
| 2     4     64     Female    BMSC       12       .  |
| 2     5     64     Female    BMSC       18       .  |
| 2     6     64     Female    BMSC       24     41.8 |
| 3     0     52     Female    ACC        0      44.3 |
|-----------------------------------------------------|
| 3     1     52     Female    ACC        3      41.4 |
| 3     2     52     Female    ACC        6      38.9 |
| 3     3     52     Female    ACC        9        .  |
| 3     4     52     Female    ACC        12       .  |
| 3     5     52     Female    ACC        18     46.8 |
|-----------------------------------------------------|
| 3     6     52     Female    ACC        24     51.1 |
+-----------------------------------------------------+
```

Figure 8.3 Database of three patients undergoing cartilage repair from a repeated measures study including a baseline assessment of PCS and up to six further assessments converted from wide to long format (part data from Nejadnik, Hui, Choong, et al., 2010)

this way before the command (**twoway connected PCS t**) of Figure 8.2(b) can be implemented. If the variables are named as (**PCS***) and (**t***), as we have just described, with the * indicating that it will be replaced by increasing non-negative numerical values, then statistical analysis packages can convert a wide file into a long file easily. Thus, the command (**reshape long PCS t, i(id)**) of Figure 8.3 converts the data of Figure 8.2(a) from wide into a long database format. The command recognizes that there are seven potential observations for each subject by creating the variable _j, which takes the values 0 to 6 and represents the differing values taken by * above. The command places '_' before the 'j' here to emphasize that this variable name is generated by the program itself and is not part of the original database. Alternatively, a name can be given by the analyst to replace _j by adding, for example, (**j(Record)**) to the reshape command. This will then name the variable for column (2) of Figure 8.3 as *Record*.

In this study the type of implant (*Implant*) received, either autologous chondrocyte (ACC) or autologous bone marrow-derived mesenchymal cells (BMSC), and the covariates *Age* and *Gender* were also recorded. In the long file format the corresponding values are repeated, as is (**id**), in all seven rows required to summarize the data from that subject.

AUTO- OR SERIAL-CORRELATION

Definition

In a cross-sectional design there is, for the particular endpoint under consideration, a single variable whose value in a subject will not depend on the magnitude of the corresponding value for any other participant in the study. In contrast, an important aspect of longitudinal designs with repeated measures is that successive observations from the same subject are unlikely to be independent. As we have previously stated, a key consideration then in planning a study involving repeated measures is the nature and strength of this correlation. In Chapter 1, *Technical details*, we introduced the correlation coefficient as a measure of the degree of association between two continuous variables and this is calculated using equation (1.16). The corresponding expression for quantifying the association between the *same* continuous measure taken on two occasions has a similar form which is

$$\rho_T(y_1, y_2) = \frac{\sum (y_{1i} - \bar{y}_1)(y_{2i} - \bar{y}_2)}{\sqrt{\sum (y_{1i} - \bar{y}_1)^2 \sum (y_{2i} - \bar{y}_2)^2}} \tag{8.2}$$

Here y_{1i} and y_{2i} represent values of two assessments of the *same* measure made on subject, i, where $i = 1, 2, \ldots, n$, $\bar{y}_1$ and $\bar{y}_2$ are the respective means at times 1 and 2, and the summation Σ is made over all n individuals. The expression is symmetric in terms of y_{1i} and y_{2i} and hence $\rho_T(y_1, y_2) = \rho_T(y_2, y_1)$. The subscript T is included here to emphasize the time element involved.

Possible patterns

The problem for the investigators is that the properties of a repeated measures design depend on ρ_T. The value of this, and how it changes with the time-interval between observations, may be hard to pinpoint.

Independent

In the special case that successive observations on the same individual can be regarded as independent then there is clearly no auto-correlation present and $\rho_T = 0$ for whichever pair of different time-points we choose to compare. Thus, the correlation matrix of Figure 8.4(a) has a diagonal which contains unity in every position (as every observation is perfectly correlated with itself) but is 0 whenever an observation is compared with a previous or subsequent one of the same (repeated) measure. In this special case, no auto-correlation has to be estimated and so the analytical process is at its simplest. For the simple linear regression model, this leads to estimates of the regression coefficients given by equations (1.8) and that for the residual standard deviation by (1.9). As the beneath and above diagonal entries of the correlation matrix of Figure 8.4(a) are symmetric (and this is true in all situations), only the half-diagonal form (given in bold) is usually presented.

Uniform or exchangeable

If the assumed auto-correlation between measurements made at any two arbitrarily chosen times, say time t_1 and time t_2, has the same value for $\rho_T(y_{t1}, y_{t2})$ whatever values of t_1 and t_2 we happen to choose, then we can write $\rho_T(y_{t1}, y_{t2}) = \rho$. As the magnitude and/or sign of ρ does not

(a) Independent

	y1	y2	y3	y4	y5	y6
y1 |	1	0	0	0	0	0
y2 |	0	1	0	0	0	0
y3 |	0	0	1	0	0	0
y4 |	0	0	0	1	0	0
y5 |	0	0	0	0	1	0
y6 |	0	0	0	0	0	1

(b) Uniform or Exchangeable

	y1	y2	y3	y4	y5	y6
y1 |	1					
y2 |	ρ	1				
y3 |	ρ	ρ	1			
y4 |	ρ	ρ	ρ	1		
y5 |	ρ	ρ	ρ	ρ	1	
y6 |	ρ	ρ	ρ	ρ	ρ	1

(c) Auto-regressive

	y1	y2	y3	y4	y5	y6
y1 |	1					
y2 |	ρ	1				
y3 |	ρ^2	ρ	1			
y4 |	ρ^3	ρ^2	ρ	1		
y5 |	ρ^4	ρ^3	ρ^2	ρ	1	
y6 |	ρ^5	ρ^4	ρ^3	ρ^2	ρ	1

(d) Unstructured

	y1	y2	y3	y4	y5	y6
y1 |	1					
y2 |	ρ_{21}	1				
y3 |	ρ_{31}	ρ_{32}	1			
y4 |	ρ_{41}	ρ_{42}	ρ_{43}	1		
y5 |	ρ_{51}	ρ_{52}	ρ_{53}	ρ_{54}	1	
y6 |	ρ_{61}	ρ_{62}	ρ_{63}	ρ_{64}	ρ_{65}	1

Figure 8.4 Examples of possible auto-correlation matrix structures arising from six equally time-spaced observations in a repeated measures study design

depend on the choice of the times we choose to compare, the correlation matrix is of the form of Figure 8.4(b). This is clearly a simple pattern but nevertheless implies that, for example, to fit a single covariate linear model we have to estimate the parameter, ρ, in addition to β_0, β_1, and σ.

Auto-regressive

In some situations it may be supposed that as the time between observations increases, the auto-correlation between observations at those times will decrease. Thus, we might assume that the auto-correlation takes the form: $\rho_T\left(y_{t1}, y_{t2}\right) = \rho^{|t_2 - t_1|}$, where $|t_2 - t_1|$ is the absolute value of the difference between t_1 and t_2, that is, whether the time difference is negative or positive we give it a positive value. Consequently, provided $|\rho_T| < 1$, $\rho_T(y_{t1}, y_{t2})$ will decline as the interval $|t_2 - t_1|$ increases. The correlation structure for the special case when there are equal intervals between successive measurements is given in Figure 8.4(c). This pattern was assumed in the analysis of changes in body-weight over time described by equation (8.1) and Figure 8.1(d) where the estimate of ρ is $r = 0.0556$. Thus, the auto-correlations, as shown in Figure 8.4(c), between measurements taken on the first day (Column y1) and the successive days (Rows y1, y2, ... , y6) would be $0.0556^{1-1} = 0.0556^0 = 1$, $\rho = 0.05556^{2-1} = 0.0556^1 = 0.05556$, $\rho^2 = 0.0556^{3-1} = 0.0556^2 = 0.003091$, ... , $\rho^5 = 0.0556^{6-1} = 0.0556^5 = 0.0000005$.

Unstructured

In this case, there is no consistent pattern over time in the auto-correlation matrix so that in the example of Figure 8.4(d) there are 15 distinct auto-correlations to estimate in addition to the regression coefficients themselves and σ. As one might imagine, this situation requires more complex algorithms to conduct the necessary calculations and, in practice, this often restricts the types of studies that can be analyzed under the unstructured assumption.

Examining patterns

One method of trying to determine the pattern of the auto-correlation matrix is to produce scatter plots of all the pairwise combinations within the data set. Thus, Figure 8.5 shows the scatter plots of the 15 pairwise comparisons that can be made of the PCS data of which part is given in Figure 8.2. This figure also includes the associated matrix of the corresponding correlation coefficients. However, in this example, because of 'missing' observations (resulting from the gaps in Figure 8.2(a)), the number of subjects contributing to the correlation estimates varies considerably. The correlations range from 0.1286 to 0.9205 (median 0.4479), and from this we may conclude that the auto-correlation matrix is not of the independent type (as all correlations are far from zero). However, these values cannot be interpreted easily as the time intervals between successive observations are not equal. The earlier assessments are spaced 3-monthly, and the later 6-monthly. Nevertheless, there is some suggestion of a decline in correlation with increasing interval, for example, the value for PCS3 against PCS6 is approximately 0.64, whereas against PCS24 is 0.25, perhaps suggesting that the underlying auto-correlation pattern may have an auto-regressive form.

FIXED-EFFECTS MODELS

Changes over time

As we have indicated by equation (8.1), the standard linear regression model has to be modified to accommodate the repeated measures design. Thus, we may have n subjects recruited with m_i repeat observations made on subject i. In the repeated measures situation including several subjects, the measurement y_i is replaced by y_{ij} as it is repeated on $j = 1$, $2, \ldots, m_i$ occasions for individual i. The least complex situation is when the number of observations per subject does not vary so $m_i = m$ for all n subjects, although in medical studies this ideal is not so often achieved. Similarly, the suffices 'ij' need to be added to t and η to give:

$$y_{ij} = \beta_0 + \beta_1 t_{ij} + \eta_{ij} \qquad (8.3)$$

Here β_0 and β_1 are the fixed, often termed population-averaged, parameters that have to be estimated with the data from all the study subjects. This implies that all subject information is combined to provide estimates of the same two parameters, β_0 and β_1. Finally, η_{ij} are the random (or error) departures of $Y_{ij} = \beta_0 + \beta_1 t_{ij}$ which we could calculate if we knew the true values of the regression model parameters. The individual values of the η_{ij} are assumed to average out at 0 over the observations from subject i but will not be independent of each other. Nevertheless, information from the different individuals concerned in the study remains independent of each other.

When describing simple linear regression we provided, in equation (1.8), the algebraic expressions for the estimates of the regression coefficients β_0 and β_1 and, in (1.9), that for the estimate of the standard deviation, σ. Alternatively expressed, the corresponding maximum

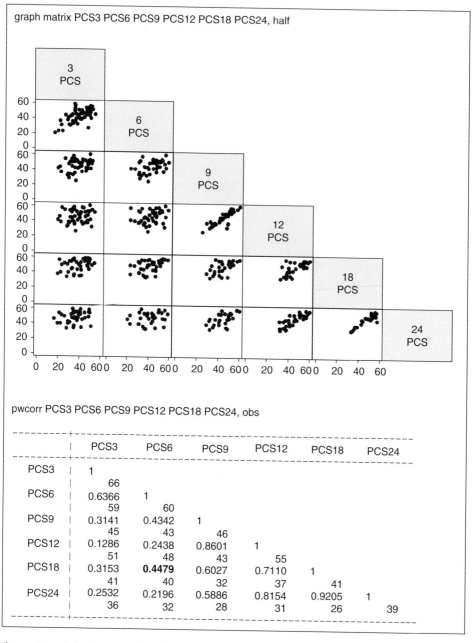

Figure 8.5 Pairwise scatter plots of successive (repeated) measures of post-surgery PCS and associated estimated auto-correlation coefficients (part data from Nejadnik, Hui, Choong, *et al.*, 2010)

likelihood equation has explicit solutions. From these, with the data on *x*, and *y* from *n* subjects, we can then calculate the corresponding estimates in a straightforward manner. Unfortunately, in the more complex situations of repeated measures, explicit expressions for the parameter estimates (additionally requiring estimates of parameters associated with the auto-correlation) are usually not available. Indeed, the likelihood equations to solve are often

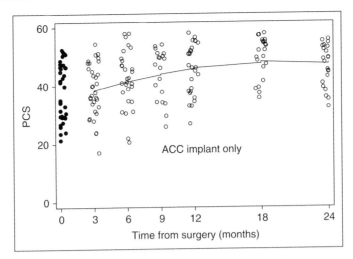

Figure 8.6 Scatter plot of baseline and successive post-implantation PCS assessments with jittering to better reveal the individual data points and a Lowess smoothed curve added to help identify the general pattern in the post-surgery values (part data from Nejadnik, Hui, Choong, *et al.*, 2010)

exceedingly complex. Fortunately, statistical packages enable the necessary calculations to be performed which then permit the corresponding models to be fitted to the data.

As is appropriate in many situations, a scatter plot of the *y*-measure against a covariate (in this case time) is often of value to help select an appropriate model. However, for the post-cartilage surgery example, PCS0 is a pre-surgical assessment and may therefore be thought of as a covariate rather than as an outcome measure. A scatter plot of the data arising from the study is given in Figure 8.6. From the fitted Lowess smoothed curve (see *Technical details* for a description of Lowess) through the successive post-surgery values there is a suggestion that PCS rose over the first 12 months and perhaps stabilized thereafter, although considerable variation is apparent. In summary, and provided we regard the baseline PCS (PCS0) as a covariate, we might initially assume a linear model for the whole post-surgery period. However, as we have indicated in Figure 8.2(b), individual profiles may differ substantially from this general pattern.

When considering the PCS data of Figure 8.6, the simplest situation arises if we think of *time* as the only covariate that we have to consider. In this case, the linear model can be written as:

$$PCS_{ij} = \beta_0 + \beta_{Time}t_{ij} + \eta_{ij} \tag{8.4}$$

One method for estimating β_0 and β_{Time} in the presence of auto-correlation is based on the population-average model using the Generalized Estimating Equation (GEE) algorithm which is implemented in Stata by using the command (**xtgee**).

Figure 8.7(a) compares the repeated measures approach to modeling the PCS post-cartilage surgery data using (**xtgee**) with the assumption of *independence* of the repeated observations with that of fitting by OLS as is used for simple linear regression. Not surprisingly these calculations give essentially the same results. The respective small differences in, for example, $SE(b_{Time})$ estimated as 0.0689 and 0.0687 arise as different computational algorithms are used by the two programs.

(a) *Linear regression model*

regress PCS t

Number of obs = 304

PCS	Coef	SE	t	p-value	95% CI
b_0	39.6959	0.8786			
b_{Time}	0.4053	0.0689	5.88	0.0001	0.2696 to 0.5409

xtgee PCS t, i(id) corr(independent)

GEE population-averaged model

Number of obs = 304, Number of groups = 68
Obs per group: min = 2 , avg = 4.5, max = 6

PCS	Coef	SE	t	p-value	95% CI
b_0	39.6959	0.8757			
b_{Time}	0.4053	0.0687	5.90	0.0001	0.2706 to 0.5399

(b) *Auto-correlated models*

Exchangeable

xtgee PCS t, i(id) corr(exchangeable) vce(boot)

Number of obs = 304, Number of groups = 68
Obs per group: min = 2, avg = 4.5, max = 6

PCS	Coef	SE	t	p-value	95% CI
b_0	39.3856	1.1986			
b_{Time}	0.4499	0.0670	6.71	0.0001	0.3185 to 0.5813

estat wcorrelation

Estimated within-id correlation matrix R:

	PCS3	PCS6	PCS9	PCS12	PCS18	PCS24
PCS3	1					
PCS6	0.4690					
PCS9	0.4690	0.4690	1			
PCS12	0.4690	0.4690	0.4690	1		
PCS18	0.4690	0.4690	0.4690	0.4690	1	
PCS24	0.4690	0.4690	0.4690	0.4690	0.4690	1

Autoregressive

xtgee PCS t, i(id) corr(autoregressive) vce(boot)

Number of obs = 37, Number of groups = 12
Obs per group: min = 2, avg = 3.1, max = 4

Note many data items omitted from this estimation

PCS	Coef	SE	t	p-value	95% CI
b_0	40.4614	2.6266			
b_{Time}	0.4657	0.4626	1.01	0.31	−0.4409 to 1.3723

Figure 8.7 Linear regression and repeated measures models to describe post-surgery PCS assessments for patients receiving autologous implantation following cartilage repair (part data from Nejadnik, Hui, Choong, *et al.*, 2010)

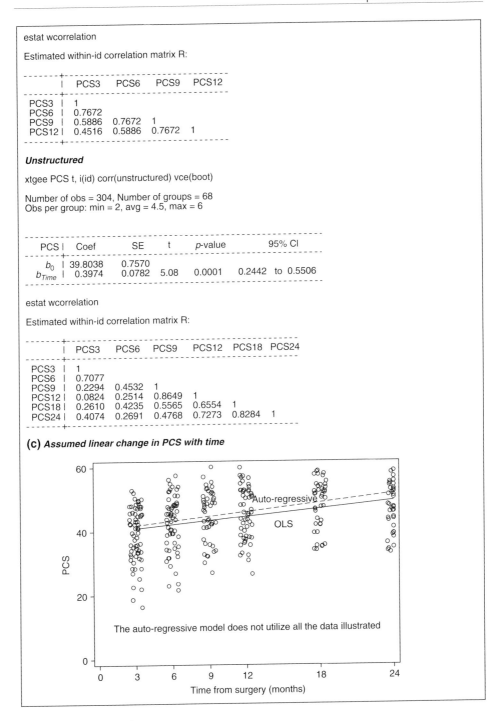

```
estat wcorrelation

Estimated within-id correlation matrix R:

-------+----------------------------------
       |  PCS3    PCS6    PCS9   PCS12
-------+----------------------------------
PCS3  |  1
PCS6  |  0.7672
PCS9  |  0.5886   0.7672   1
PCS12 |  0.4516   0.5886   0.7672   1
-------+----------------------------------
```

Unstructured

xtgee PCS t, i(id) corr(unstructured) vce(boot)

Number of obs = 304, Number of groups = 68
Obs per group: min = 2, avg = 4.5, max = 6

```
----------------------------------------------------------------
  PCS |   Coef      SE      t    p-value        95% CI
------+---------------------------------------------------------
 b₀  | 39.8038   0.7570
 b_Time | 0.3974   0.0782  5.08   0.0001   0.2442  to  0.5506
----------------------------------------------------------------
```

estat wcorrelation

Estimated within-id correlation matrix R:

```
-------+------------------------------------------------------
       |  PCS3    PCS6    PCS9   PCS12  PCS18  PCS24
-------+------------------------------------------------------
PCS3  |  1
PCS6  |  0.7077
PCS9  |  0.2294   0.4532   1
PCS12 |  0.0824   0.2514   0.8649   1
PCS18 |  0.2610   0.4235   0.5565   0.6554   1
PCS24 |  0.4074   0.2691   0.4768   0.7273   0.8284   1
-------+------------------------------------------------------
```

(c) *Assumed linear change in PCS with time*

Figure 8.7 (Continued)

However, with the *exchangeable* assumption of Figure 8.7(b), there are now noticeable differences, for example, b_{Time} has now changed from 0.4053 to 0.4499 indicating a marginally greater increase in PCS over time. Nevertheless, whichever method of fitting the model is chosen, the slope is statistically significantly different from zero with p-value <0.0001 in each case. In this situation, and following the command (**xtgee PCS t, i(id) corr(exchangeable)**), the command (**estat wcorrelation**) of Figure 8.7(b) provides an estimate of the common auto-correlation as 0.4690, which is close to the median value of 0.4479 given in Figure 8.5.

Earlier we conjectured that the auto-correlation may take the auto-regressive form. After making this assumption in Figure 8.7(b), the estimates of $b_0 = 40.4614$ and $b_{Time} = 0.4657$ do not differ markedly from the earlier calculations. However, because of gaps in the data, in order to fit the model with the auto-regressive assumption, the program had to exclude many study participants and so the $SE(b_{Time}) = 0.4626$ is much larger than that estimated by the other models. A further consequence is that the estimation process is automatically confined (in this example) to the first four post-operative assessments. This estimates the auto-correlation between two successive measures three months apart as $r_3 = 0.7672$, those six months apart as $r_6 = 0.7672^2 = 0.5886$ and $r_9 = 0.7672^3 = 0.4516$. The difference between the estimates provided by the auto-regressive auto-correlation and the OLS estimates of the linear regression equation are shown in Figure 8.7(c), and are not very major as the same general trend of increasing PCS over time is demonstrated. Nevertheless, it is important to note that assuming the auto-correlation structure is auto-regressive reduces the number of groups (here patients useful for modeling purposes) from 68 to only 12 so that the associated $SE(b_{Time}) = 0.4626$ is seriously inflated compared with the estimates obtained when other auto-correlation structures are utilized.

Finally, if one assumes the auto-correlation is unstructured the regression model estimates become $b_0 = 39.8038$, $b_{Time} = 0.3974$ and $SE(b_{Time}) = 0.0782$. The 15 auto-correlation coefficients range in value from 0.0824 to 0.8649 with a median of 0.4532.

The calculations of the standard errors of the regression coefficients from data in a repeated measures design are quite sensitive to the assumptions made when defining the model to fit. Thus, as we outline in Chapter 5, *Over-dispersion and robust estimates*, robust methods of estimating these quantities are therefore recommended. In this example, we have used bootstrap estimates by adding (**vce(boot)**) to all but the (**corr(independent)**) command of Figure 8.7(a), although the options available are likely to differ between different software packages.

Comparing groups

In a certain sense, we are not so interested in how the PCS measure changes with time, although if increasing values of physical performance indicate improvement for the patient then this is, of course, important. What we need to know in a comparative clinical study is whether the particular method of implantation by autologous BMSC or by ACC given to the patient influences the outcome. So the model we now have to consider for comparing two treatments is:

$$y_{ij} = \beta_0 + \beta_{Time} t_{ij} + \beta_{Implant} Implant_i + \eta_{ij} \tag{8.5}$$

where $Implant_i = 0$ (ACC) or 1 (BMSC) depending on the implant concerned.

For illustrative reasons we assume that the auto-correlation has the exchangeable form as this uses all the data available. This model is fitted using the command (**xtgee PCS t**

`Implant i(id) corr(exchangeable) vce(boot))`, and the results are given in Figure 8.8. This estimates the PCS score difference between implants as $b_{Implant}=0.9057$, which is not statistically significant in this case (p-value$=0.55$) with changes over time (p-value$=0.0001$) increasing by an estimated $b_{Time}=0.4515$ units per month.

The calculation of the auto-correlation involves calculating the residuals of the individual data values from that estimated by the fitted model. If there is a different model for each implant, then residuals are calculated by comparing observed values with those predicted by the associated implantation group. When there is a substantial difference between groups, the corresponding residuals will be much smaller in magnitude than those calculated assuming no difference between groups. In such a case the estimated auto-correlations may be substantially changed. In our situation, however, the estimated difference between implants is small with an associated auto-correlation of $r=0.4715$, which is not very different from 0.4690 obtained earlier in Figure 8.7(b).

Although in equation (8.5) the 'time' and 'implant' can be thought of as covariates, and the fitting process regards these as such, it is better to think of these variables as features of the design. So, as we describe in Chapter 7, we designate these as design- or D-variables rather than simply covariates. Also it may be better to write the model in the reordered format as: $y_{ij}=\beta_0+\beta_{Implant}Implant_i+\beta_{Time}t_{ij}+\eta_{ij}$, to emphasize that, of the two D-variable parameters concerned, $\beta_{Implant}$ is the major focus. In practice there will be occasions when $\beta_{Time}=0$ but, nevertheless, there may be a statistical difference between groups.

We noted earlier, that the baseline (pre-surgery) PCS measure (PCS0) may be considered a covariate as subsequent values may be influenced by these initial recordings. Thus, a patient with high PCS0 might be anticipated to have higher post-surgery values than one with low PCS0. In this situation model (8.5) may be extended to become:

$$PCS_{ij} = \beta_0 + \beta_{Implant}Implant_i + \beta_{Time}t_{ij} + \beta_{PCS0}PCS0_i + \eta_{ij} \qquad (8.6)$$

in which we regard the PCS0 as a known, or at least a very probable, K-covariate.

The results of fitting this extended model are shown in Figure 8.9. After adjusting for baseline PCS, the estimated difference between implants is now decreased in magnitude to 0.5074 and remains statistically not significant (p-value$=0.72$). Nevertheless, a value of $C=0.5074/0.9057=0.6$ in magnitude would be regarded as a statistically important change in the estimate, but, as the estimated effect size remains small, this change too would have little clinical impact. The estimated regression coefficient for time is essentially unchanged, and the associated (exchangeable) auto-correlation is estimated as 0.4213.

In general terms, more covariates could be added to the model, for example, it may be thought that male and female patients may have quite different experiences and their relative numbers in each implant group may affect the magnitude of the estimated difference between them. However, as we have seen, in order to fit repeated measures models there have to be sufficient data available to ensure that the resulting estimates are reliably estimated. This is almost certainly not the case with some of our illustrative analyses where, because of paucity of the data for the models we wish to describe, estimates of some of the regression coefficients have very large standard errors and hence there are extremely wide confidence intervals for the corresponding parameters. In general, longitudinal studies of whatever type require extra care with their design and implementation to ensure that *all* the data required (often of a large volume) are indeed collected by the investigating team.

```
tabulate Implant

---------+----------
Implant  |  Freq
---------+----------
    ACC  |   34
   BMSC  |   34
---------+----------
  Total  |   68
---------+----------
```

```
xtgee PCS t Implant, i(id) corr (exchangeable) robust
```

GEE population-averaged model

Number of obs = 304, Group variable: id, Number of groups = 68
Obs per group: min = 2, avg = 4.5, max = 6

PCS	Coef	Robust SE	z	p-value	[95% CI]
b_0	38.9194	1.4169			
$b_{Implant}$	0.9057	1.5307	0.59	0.55	−2.0944 to 3.9057
b_{Time}	0.4515	0.0689	6.55	0.0001	0.3165 to 0.5865

```
estat wcorrelation
```

	PCS3	PCS6	PCS9	PCS12	PCS18	PCS24
PCS3	1					
PCS6	0.4715	1				
PCS9	0.4715	0.4715	1			
PCS12	0.4715	0.4715	0.4715	1		
PCS18	0.4715	0.4715	0.4715	0.4715	1	
PCS24	0.4715	0.4715	0.4715	0.4715	0.4715	1

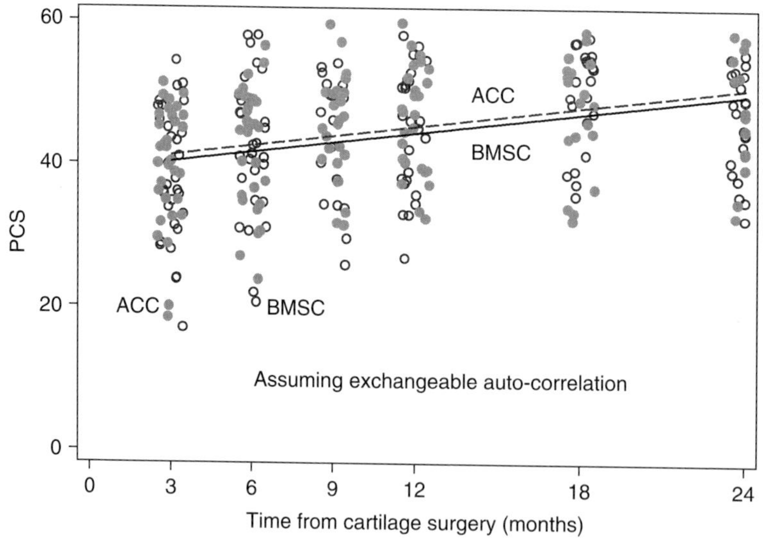

Figure 8.8 The effect of type of autologous implantation, ACC or BMSC, on post-surgery PCS score levels accounting for assumed linear changes over time (part data from Nejadnik, Hui, Choong, *et al.*, 2010)

```
xtgee PCS Implant t PCS0, i(id)  corr(exchangeable) robust
```

PCS	Coef	SE	z	p-value	[95% CI]
b_0	27.6156	3.3109			
$b_{Implant}$	0.5074	1.3991	0.36	0.72	−2.2348 to 3.2497
b_{Time}	0.4514	0.0688	6.56	0.0001	0.3165 to 0.5862
b_{PCS0}	0.2963	0.0809			

```
estat wcorrelation
```

	PCS3	PCS6	PCS9	PCS12	PCS18	PCS24
PCS3	1					
PCS6	0.4213	1				
PCS9	0.4213	0.4213	1			
PCS12	0.4213	0.4213	0.4213	1		
PCS18	0.4213	0.4213	0.4213	0.4213	1	
PCS24	0.4213	0.4213	0.4213	0.4213	0.4213	1

Figure 8.9 Testing the effect of implant received on subsequent PCS score levels accounting for assumed linear changes over time and adjusting for baseline PCS values (part data from Nejadnik, Hui, Choong, et al., 2010)

Multi-level models

Regression models like equation (8.5) and (8.6) can be thought of as consisting of two levels. One level (Level-1) corresponds to changes over time within each subject, while the second (Level-2) describes the between subject variation. Thus, these equations are referred to as 2-Level models. In Chapter 11 we describe, although in a quite different context, a 3-level model. In general these so-called hierarchical models can have multiple levels.

MIXED-EFFECTS MODELS

Random effects

If we return to equation (8.3), then this is a rather simplified version of the model for a repeated measures design in that it assumes every subject has the same underlying population-averaged model with parameters β_0 and β_1. Thus, apart from random variation which may obscure the underlying pattern, every individual is assumed to be following the same model trajectory over time. However, often a more realistic assumption is that each subject, i, has their own trajectory implying that each has his or her own personal values of the regression coefficients. In this situation each individual has their own fixed-effects model, which for subject, i is:

$$y_{ij} = \beta_{0i} + \beta_{Time,i}t_{ij} + \eta_{ij}$$ (8.7)

with repeated measures taken on $j = 1, 2, \ldots, m_i$ occasions.

The difficulty now is that β_{0i} and $\beta_{Time,i}$ have to be estimated for each subject from the m_i observations made, so that with say 100 subjects, 200 model parameters would need to be estimated. In addition, if there are relatively few repeated measures for some subjects the associated parameter estimates will not be very reliable.

To overcome these difficulties, random-effects models may be assumed. In such a model, the individual β_{0i} are assumed to follow a Normal distribution with a mean value of β_0^* and standard deviation of σ_0^*. The * is added here as a reminder that, for example, the random-effects β_0^* differs in nature from β_0 of the fixed-effect model. Similarly, we also have the parameter β_{Time}^* and the standard deviation, σ_{Time}^*, for the change with time component of the regression model. The model corresponding to (8.7) is now written as:

$$y_{ij} = \beta_0^* + \beta_{Time}^* t_{ij} + \eta_{ij}^* \tag{8.8}$$

where η_{ij} of (8.7) is replaced by η_{ij}^* (which contains elements of η_{ij}) with standard deviation denoted $\sigma_{Residual}^*$. However, within $\sigma_{Residual}^*$ are also the components of the variation summarized by σ_0^* and σ_{Time}^*. This random-effects model reduces the number of regression coefficients to two once more (β_0^* and β_{Time}^*), but with two additional parameters, σ_0^* and σ_{Time}^*, to be estimated. However, this is far fewer than would be the case with model (8.7).

Random and fixed effects components

A situation that often arises is when some of the terms in a repeated measures model may be considered as random, whereas others are fixed. In such cases the regression models are then referred to as mixed-models. For example, it is clear from the PCS0 data of Figure 8.6 that pre-surgery measures indicate a wide range of PCS scores at this stage. Thus, it may be no surprise, therefore, that the subjects concerned may have distinct subsequent score profiles. One possibility is that the intercept, β_0, may be thought of as a random effect, but all have a common (fixed-effect) time profile, β_{Time}. In this case the model becomes:

$$y_{ij} = \beta_0^* + \beta_{Time}^* t_{ij} + \zeta_{ij}^* \tag{8.9}$$

Here, η_{ij}^* is replaced by ζ_{ij}^* which has only two components, corresponding to $\sigma_{Residual}^*$ and σ_0^*, rather than three in the full random-effects model of (8.8).

If we fit this model with an unstructured auto-correlation assumption to the PCS data, then the command takes the form (**xtmixed PCS t || id: covariance(unstructured) robust**) and the results are given in Figure 8.10(a). The random effects estimate of the intercept, $b_0^* = 39.3933$ with standard deviation $s_0^* = 5.4599$. This suggests that individual patient intercept values range from approximately $39.3933 - 1.96 \times 5.4599$ to $39.3933 + 1.96 \times 5.4599$ or 28.69 to 50.09. This range covers much of the range of PCS0 scores of 22.7 to 53.2.

The OLS estimate of the slope of $b_{Time} = 0.4053$ given in Figure 8.10(b) is less than the fixed-effects estimate of $b_{Time} = 0.4487$ in the mixed model of Figure 8.10(a).

If we further assume that both intercept and slope are random effects, then the model of (8.8) is relevant and this is fitted using the command (**xtmixed PCS t || id: t**). The associated output is summarized in Figure 8.11. The random effects $b_0^* = 39.4156$ with standard deviation $s_0^* = 6.7723$, indicating individual intercept values ranging from $39.4156 - 1.96 \times 6.7723 = 26.14$ to $39.4156 + 1.96 \times 6.7723 = 52.69$. This now covers a wider range of PCS than the model with only the intercept as a random effect. Further,

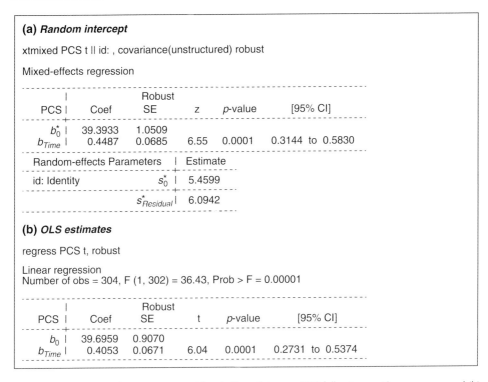

Figure 8.10 (a) Random intercept and fixed-effect of time on PCS following cartilage surgery, and (b) the corresponding OLS model (part data from Nejadnik, Hui, Choong *et al.*, 2010)

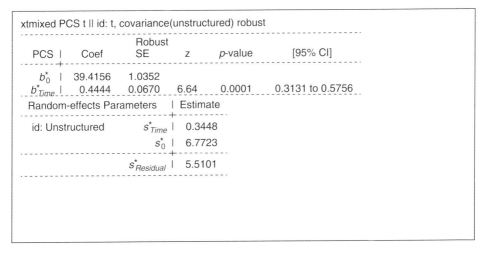

Figure 8.11   Random-effects model for intercept and slope for testing the effect of time on PCS post-cartilage surgery (part data from Nejadnik, Hui, Choong *et al.*, 2010)

the random-effects slope ranges over $0.4444 \pm 1.96 \times 0.3448$ or -0.2314 to $+1.1202$ PCS units of change per month. Thus, although the average profile indicates an increasing PCS score over time post-surgery, the negative values of some of the (individual) slopes indicate that there are clearly patients whose PCS levels decline over the study period.

Comparing implants

xtmixed PCS Implant t II id: t, covariance(unstructured) robust

PCS		Coef	Robust SE	z	p-value	[95% CI]
b^*_0	38.9814	1.3996			
$b_{Implant}$	0.8388	1.5388	0.55	0.59	−2.1771 to 3.8548
b^*_{Time}	0.4463	0.0672	6.64	0.0001	0.3145 to 0.5781

Random-effects Parameters	Estimate
s^*_0	6.7508
s^*_{Time}	0.3442
$s^*_{Residual}$	5.5099

Figure 8.12   Comparing implants with respect to PCS: mixed-model for random-effects intercept and slope and fixed-effect implant difference (part data from Nejadnik, Hui, Choong *et al.*, 2010)

However, the major focus of this study is to compare the relative efficacy of the two implants so an appropriate model to consider is the following one with a fixed effect for implant difference but random intercepts and slope:

$$PCS_{ij} = \beta^*_0 + \beta_{Implant}Implant_i + \beta^*_{Time}t_{ij} + \zeta^*_{ij} \tag{8.10}$$

The residual term denoted ζ^*_{ij} will have components concerned with σ^*_0 and σ^*_{Time} as well as residual variation. The results of fitting (8.10) to the PCS data are summarized in Figure 8.12 and give the estimated difference between implants as $b_{Implant}=0.84$ units (95% CI −2.18 to +3.85, p-value=0.59), the magnitude of which is unlikely to be of any clinical importance.

Binary endpoints

Viardot-Foucault, Prasath, Tai, *et al.* (2011) report the outcome following fertility treatment given to women who were seeking help in achieving conception. This study has a repeated measures design in which, on a woman-by-woman basis, following each cycle of treatment the endpoint was whether or not a successful pregnancy ensued. The repeated endpoint variable 'subsequent pregnancy' (Yes or No) is clearly a binary variable. However, there is no record of the time intervals between cycles. As a consequence, 'time' is the ranking of 1, 2 or 3 of the treatment cycle received. Some of the results are summarized in the wide file format of Figure 8.13(a), which includes a selection of individuals and their covariates at first presentation: age (*Age0*), endometrial thickness (*End0*) and numbers of mature follicles (*Foll0*) assessed at their first visit. Thus, for example, Patient id=26 was aged 40.5 years, endometrial thickness 7–7.9 mm, mature follicles 0, and had a single cycle of treatment but failed to achieve a pregnancy. She did not return for subsequent treatment and so is denoted as Sequence '0--', where '0' denotes 'fail' and '-' no treatment given. In contrast, Patient id=54 was aged 37.8 years, endometrial thickness of 8 mm or more, with 0 mature follicles also failed after the first cycle but subsequently received two more cycles and had a successful pregnancy on each occasion. Her sequence is denoted '011' in which '1' denotes 'success'. The women are classified by sequence type in Figure 8.13(b) and the vast majority (358+115+12=485 or 80.6%) failed after receiving one, two or three cycles of treatment. Nevertheless, 117 (19.4%) achieved at least one successful pregnancy.

Just as for the continuous endpoint variable situation, the wide file has to be converted to the long format for the repeated measures analysis. Part of this long file is shown in Figure 8.13(c). In this case because all the 'time' intervals are equal, the computer generated variable (_j) created by converting the wide file to long format exactly mirrors the covariate cycle (*Cyc*).

The simplest mixed model to consider for these data is that analogous to equation (8.9) and involves only time but now expressed in terms of the cycles of treatment received. Hence the corresponding logistic model is

$$\text{logit}(y_{ij}) = \beta_0^* + \beta_{Cycle}Cyc_{ij} + \eta_{ij} \tag{8.11}$$

where y_{ij} is a binary variable taking values 0 or 1. This is fitted assuming a random intercept, β_0^* (rather than fixed β_0) and a fixed slope, β_{Cycle}, using the mixed model command (**xtmelogit**) and assuming an unstructured auto-correlation. The full command (**xtmelogit Preg Cyc || (id):, covariance(unstructured)**) gives the results of Figure 8.14(a).

(a) Wide file format

list id Age0 End0 Foll0 Cyc1 Preg1 Cyc2 Preg2 Cyc3 Preg3 Sequence

id	Age0	End0	Foll0	Cyc1	Preg1	Cyc2	Preg2	Cyc3	Preg3	Sequence
26	40.5	7.0−7.9	0	1	0	.	.	.	.	0--
30	40.3	8+	0	1	1	.	.	.	.	1--
46	39.8	7.0−7.9	2	1	0	.	.	.	.	0--
47	39.0	<=6.9	2	1	0	2	0	.	.	00-
50	36.9	8+	2	1	0	2	0	.	.	00-
52	37.6	8+	1	1	0	2	0	3	0	000
54	37.8	8+	0	1	0	2	1	3	1	011
56	37.8	8+	2	1	0	.	.	.	.	0--
60	36.4	8+	0	1	0	2	1	.	.	01-
69	35.3	7.0–7.9	0	1	1	2	0	3	0	100

(b) Alternative sequences of treatment received and outcome

tabulate Sequence

Sequence	Freq.	Percent
0--	358	59.47
00-	115	19.10
000	12	1.99
001	1	0.17
01-	20	3.32
010	2	0.33
011	1	0.17
1--	77	12.79
10-	7	1.16
100	2	0.33
101	1	0.17
11-	4	0.66
110	2	0.33
Total	602	100.00

Figure 8.13 Repeated measures study of conception outcome following sessions at an assisted pregnancy clinic (part data from Viardot-Foucault, Prasath, Tai, *et al.*, 2011)

```
(c) Long file format

reshape long Preg, id

list id _j Age0 End0 Foll0 Cyc Preg Sequence
+-------------------------------------------------------+
| id   _j   Age0     End0    Foll0   Cyc   Preg Sequence |
|-------------------------------------------------------|
| 26    1   40.5    7.0-7.9     0      1      0    0--    |
| 30    1   40.3        8+      0      1      1    1--    |
| 46    1   39.8    7.0-7.9     2      1      0    0--    |
| 47    1   39        <=6.9     2      1      0    00-    |
| 47    2   39        <=6.9     2      2      0    00-    |
|-------------------------------------------------------|
| 50    1   36.9        8+      2      1      0    00-    |
| 50    2   36.9        8+      2      2      0    00-    |
| 52    1   37.6        8+      1      1      0    000    |
| 52    2   37.6        8+      1      2      0    000    |
| 52    3   37.6        8+      1      3      0    000    |
|-------------------------------------------------------|
| 54    1   37.8        8+      0      1      0    011    |
| 54    2   37.8        8+      0      2      1    011    |
| 54    3   37.8        8+      0      3      1    011    |
| 56    1   37.8        8+      2      1      0    0--    |
| 60    1   36.4        8+      0      1      0    01-    |
|-------------------------------------------------------|
| 60    2   36.4        8+      0      2      1    01-    |
| 69    1   35.3    7.0-7.9     0      1      1    100    |
| 69    2   35.3    7.0-7.9     0      2      0    100    |
| 69    3   35.3    7.0-7.9     0      3      0    100    |
+-------------------------------------------------------+
```

Figure 8.13 (Continued)

The estimated slope $b_{Cycle}=0.1108$ corresponds to an $OR=\exp(0.1108)=1.12$ suggesting that the probability of obtaining a pregnancy increases with increasing number of cycles. However, the result is far from being statistically significant with (**testparm   Cyc**) giving the p-value$=0.62$. If both the intercept and slope are assumed to be random effects as in Figure 8.14(b), then $b^*_{Cycle} = 0.3558$ with a large $SD(b^*_{Cycle})=0.3928$. This suggests that the individual slopes vary between $0.3558 \pm (1.96\times0.3928)$ or from −0.41 to 1.13, thereby indicating no systematic pattern of change over the cycles.

The number of pregnancies achieved in relation to the endometrial thickness ($End0$) determined from each woman immediately prior to the first cycle of infertility treatment is summarized in Figure 8.15(a) so that, for example, $(10+1)=11$ women conceived (13.6%) at some stage with endometrial thickness at first presentation of $\leq$ 6.9 mm and $(82+4)=86$ (21.2%) when thickness was ≥ 8 mm. The associated model takes the form

$$\text{logit}(y_{ij}) = \beta^*_0 + \gamma_{End0}End0_i + \beta^*_{Cycle}Cyc_{ij} + \eta_{ij} \tag{8.12}$$

However, although $End0$ is a 3-level ordered categorical covariate, a more cautious approach to analysis may first consider this as unordered and therefore the associated parameter, γ_{End0}, in equation (8.12) will be replaced by two parameters corresponding to the dummy variables that will need to be created.

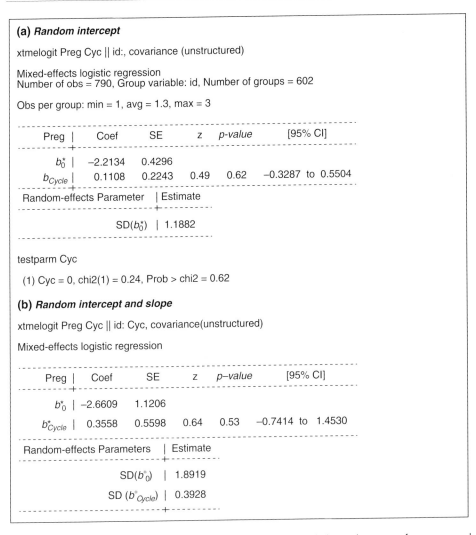

Figure 8.14 (a) Random intercept and (b) random intercept and slope alternatives for a repeated measures logistic model for conception outcome on cycle of treatment at an assisted pregnancy clinic (part data from Viardot-Foucault, Prasath, Tai, et al., 2011)

Assuming that the intercept and the slope parameter for *Cyc* are random effects, but those for the unordered categorical covariate *End*0 are fixed effects, then the repeated measures command for model (8.12) uses the mixed model command, the full details of which are shown in Figure 8.15(b) together with the corresponding output. Thus, the *OR* comparing those of thickness 7.0–7.9 mm with those of thickness ≤ 6.9 mm is 1.5415 (*p*-value = 0.37). If the endometrial thickness categories could be regarded as ordered categorical on a numerical scale of 0, 1 and 2 (say), this would imply that those of category 8.0+ mm would then have an *OR* of approximately $1.5415^2 = 2.41$. However, the actual *OR* = 1.9369 is not close to this and therefore suggests that it would not be appropriate to simplify the model using an equal interval numerical scale for *End*0.

(a) Number of pregnancies by first presentation endometrial thickness

tabulate End0 nPreg

```
---------+----------------------+------+----------+
         |                      |      |  Ever    |
         |        nPreg         |      | Pregnant |
End0Map  |   0     1     2  |  Total  |   (%)    |
---------+----------------------+------+----------+
  <=6.9  |  70    10     1  |   81    |   13.6   |
 7.0-7.9 |  96    17     3  |  116    |   17.2   |
    ≥8   | 319    82     4  |  405    |   21.2   |
---------+----------------------+------+----------|
  Total  | 485   109     8  |  602    |   19.4   |
---------+----------------------+------+----------+
```

(b) Fixed effect – unordered categorical variable endometrial thickness – Random – intercept and slope for cycle

xi : xtmelogit Preg i.End0 Cyc || id: Cyc, covariance (unstructured)

Mixed-effects logistic

Preg	Coef	SE	z	p-value	[95% CI]
b_0^*	−3.0786	1.1701			
b_{Cycle}^*	0.2841	0.5647	0.50	0.62	−0.8227 to 1.3909
$End0_{\leq 6.9}$	0				
$End0_{7-7.9}$	0.4327	0.4840	0.89	0.37	−0.5158 to 1.3813
$End0_{\geq 8}$	0.6611	0.4220	1.57	0.12	−0.1660 to 1.4882

Random–effects Parameters	Estimate
id: Unstructured	
SD (b_0^*)	1.6819
SD (b_{Cycle}^*)	0.2577

Preg	OR	SE
$End0_{\leq 6.9}$	1	
$End0_{7-7.9}$	1.5415	0.7460
$End0_{\geq 8}$	1.9369	0.8174
Cyc	1.3286	0.7503

Figure 8.15   Influence of endometrial thickness at first presentation from a repeated measures study of the conception outcome following sessions at an assisted pregnancy clinic (part data from Viardot-Foucault, Prasath, Tai, et al., 2011)

The number of pregnancies achieved in relation to the number of mature follicles at first presentation is summarized in Figure 8.16(a) so that, for example, 57 women (18.0%) conceived at some stage with no mature follicles at first presentation and 14 (26.9%) when there were three or more. The associated mixed model command with fixed effect for *Foll0* and random effects for the constant and *Cyc* is given in Figure 8.16(b). The estimated $OR = 1.2040$ (95% CI 0.9629 to 1.5054, p-value = 0.10) is relatively large but is not statistically significant, as is confirmed using the (**testparm Foll0**) command.

(a) *Number of pregnancies by number of mature follicles at first presentation*

tabulate Foll0 nPreg

```
--------+-----------------------------+-------+-----------+
        |                             |       |   Ever    |
        |           nPreg             |       | Pregnant  |
 Foll0  |     0          1         2  | Total |    (%)    |
--------+-----------------------------+-------+-----------+
    0   |   260         54         3  |  317  |   18.0    |
    1   |    65         12         1  |   78  |   16.7    |
    2   |   122         30         3  |  155  |   21.3    |
    3   |    38         13         1  |   52  |   26.9    |
--------+-----------------------------+-------+-----------+
 Total  |   485        109         8  |  602  |   19.4    |
--------+-----------------------------+-------+-----------+
```

(b) *Single numerical covariate – number of mature follicles*

xtmelogit Preg Foll0 Cyc || id: Cyc, covariance (unstructured)

Mixed-effects logistic regression

```
----------------------------------------------------------------------
     Preg  |    Coef      SE       z    p-value        [95% CI]
-----------+----------------------------------------------------------
     b₀*    |  -2.4484   1.0209
  b*Cycle  |   0.1499   0.5792   0.26    0.80    -0.9854 to 1.2851
  bFoll0   |   0.1856   0.1140   1.63    0.10    -0.0378 to 0.4091
-----------+----------------------------------------------------------
     Preg  |     OR       SE       z    P>|z|          [95% CI]
-----------+----------------------------------------------------------
      Cyc  |   1.2040   0.6727   1.63    0.10     0.9629 to 1.5054
    Foll0  |   1.1617   0.1372
----------------------------------------------------------------------
 Random-effects Parameters | Estimate
---------------------------+------------
id : Unstructured          |
            SD(b₀*) | 1.2819
        SD(b*Cycle) | 0.0632
--------------------------------------------
```

testparm Foll0
(1) Foll0 = 0, chi2(1) = 2.65, Prob > chi2 = 0.10

(c) *Testing for linearity*

gen SQFoll0 = Foll0*Foll0

reshape long Preg Cyc, i(id)

xtmelogit Preg Foll0 SQFoll0 Cyc || id: Cyc, covariance (unstructured)

Mixed-effects logistic

```
------------------------------------
     Preg  |    Coef      SE
-----------+------------------------
     b₀*    |  -2.4756   1.0214
  b*Cycle  |   0.1847   0.5658
  bFoll0   |  -0.0676   0.3926
 bSQFoll0  |   0.1002   0.1490
------------------------------------
```

testparm SQFoll0

(1) SQFoll0 = 0, chi2 (1) = 0.45, Prob > chi2 = 0.50

Figure 8.16 Influence of the number of mature follicles at first presentation from a repeated measures study of outcome following sessions at an assisted pregnancy clinic (part data from Viardot-Foucault, Prasath, Tai, *et al.*, 2011)

However, there is a suggestion that the proportions ever pregnant in Figure 8.16(a) are very similar when the number of mature follicles is 0 or 1 and then rises when the numbers increase. This suggests it may be appropriate to merge the first two groups or to check whether a more complex model is required to better summarise these data.

If the latter option is taken, the squared term *SQFoll0* of Figure 8.16(c) is first created. This has to be generated using the wide format database which, once obtained, must then be reshaped into the long format. Following this, the quadratic model is fitted by means of (**xtm-elogit Preg Foll0 SQFoll0 Cyc || id: Cyc, covariance(unstructured)**)). Testing the quadratic term using the (**testparm SQFoll0**) command does not reject the null hypothesis that the quadratic regression coefficient is zero (*p*-value=0.50), and hence the more complex model is not likely to be justified.

In practice, if both the number of mature follicles and the endometrial thickness are both considered as potentially important covariates then the model can be extended to include them both. As 'time' is a key aspect of all these models it is usually advisable to always include it in the modeling process and (even if not statistically significant) in all circumstances describe the details of its effect in the subsequent study report.

SUBJECT-SPECIFIC VERSUS POPULATION-AVERAGED MODELS

In the section *Fixed-effects models*, we described how repeated measures data may be analyzed for a continuous outcome variable such as PCS score using the population-averaged model based on the GEE algorithm. Although not specifically illustrated, the GEE procedure may also be similarly implemented for the analysis of binary endpoints, such as a successful pregnancy. In general, the estimated regression coefficients for the random-intercept or mixed effects logistic models such as those of Figure 8.14(a) and Figure 8.14(b) will be more extreme (further from the null value of 0) than those fitted by the GEE model of Figure 8.17 with command (**xtlogit Preg Cyc, pa vce(robust)**)). Such discrepancies arise because the GEE logistic regression models fit the overall population-averaged probabilities, whereas the random effects or mixed effects logistic regression models fit subject-specific probabilities of individuals (Rabe-Hesketh and Skrondal, 2008). Thus in the random-intercept model of Figure 8.14(a), we can interpret the $OR=\exp(0.1108)=1.12$ for cycle, as a 12% increase in odds of pregnancy per increase in treatment cycle for each patient. On the other hand, the estimated population-averaged $OR=\exp(0.0876)=1.09$,

```
xtlogit Preg Cyc, pa vce(robust)

GEE population-averaged model
Number of obs = 790,        Group variable: id,         Number of groups = 602
Link : logit,               Family : binomial,          Correlation: exchangeable
--------------------------------------------------------------------------------------
               |              Robust
         Preg  |    Coef       SE        z     p-value          [95% CI]
---------------+----------------------------------------------------------------------
          b₀   |  -1.7742    0.2494
       b_Cycle |   0.0876    0.1807     0.49     0.63      -0.2665 to 0.4418
--------------------------------------------------------------------------------------
```

Figure 8.17 Population-averaged logistic regression model for conception outcome on cycle of treatment at an assisted pregnancy clinic (part data from Viardot-Foucault, Prasath, Tai, *et al.*, 2011)

suggests a 9% increase in odds of pregnancy per increase in treatment cycle amongst the women who attended the assisted pregnancy clinic.

TECHNICAL DETAILS

Analytical options

It should be recognized that there are many analytical options available for summarizing repeated measures designs. As ever, the models chosen should reflect the key questions posed by the design. Nevertheless, once the appropriate model(s) is determined, there are still options with respect to the choice of the auto-correlation structure and the type of robust estimator of the corresponding standard errors. Choices for these may be guided by experience gained from the analysis of previous studies.

One should also be aware that different software packages may offer different analytical options and, further, that approaches are constantly under refinement and new statistical development is continually in progress.

In some of our examples, the results from using models allowing for a specific auto-correlation structure have not differed a great deal from those using an independence assumption. However, even though this may often be the case for the estimated regression coefficients, the extent of agreement is likely to be very data specific. In general, if the auto-correlations are high then the differences will generally be larger. Despite the lack of major differences in the estimates of the regression coefficients, we have shown how the corresponding estimated standard errors (SE) may differ depending on the auto-correlation structure assumed. We also recommend that robust methods should always be used to obtain the standard errors.

Lowess

The Locally Weighted Scatterplot Smoothing (Lowess) curve estimated in Figure 8.6 ignores the auto-correlation structure of the data concerned. The process begins at the left-hand extremity of the scatter plot by identifying a window in time (say one month – more precisely 30 days) and calculates the mean value (although there are other possibilities) of all the PCS assessments made within that time-frame. The process closes, by calculating the mean of all the assessments falling in the last month (at about four years) of observation. In between these two extremes, the month window moves from left to right observation time-point by time-point continually (by dropping the former and adding the latter) calculating all the corresponding means. The means once calculated are then plotted to produce the smooth Lowess. If the width of the window (termed the bandwidth) is too small, then very few points will be in each window and the resulting plot will not be very smooth. In contrast, if the bandwidth is too large then this may smooth out entirely the underlying pattern. Clearly, in our PCS example with very large 'gaps' in the data, some refinement of this methodology is required. A more detailed account of Lowess is given by Diggle, Liang and Zeger (1994).

9   Regression Trees

SUMMARY

This chapter describes the use of regression trees to help identify, among patients with a particular disease or condition, homogeneous subgroups each with an identifiable but different prognosis. The aim of establishing the groups is to tailor subsequent treatment and/or care in order to improve the ensuing outcome. The classification consists of a tree-like structure beginning with a single mother or root node which is split into branches to form intermediate and/or terminal nodes referred to variously as offspring nodes, daughter or son nodes, or leaf. The root node represents all patients in the study, whereas the offspring nodes correspond to (relatively) homogeneous subgroups of patients that are identified based on specific covariate information. Subsequently, as the tree evolves, the nodes become increasingly more homogeneous, thereby identifying important segments of the data. Details of how the tree growing process is curtailed, using a tree pruning procedure, as well as difficulties associated with the regression tree approach are included.

INTRODUCTION

A key objective of many medical studies is to define a set of clinical criteria to identify patients with a specific disease condition who, at diagnosis, are predisposed to be at differential risk of recovery. Thus, *Example 1.7* identified, among 8,800 young patients with neuroblastoma (NB), a regression tree of 20 terminal nodes. One terminal node of the section of the tree shown in Figure 1.13 arises from a split of the mother node of 8,800 patients into a left daughter of 5,131 patients who are INSS stage 1, 2, 3, or 4S, and then a further split creates a granddaughter node comprising 162 patients who are either ganglio-neuroma (GN), maturing ganglioneuroblastoma (GNB) or intermixed. This terminal node has a 5-year event-free survival (EFS) of 97% and an overall survival (OS) of 98%, and hence defines a subgroup of patients with excellent prognosis.

Standard regression models such as those we have described so far in this text are commonly used to generate decision rules for classifying patients into clinically relevant

Regression Methods for Medical Research, First Edition. Bee Choo Tai and David Machin.
© 2014 Bee Choo Tai and David Machin. Published 2014 by John Wiley & Sons, Ltd.

categories. For example, Tan, Law, Ng and Machin (2003) used a Cox proportional hazards approach to establish a prognostic model to identify patients with hepatocellular carcinoma (HCC) of low-, medium- and high-risk with associated 6-month survival probabilities of 43%, 21% and 3%, respectively. Specifically, they studied 11 potential covariates from which three: Zubrod score (0, 1, >2 or unknown), Ascites (Absent, Present or unknown), and serum alpha-fetoprotein (AFP, μg/L) level, were selected to form a simple prognostic model. The aim was to facilitate the management of such patients by adopting a risk-based strategy for the choice of their subsequent treatment. However, this type of model (although this need not be the case) does not take note of the influences of possible interactions between some of the covariates concerned. Thus, the HCC model assumes that, for one particular patient group (say those with Zubrod score=0), the influence of another covariate (say the presence of Ascites) will have precisely the same negative effect as in each of the other Zubrod score groups.

In contrast, the Classification And Regression Tree (CART) methodology, initially proposed by Breiman, Freedman, Olshen and Stone (1984), generates clinical decision rules without requiring any model assumptions. The Classification aspect of the method deals with outcome variables which are binary, such as whether or not a patient has hypertension, or are categorical in nature. In contrast, Regression Tree usually refers to situations where the outcome of concern is continuous such as diastolic blood pressure (DBP) recorded in mmHg. However, the technique may be extended to outcomes which are count or time-to-event in nature, for example, the number of fracture patients attending Accident & Emergency Departments over a period of time in several hospitals, or the survival time of children following a diagnosis of NB.

ILLUSTRATIVE EXAMPLE

Lee, Tai, Soon, *et al*. (2010) used a set of intravascular ultrasound-derived anatomic criteria (covariates) to identify patients likely to have functionally significant stenoses as assessed by low fractional flow reserve (FFR). A binary outcome of FFR<0.75 or 75% (termed LowFFR) indicates that the blockage is severe enough to obstruct blood flow. They assessed FFR in all patients and, among the anatomic criteria recorded, plaque burden (PB, %), minimum lumen area (MLA, mm^2) and lesion length (LL, mm) were then used to construct a classification tree in the form of Figure 9.1. The principal covariate was established as the PB. The values of this covariate were then divided to define daughter nodes using a cut-point of<79.09%, which identified a group of 39 (45.9%) patients with a low PB and among this group (Node *A* - a terminal node) only 1 (2.6%) was identified as LowFFR. In contrast, 32/46 (69.6%) in the group with high PB (Node II) were regarded as LowFFR.

This latter group of 46 patients was then subdivided on the basis of the lesion (MLA). This identified 9 with an area$\geq$2.25 mm^2 of which, in this second terminal node *B*, 1 (11.1%) had LowFFR. The 37 with area<2.25 mm^2 were then further subdivided by a cut-point of 12.55 mm for their lesion length (LL) to define terminal node *C* with 26/27 (96.3%) and terminal node *D* with 5/10 (50.0%) LowFFR, respectively.

The classification tree has two intermediate (nodes II and III) and four terminal nodes (*A*, *B*, *C*, *D*). The latter are each given their designated class as good, intermediate or poor prognosis. Terminal node *D* is designated *Intermediate*, although the actual proportions of Low and High are equal.

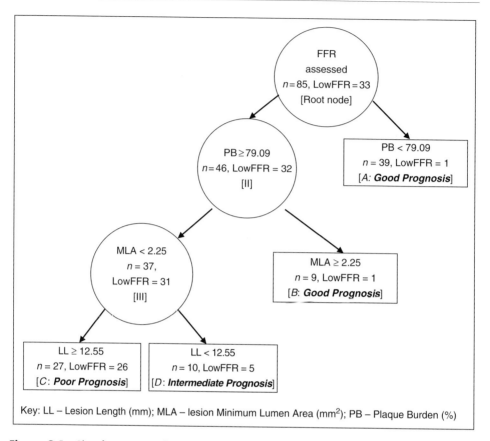

Key: LL – Lesion Length (mm); MLA – lesion Minimum Lumen Area (mm²); PB – Plaque Burden (%)

Figure 9.1 Classification tree obtained from identifying significant risk factors of low fractional flow reserve (LowFFR) and their respective cut-points to define Good and Poor prognostic groups in patients having undergone non-urgent coronary angiography (part data from Lee, Tai, Soon, *et al.*, 2010)

Thus, the four eventual leaves, [A], [B], [D], and [C], of the classification tree of Figure 9.1, identify groups with LowFFR of 2.6, 11.1, 50.0, and 96.3%, respectively.

TREE BUILDING

The tree growing process is a binary recursive partitioning procedure which divides, for example, the root node (the upper circular disc of Figure 9.1) and subsequent non-terminal offspring nodes (the other circular discs) into further terminal or non-terminal offspring nodes repeatedly. Each split is evaluated to maximize the discriminant ability of each covariate given the previous splits. The criterion used to make the splits varies with the type of outcome variable concerned.

The process therefore involves identifying the principal covariates concerned, ranking these, and then dividing each ranked covariate into two groups on some basis. Within each of the daughter nodes thereby created, consideration has now to be given as to whether other covariate information can be used to create more branches or if the branch is to remain a single stem and hence be designated a terminal node or leaf. Once this process is completed, further branches from the intermediate nodes may or may not need to be developed.

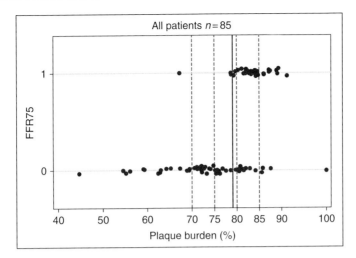

Figure 9.2 Scatter plot of the binary variable FFR75 against plaque burden (PB) in patients who had undergone non-urgent coronary angiography (part data from Lee, Tai, Soon, *et al.*, 2010)

Binary outcome

As we have noted, in the study of Lee, Tai, Soon, *et al.* (2010), those patients with FFR<75% (LowFFR) were considered to have functionally significant lesions, and were coded FFR75=1. The remainder, with FFR≥75%, were coded FFR75=0. Thus, the continuous endpoint FFR is converted to one of a binary form.

Continuous covariates

Figure 9.2 shows a scatter plot of FFR75 against plaque burden (PB) from which it can be seen that the majority with FFR75=1 have a high PB, with only a few patients with PB less than 80% giving a clear indication that daughter nodes might be created by a division close to this value. In contrast, PB has a wider range of values in those with FFR75=0.

In order to distinguish overlapping observations in the horizontal directions of FFR75 equal to 0 and 1, some jittering of the plotting positions of the data points has been used. However, such a process also induces jitter in the vertical direction and so this graph (and others in this chapter) appears to imply that non-integer values are possible. This is not the case; FFR75 can only take either of the two possible values of 0 or 1.

The process of identifying where a cut should be made to define two daughters proceeds along the following lines. In general, if the covariate x is a continuous variable taking n distinct values $(x_1, x_2, \dots, x_n)$ these can be ranked from smallest to largest to give $(x_{[1]}, x_{[2]}, \dots, x_{[n]})$. For example, for the 85 patients of Figure 9.2 there are, potentially at least, 85 distinct values of PB that can be ranked from smallest to largest. Each of these ordered values will have an associated endpoint value; in this case 0 or 1 of the binary endpoint FFR75.

Suppose one starts cutting the covariate values into two segments beginning with a cut-point between $x_{[1]}$ and $x_{[2]}$, then the first group (left-hand) would comprise a single individual and the second group (right-hand) the remaining $n-1$ individuals. Moving along the ranking sequence, a second cut between $x_{[2]}$ and $x_{[3]}$ is possible, which then has a left group of 2 individuals and a right group comprising the remaining $n-2$. This process can be repeated until the final cut between $x_{[n-1]}$ and $x_{[n]}$ has the left group with $n-1$ individuals and the final right group 1 individual. This process results in $G=n-1$ cut-points or different divisions of the data into two groups.

In practice, some of the n observations may have the same covariate value so that when they are ranked there may only be $m \leq n$ distinct values remaining. Further, it is not sensible to cut in the region where the two distributions of PB for FF75 equal to 0 and 1 do not overlap. Thus, Figure 9.2 indicates that cuts in PB below about 65% would not be considered. In such circumstances the value of G will be further reduced.

Nevertheless, the creation of the G divisions proceeds in the way just described. Once the divisions of Left and Right groups have been identified, a decision as to which of these is optimal for the cut has to be made. We use the notation Left and Right daughters while explaining and developing the regression trees although this notation may not concur with the relative positions of the nodes in the final regression tree presented schematically.

One systematic way of making the decision is based on the proposal by Zhang, Holford and Bracken (1996) to use the so-called entropy or information criterion for what is termed the impurity. This is defined by:

$$i_{Root} = -Q_{Root}\log Q_{Root} - (1-Q_{Root})\log(1-Q_{Root}) \tag{9.1}$$

where Q_{Root} is the proportion of patients with the characteristic of concern within the root node in question.

The optimum cut-point is then determined by next calculating at every possible cut-point, x_g, the impurities

$$i_{Left} = -Q_{Left}\log Q_{Left} - (1-Q_{Left})\log(1-Q_{Left})$$

and

$$i_{Right} = -Q_{Right}\log Q_{Right} - (1-Q_{Right})\log(1-Q_{Right})$$

$$(9.2)$$

Here Q_{Left} is the proportion of patients with the characteristic of concern in the Left node category defined by a cut-point at x_g, and Q_{Right} is similarly defined.

The optimum cut-point is determined as that which maximizes the reduction in impurity

$$\Delta = i_{Root} - P_{Left}i_{Left} - P_{Right}i_{Right} \tag{9.3}$$

where P_{Left} and P_{Right} are the proportions of the total number of subjects in the Left and Right groups defined by the split.

For the root node of Figure 9.1, comprising all patients who had undergone non-urgent coronary angiography, $Q_{Root}=33/85=0.3882$. Thus, from equation (9.1), $i_{Root} = -0.3882 \times \log(0.3882) - (1 - 0.3882) \times \log(1 - 0.3882) = 0.6679$.

For each of the G cuts, the proportions with the endpoint of interest Q_{Left} and Q_{Right} are obtained and hence i_{Left} and i_{Right} of equation (9.2) calculated. A selection of values of $i(g)$ for the patients who had undergone non-urgent coronary angiography is given in Figure 9.3. In this example, if we denote PB by x, then the minimum value is $x_{[1]}=44.00$, the maximum $x_{[85]}=99.51$. If the cut is made at 70%, a convenient point between $x_{[15]}=69.88$ and $x_{[16]}=70.30$, then $Q_{Left}=1/15=0.0667$ and $Q_{Right}=(0+3+17+12)/(13+17+23+17)=32/70=0.4571$ with corresponding values of $i_{Left}=0.2450$ and $i_{Right}=0.6895$. The proportions of the total number of patients in each group are $P_{Left}=15/85=0.1765$ and $P_{Right}=1-P_{Left}=0.8235$. Using equation (9.3), these lead to $\Delta=i_{Root} - P_{Left}i_{Left} - P_{Right}i_{Right}=0.6679 - (0.1765 \times$

FFR75	<69.99	70–74.99	Plaque burden, PB (%) 75–79.99	80–84.99	85+	Total
0	14	13	14	6	5	52
1	1	0	3	17	12	33
Total	15	13	17	23	17	85
P_g	0.0667	0.0000	0.1765	0.7391	0.7059	0.3882

Total entropy: $i_{Root}=0.6679$

Split						
Q_1 $i(1)$ $P_{Left}\,/\,P_{Right}$	1/15=0.0667 0.2450 15/85=0.1765		32/70=0.4571 0.6895 70/85=0.8235			0.0569
Q_2 $i(2)$ $P_{Left}\,/\,P_{Right}$	1/28=0.0357 0.1540 28/85=0.3294		32/57=0.5614 0.6856 57/85=0.6706			0.1572
Q_3 $i(3)$ $P_{Left}\,/\,P_{Right}$	4/45=0.0889 0.3000 45/85=0.5294		29/40=0.7250 0.5882 40/85=0.4706			0.2323
Q_4 $i(4)$ $P_{Left}\,/\,P_{Right}$	21/68=0.3088 0.6181 68/85=0.8000		12/17=0.7059 0.6058 17/85=0.2000			0.0524

Optimal Cut PB ≥ 79.09						
Q_{Left}	Q_{Right}	i_{Left}	i_{Right}	P_{Left}	P_{Right}	$\Delta_{Maximum}$
0.0256	0.6957	0.1192	0.6145	0.4588	0.5412	0.2806

Figure 9.3 Illustration of the type of calculations required to obtain Δ from information on the relationship between the binary variable FFR75 and the continuous covariate plaque burden in patients who had undergone non-urgent coronary angiography (part data from Lee, Tai, Soon, et al., 2010)

0.2450) − (0.8235 × 0.6895)=0.0569. In the four cuts of PB at 70%, 75%, 80% and 85% illustrated in Figures 9.2 and 9.3, that with the maximum value of equation (9.3) is the cut at PB < 80% with $\Delta_{Maximum}$ =0.2323.

In general, a potential cut-point of a covariate is taken as the mid-point of two successive ranked values. For the covariate PB in this example, there are $G=67$ potential cuts. The 'best' of these is identified by examining the profile of Δ over the range of PB values shown in Figure 9.4. The maximum Δ arises when PB=79.09%, at which point Q_{Left}=0.0256, Q_{Right}=0.6957, i_{Left}=0.1192, i_{Right}=0.6145, P_{Left}=0.4588, P_{Right}=0.5412 and Δ_{PB}(79.09)=0.2806.

First level

In general, there will be more than a single candidate covariate to consider in order to establish the first of the daughter nodes emerging from the mother root node. Thus, the study of Lee, Tai, Soon, *et al.* (2010) also includes the covariates MLA and LL. The scatter plot of FFR75 against each of these is shown in Figure 9.5. It is immediately clear from Figure 9.5(b)

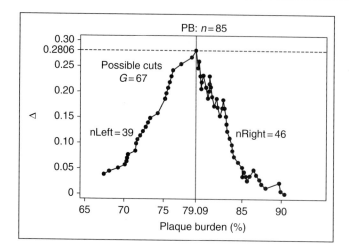

Figure 9.4   Binary FFR75: Scatter plot of Δ against plaque burden (PB) in patients who had undergone non-urgent coronary angiography (part data from Lee, Tai, Soon, *et al.*, 2010)

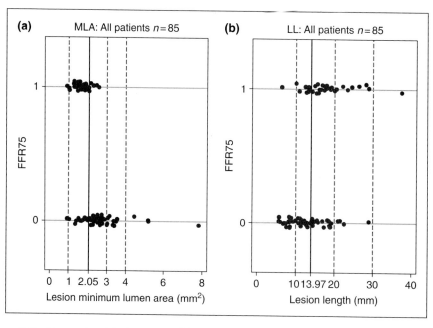

Figure 9.5   Scatter plot of the binary variable FFR75 against (a) lesion minimum lumen area (MLA) and (b) lesion length (LL) in patients who had undergone non-urgent coronary angiography (part data from Lee, Tai, Soon, *et al.*, 2010)

that LL is unlikely to be a good candidate for the first split as there is considerable overlap in values of LL in the two groups, ranging from 5.22 to 27.77 mm when FFR75=0, and 7.17 to 38.32 mm when FFR75=1.

In contrast, MLA may well be a competitor to PB for establishing the first cut as the distribution of MLA within FFR75=1 is relatively restricted, whereas that when FFR75=0 takes a wide range of values.

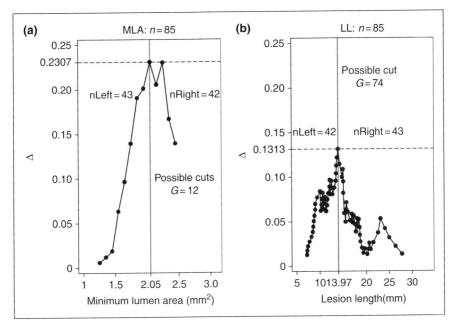

Figure 9.6 Binary FFR75: Scatter plots of the Δ against (a) lesion minimum lumen area and (b) lesion length in patients who had undergone non-urgent coronary angiography (part data from Lee, Tai, Soon, et al., 2010)

To determine which of several candidate covariates is to provide the first split for the classification tree, equation (9.3) is evaluated for each cut within each of the covariates and the corresponding $\Delta_{Maximum}$ are determined. From these, the covariate with the largest $\Delta_{Maximum}$ is chosen for the first split.

It is clear from Figure 9.5(a) that once MLA exceeds about $3\,\text{mm}^2$, the corresponding patients all have FFR75=0 so the effective number of covariate cut-points (essentially created to distinguish the binary 0 and 1 FFR75 groups) is thereby reduced. Also, among the 85 patients there are only 28 distinct recorded values of MLA. Together these have contributed to the reduction in effective number of cut-points from $n-1=84$ to $G=12$. In contrast, among the overlapping values in the distributions of LL in the two FFR75 groups, there are $G=74$ relevant cut-points.

The profiles of the different values of Δ for the covariates MLA and LL are shown in Figure 9.6. The corresponding values of $\Delta_{Maximum}$ are $\Delta_{MLA}(2.05)=0.2307$ and $\Delta_{LL}(13.97)=0.1313$. Both of these are lower than $\Delta_{PB}(79.09)=0.2806$, and thereby confirm the choice of PB for the first cut.

There are two local maxima in Figure 9.6(a) with a smaller Δ value between them. The three consecutive values are Δ_{MLA} $(2.05)=0.2307$, Δ_{MLA} $(2.15)=0.2055$, and Δ_{MLA} $(2.25)=0.2301$, with the latter cut having a value only 0.0006 less than the maximum. Thus, there may be some concern as to how appropriate is a cut-point at $2.05\,\text{mm}^2$. This situation underlines the problems associated with using an automated cut-procedure without some graphical back-up. However, as the first cut is to be made on the basis of PB, a cut in the rather ambiguous situation of MLA is avoided at this stage of the process.

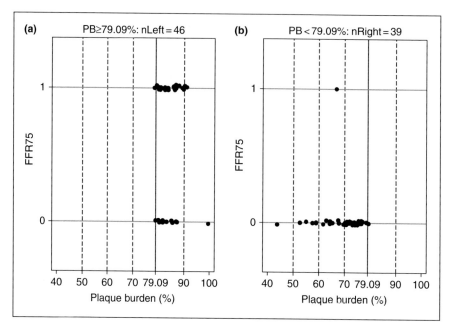

Figure 9.7   Scatter plot of the binary variable FFR75 against plaque burden (PB) within the Left (a) and Right (b) daughter nodes defined by a PB cut-point of 79.09% in patients who had undergone non-urgent coronary angiography (part data from Lee, Tai, Soon, et al., 2010)

Second and subsequent levels

Once the first daughter nodes are identified, each of these can then be thought of as the next generation mother or root nodes, which in turn can then be potentially split into their daughter nodes to create granddaughters. Although the root node has been split on the basis of PB, nevertheless this covariate remains a potential for use as a further split within the first Left and Right daughter nodes that have been created. However, Figure 9.7(b) suggests that such a partition is unlikely to be useful in further dividing the Right daughter as there is only one subject with FFR75=1. Indeed, in this situation with only a single patient in the FFR75=1 group, the remaining covariates need not be considered. In consequence, this node is now dubbed a 'Terminal node' as no more splitting will occur.

In contrast, there remains the potential to split the Left daughter and so it is considered (at this stage) as an 'Intermediate' node (denoted II in Figure 9.1). In this node the distributions of PB in Figure 9.7(a) remain overlapping in the FFR75 groups, and so once more LL and MLA compete with PB to define the next cut-point. Of course, if the result is that PB is then chosen to make a binary split in this subgroup, then effectively (in this example) the whole range of PB values will then be divided into 3 categories. So although the splitting process is binary, succeeding splits may cause a continuous or ordered categorical covariate to be eventually segmented into more than a single divisions.

As the values for PB are restricted to ≥79.09% in the Left daughter (Node II), as shown in Figure 9.8(a) and (b), the corresponding range of values of the other covariates, MLA and LL, for subsequent splits will now be constrained to the values of those patients who are included within the (new) mother node concerned. Thus, for MLA the range of values for those with FFR75=0 has now been reduced from 1.2-7.6 to 1.2-4.9 mm², although that for

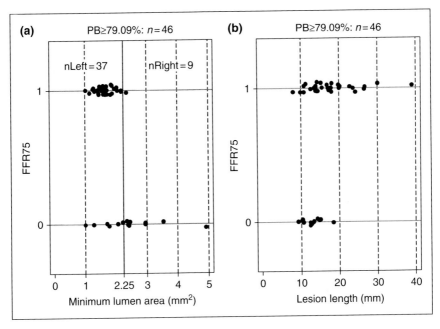

Figure 9.8 Scatter plot of the binary variable FFR75 against (a) lesion minimum lumen area and (b) lesion length within the Intermediate Node II defined by plaque burden ≥ 79.09% in patients who had undergone non-urgent coronary angiography (part data from Lee, Tai, Soon, *et al.*, 2010)

FFR75 = 1 remains as 1.2-2.5 mm^2. Correspondingly for LL, the range of values for those with FFR75 = 0 has now been reduced from 5.22–27.77 to 8.68–19.96 mm, although that for FFR75 = 1 remains as 7.17–38.32 mm. It turns out that MLA is chosen for the next split at a value of 2.25 mm^2 as indicated in Figure 9.8(a).

As an example of subsequent splitting we consider the Intermediate Node III of Figure 9.1, defined by PB ≥ 79.09% and MLA < 2.25 mm^2, and comprising $n = 37$ patients. In which case Figure 9.9(a) indicates how this node might be further split into two daughters on the basis of values of LL, and Figure 9.9(b) indicates that $\Delta_{LL}(12.55) = 0.1403$ defines the associated division.

The processes just described were implemented by writing 'one-off' computer code in Stata. This was very time consuming and, more importantly, is not suitable for other examples. However, within the statistical program *R* there is a routine, termed *rpart*, described by Therneau and Atkinson (2011), which can be used to construct classification trees. The program identifies '*son*' rather than '*daughter*' nodes. Thus, Figure 9.10 illustrates the computer code and (annotated) output from *R* which reproduces all the nodes of Figure 9.1. To obtain the classification tree, the method 'class' is specified if the outcome is a categorical variable of two or more groups—in our case FFR75 is binary. The statement (**data = Lee_Binary**) refers to the name of the data file to be used for the calculations. Further, the statement (**FFR75 ~ PB + MLA + LL**) identifies the endpoint variable of concern as FFR75 and, following (~), that the covariates to be examined are PB, MLA and LL. In addition to the primary nodal cut-points chosen, the program also ranks 'second-choice cuts' at each stage. Thus, for the Intermediate Node III, although the primary cut is made at LL < 12.55 mm, the program suggests a second-choice of PB < 80.615% and a third option of MLA < 1.95 mm^2.

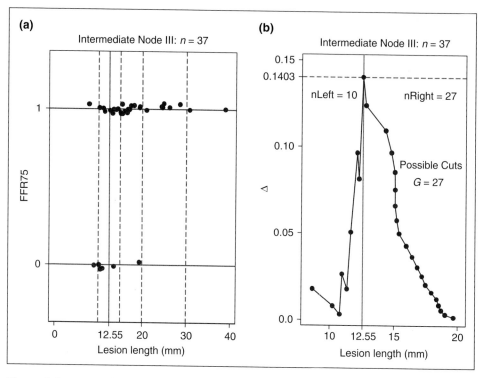

Figure 9.9 Scatter plots of (a) the binary variable FFR75 and (b) Δ against LL within the Intermediate Node III defined by PB ≥ 79.09% and MLA<2.25 mm² in patients who had undergone non-urgent coronary angiography (part data from Lee, Tai, Soon, et al., 2010)

Binary and categorical covariates

If a binary covariate is involved, then $G=1$ as only one split is possible and hence only a single Δ can be obtained. To decide if this is sufficiently large to form daughter nodes, it can be compared with $\Delta_{Maximum}$ from the other covariates concerned. In situations where ordered categorical covariates are involved, these may be treated for calculation purposes as if they are continuous as this case parallels the upper section of Figure 9.3, which essentially regards PB as a categorical covariate of $n=5$ groups with $G=4$ possible cut-points. Even if the covariate is an unordered (nominal) categorical variable, the same procedures can apply. As a potential risk factor, and in which case the four blood groups A, B, O and AB can be organized into two groups in seven different ways: These groups are: [A: B+O+AB], [B: O+AB+A], [O: AB+A+B], [AB: A+B+O], [A+B: O+AB], [A+O: AB+B], and [A+AB: B+O]. For each of these groupings, calculations for Δ can be made so that the optimum covariate, and the associated cut to define the daughter nodes, can be established.

Continuous outcome

When the outcome variable, y, is continuous, it does not necessarily follow that if the covariate x is placed in rank order then the associated y will also follow that same rank order. Thus, if FFR is retained on a continuous scale, then the scatter plot of FFR against PB in Figure 9.11 indicates that this is indeed the situation for this example.

(a) *Command*

rpart(formula = FFR75 ~ PB + MLA + LL, data = Lee_Binary, method = "class")

(b) *Output*

Root Node: 85 observations

   class counts: 33   52
   left son (46 obs) right son (39 obs)

   Primary splits:
       PB **< 79.09** to the right
       MLA < 2.05
       LL   < 13.97

Intermediate Node II: 46 observations

   class counts: 32   14
   left son (37 obs) right son (9 obs)

   Primary splits:
       MLA < 2.25 to the left
       LL   < 13.97
       PB   < 82.555

Terminal Node *A*: 39 observations

   class counts: 1   38

Intermediate Node III: 37 observations

   class counts: 31   6
   left son (27 obs) right son (10 obs)

   Primary splits:
       LL **< 12.55** to the right
       PB   < 80.615
       MLA < 1.95

Terminal Node *B*: 9 observations

   class counts: 1   8

Terminal Node *C*: 27 observations

   class counts: 26   1

Terminal Node *D*: 10 observations

   class counts: 5   5

Figure 9.10 Binary FFR75: Edited and annotated *R* commands and output for the full classification tree considering MLA, PB and LL (part data from Lee, Tai, Soon, *et al.*, 2010)

As with a binary outcome, in order to establish the cut-point of the covariate so as to create two daughter nodes, a reduction in impurity is calculated. One means of determining this is to compare the total sums of squares from all the patients within the (root) node, with those obtained from the sum of the corresponding total sums of squares within each of the potential Left and Right daughter nodes. Thus, the process begins with all the data, within the (root) node concerned, to obtain the total sum of squares

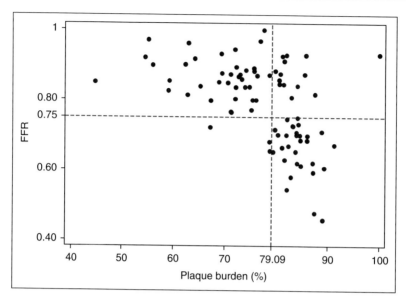

Figure 9.11   Scatter plot of continuous FFR against PB in patients who had undergone non-urgent coronary angiography (part data from Lee, Tai, Soon, *et al.*, 2010)

$$SS_{Root} = \sum_i [y_i - \overline{y}_{Root}]^2 \tag{9.4}$$

For the data of Figure 9.11, $n_{Root}=85$, $\overline{y}_{Root} = 0.7854118$, and $SS_{Root}=10.0520868$, where for brevity we have replaced FFR by y. (More decimal places are retained here than is usual in most contexts as it is difficult to be sure how much precision will be required in order to establish a cut.)

This is followed by calculating at each of the G potential cut-points the quantities

$$SS_{Left} = \sum_i [y_i - \overline{y}_{Left}]^2 \text{ and } SS_{Right} = \sum_i [y_i - \overline{y}_{Right}]^2 \tag{9.5}$$

Finally, the change in impurity for a continuous endpoint is:

$$\Delta = SS_{Root} - SS_{Left} - SS_{Right} \tag{9.6}$$

After some algebra this can be alternatively expressed as:

$$\Delta = n_{Left}\overline{y}^2_{Left} + n_{Right}\overline{y}^2_{Right} - n_{Root}\overline{y}^2_{Root} \tag{9.7}$$

The split is eventually made at the point for which Δ is the maximum.

First level

For illustration, we consider the $n_{Root}=85$ subjects in the initial root node of Figure 9.1. If the cut-point is made after the observation whose covariate PB is ranked seventh, that is at $PBCut_{[7]}=62.49\%$, then $n_{Left}=7$ and $n_{Right}=85-7=78$. The corresponding means of the two potential nodes are $\overline{y}_{Left} = 0.8785714$ and $\overline{y}_{Right} = 0.7770513$, respectively. Consequently,

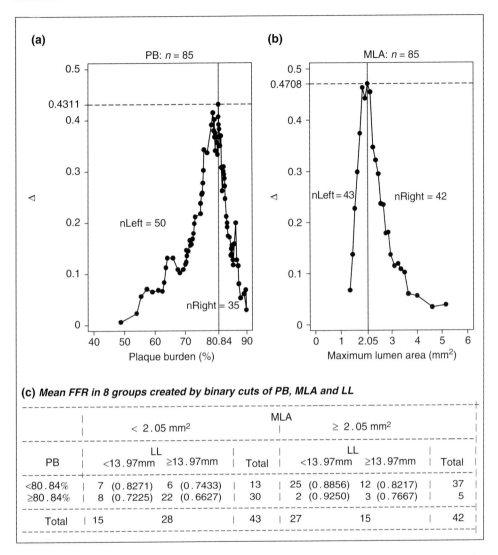

Figure 9.12 Scatter plots of Δ in patients who had undergone non-urgent coronary angiography obtained using the continuous variable FFR against (a) PB and (b) MLA, and (c) the mean FFR in the 8 groups defined by the binary cuts of PB, MLA, and LL (part data from Lee, Tai, Soon, *et al.*, 2010)

$\Delta=7\times(0.8785714)^2+78\times(0.7770513)^2-85\times(0.7854118)^2=0.066200$. If, however, the split is made at $PBCut_{[78]}=87.45\%$, the two potential nodes have $\bar{y}_{Left}=0.7946154$ and $\bar{y}_{Right}=0.6828571$, respectively, and $\Delta=78\times(0.7946154)^2+7\times(0.6828571)^2-85\times(0.7854118)^2=0.080226$. Had the split been at a PB=79.09%, as when the binary endpoint FFR75 was used in Figure 9.1, then this corresponds to $n_{Left}=39$, $n_{Right}=85-39=46$, with $\bar{y}_{Left}=0.8612821$, $\bar{y}_{Right}=0.7210870$ and $\Delta=39\times(0.8612821)^2+46\times(0.7210870)^2-85\times(0.7854118)^2=0.414830$.

In the above example $\Delta_{PB}(79.09)=0.4148$ and is clearly larger than the other illustrated values of 0.0662 and 0.0802, so this indicates that we might choose the optimum cut-point to be in the region of PB=79.09% just as when the binary variable FFR75 was the endpoint of concern. In fact, the full profile of Δ given in Figure 9.12(a) shows that the maximum of

Δ corresponds to PB=80.84%, with 50 patients having a value less than this and the remaining 35 greater or more, although the profile of values of Δ in the region of $\Delta_{PB}(80.84)=0.4311$ is very irregular.

The Δ profile for MLA in Figure 9.12(b) indicates a larger $\Delta_{MLA}(2.05)=0.4708$, than $\Delta_{PB}(80.84)=0.4311$; whereas that for LL (not illustrated) is $\Delta_{LL}(13.97)=0.3115$. These

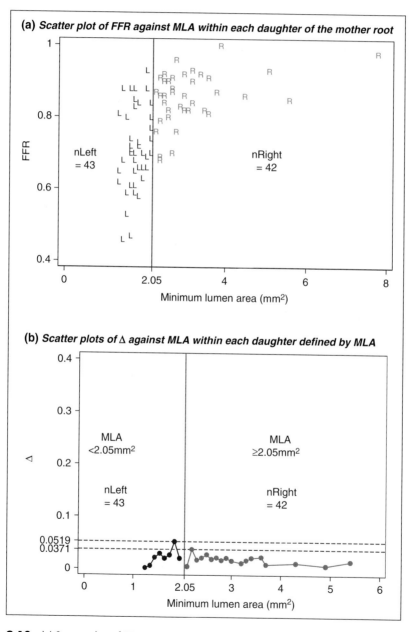

Figure 9.13 (a) Scatter plots of FFR against MLA within two daughter nodes defined by the cut of MLA at 2.05 mm² and (b) the corresponding Δ profiles for MLA within these daughters in patients who had undergone non-urgent coronary angiography (part data from Lee, Tai, Soon, et al., 2010)

maxima suggest, in contrast to the binary FFR75 situation, that the first cut to establish the two daughters should be made using MLA.

Second and subsequent levels

Once the potential primary cuts are established, one approach is to form prognostic groups on the basis of all combinations of these possible cuts of the mother root. In which case, there would be $2^3=8$ potential risk groups. The number of patients in each of these groups is indicated in Figure 9.12(c). This shows, for example, that there are seven patients who are the 'Left' cuts of all the three covariates concerned and have mean FFR $=0.8271$, and there is a second group of 12 with very similar mean FFR $=0.8217$. The next step would be to merge these two groups into a single category of 19 patients with mean 0.8237. Thus the number of groups is reduced from 8 to 7, and such a merging may be taken further.

The aim of a regression tree approach is also to reduce the final number of groups but with a splitting (rather than combining) process that preserves the homogeneity with respect to FFR. Thus, once two daughter nodes are established, in this case by using MLA $<2.05 \, mm^2$ as the cut-point, then each of these become new mother nodes and will then be examined to see if, when considering the same and the other covariates, any one of these establishes the basis for a subsequent split within the respective node.

Thus, the structure of the change in impurity, as defined by either equation (9.6) or (9.7), applies equally to all the nodes of the Intermediate type created after the first split. The splitting process is applied if necessary at each level, and continues until each node becomes Terminal.

The scatter plot of FFR against MLA in Figure 9.13(a) shows little variation in FFR among those in the Right daughter node despite a broad range of values of MLA above $2.05 \, mm^2$. In contrast, there is much greater variation in FFR from 0.46 to 0.93 in the Left daughter section, but little variation in MLA values. Both segments indicate that there is little potential for further spilt of MLA. This is confirmed by Figure 9.13(b), which shows little variation in the values of Δ in both the Left and Right daughter nodes, peaks of small magnitude at $\Delta_{MLA}(1.85)=0.0519$ and $\Delta_{MLA}(2.25)=0.0371$ respectively.

In contrast, Figure 9.14 suggests that there is some potential to divide the Left daughter node with respect to the covariate PB with a peak at $\Delta_{PB}(79.09)=0.1805$. Although not illustrated, LL has profiles of Δ all with values below 0.1, although splits at 15.01 and 17.12 mm are indicated within the Left and Right daughters.

The analysis using R statistical software of the continuous variable FFR from Lee, Tai, Soon, et al. (2010) suggests, in Figure 9.15, the rank order selection of the potential primary splits at the root (Root Node I) are MLA <2.05, PB <80.84 and LL <13.97. Thus, the split at MLA <2.05 produces left and right daughter nodes with mean FFR of 0.7119 and 0.8607. The R routine then designates the right daughter as a terminal node [Node A]. In contrast, the left node is deemed *Intermediate* [Node II] and the rank order selection of the potential splits is PB <79.09, LL <15.005 and MLA <1.85. The split is then made using PB to identify daughter nodes B and C with mean FFR of 0.6785 and 0.8378, respectively, and both are designated *Terminal*. The final regression tree is summarized in Figure 9.16(a). The box-whisker plot of Figure 9.16(b) emphasizes that although there is a clear difference in mean FFR between the three terminal nodes, there remains considerable overlap in terms of individual patient values.

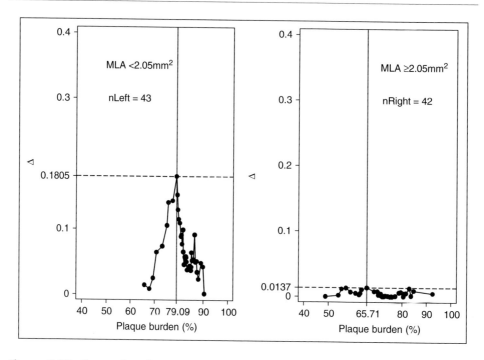

Figure 9.14   Scatter plots of Δ against PB, within the nodes defined by a cut at MLA=2.05 mm², in patients who had undergone non-urgent coronary angiography (part data from Lee, Tai, Soon, et al., 2010)

Time-to-event outcome

When the outcome is time-to-event, such as those examples discussed in Chapter 6, the choice of where to split from successive left to right cuts of the covariate concerned can be made on the basis of an appropriate statistical procedure such as the logrank test used by LeBlanc and Crowley (1993). However, to link the methodology closer to the context of this book, we use Cox regression to test the significance of the difference between survival times of the potential daughters to determine the optimal split as did Cohn, Pearson, London, et al. (2009).

In the study by Chong, Tay, Subramaniam, et al. (2009), discussed in Chapter 6, patients resident in a long-stay psychiatric hospital were examined on a census day when their demographic data and clinical details were recorded. The patients were then followed for up to an 8-year period post census to determine their subsequent survival time. To illustrate the creation of a regression tree using time-to-event data, their gender, ethnicity, age and diagnosis of tardive dyskinesia (TD) (Absent, Mild or Definitive) are used and these are summarized in Figure 9.17 where, for example, the hazard ratio for gender, $HR=1.86$, suggests a greater mortality among the males albeit not statistically significant (p-value$=0.069$). As we are focusing on a binary split for the unordered categorical variable *Ethnicity* of Figure 9.17, each HR represents one ethnic group versus the other two combined. For a similar reason, those for the ordered categorical variable *Age* compare the cumulative number from the youngest patient in the study to the oldest within a category, with all those in the immediate older age categories. Thus, $HR=2.85$ compares the age categories 29–49 and 50–59 combined

Commands

Regression tree:
rpart(formula = FFR ~ ., data = Lee_Continuous)

Variables actually used in tree construction:
[1] LL MLA PB

Output

Root Node I: 85 observations

Mean = 0.7854, SD = 0.1190

left son (43 obs) right son (42 obs)

Primary splits:

MLA < 2.05 to the left

PB   < 80.84

LL   < 13.97

Intermediate Node II : 43 observations

Mean = 0.7119, SD = 0.1094

left son (34 obs) right son (9 obs)

Primary splits:

PB   < 79.09 to the right

LL   < 15.005

MLA < 1.85

Terminal Node *A* : 42 observations

Mean = 0.8607, SD = 0.0719

Terminal Node *B* : 34 observations

Mean = 0.6785, SD = 0.0940

Terminal Node *C* : 9 observations

Mean = 0.8378, SD = 0.0614

Figure 9.15   Final nodes for the regression tree considering MLA, PB, and LL for the continuous variable FFR determined using R (part data from Lee, Tai, Soon, *et al.*, 2010)

with all in the two older categories 60-69 and 70-105 years. A similar structure is used for the ordered categories of Absent, Mild and Definitive TD.

In order to establish a regression tree starting from the root of 605 patients, the covariate providing the cut with highest z-statistic (and hence smallest p-value) determines the daughter nodes. The largest *HR* in Figure 9.17, perhaps not surprisingly, suggests the covariate *Age* with a cut at 70 is of primary importance. This then identifies a Left node of 481 (79.5%) and a Right node of the remaining 124 (20.5%) individuals. The corresponding Kaplan-Meier (K-M) estimates of the cumulative death rates (CDR) for the two age groups selected are shown in Figure 9.18. The respective 5-year rates for the younger and older age groups are 3.33% and 11.29%, respectively.

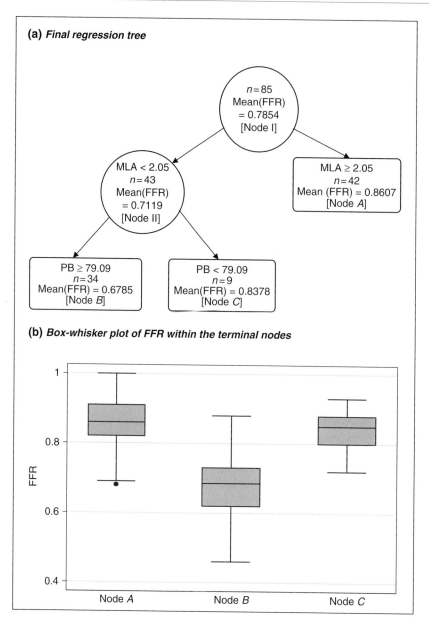

Figure 9.16 (a) The regression tree considering MLA, PB, and LL for the continuous variable FFR and (b) box-whisker plot of the individual patient FFR values within each terminal node (part data from Lee, Tai, Soon, et al., 2010)

After examining the covariates within each daughter node determined by *Age* in Figure 9.19, it seems apparent that the Left daughter might be further partitioned by creating nodes from the binary split of Absent/Mild versus Definitive TD as the corresponding $HR=2.86$ and p-value$=0.00067$. The respective 5-year CDRs are 2.53% and 4.85%. In contrast, further division of the Right node does not seem likely as all p-values>0.05. The

		Alive	Dead	Cut	HR	Cox z-statistic	p-value
Gender	Female (F)	130	10				
	Male (M)	403	62	F v M	1.86	1.82	0.069
Ethnicity	Chinese (C)	473	65	I+M v C	1.14	0.32	0.748
	Indian (I)	10	4	Ma+C v I	2.78	1.99	0.047
	Malay (Ma)	50	3	C+I v Ma	0.45	−1.36	0.174
Age (years)	29–49 (A1)	99	7	1	1	–	–
	50–59 (A2)	169	11	A1 v A2+A3+A4	2.01	1.76	0.079
	60–69 (A3)	171	24	A1+A2 v A3+A4	2.85	3.84	0.00012
	70–105 (A4)	**94**	**30**	A1+A2+A3 v A4	**3.17**	**4.82**	**0.00005**
Tardive	Absent (Ab)	295	23		1	–	–
dyskinesia	Mild (Mi)	42	5	Ab v Mi+De	2.42	3.49	0.00049
	Definitive (De)	196	44	Ab+Mi v De	2.46	3.72	0.00020

Figure 9.17 Gender, ethnicity, age and presence or otherwise of tardive dyskinesia in psychiatric patients and associated hazard ratios (part data from Chong, Tay, Subramaniam, *et al.*, 2009)

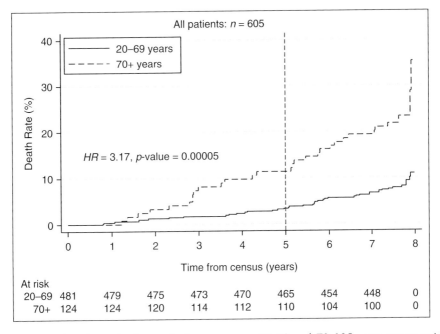

Figure 9.18 Cumulative death rates in the age groups 20–69 and 70–105 years among resident psychiatric patients (part data from Chong, Tay, Subramaniam, *et al.*, 2009)

cumulative K-M curves of Figure 9.20(a) with respect to the binary division of TD show a clear division in failure rates within the younger patients.

Potentially these nodes could be further divided into daughter nodes, although in this example no further division appeared warranted. The final tree comprising three terminal nodes with CDRs of 2.53, 4.85 and 11.29%, respectively, is summarized in Figure 9.20(b).

		Alive	Dead		HR	z-statistic	p-value
				Left Node < 70 years			
Gender	Female (F)	99	5				
	Male (M)	340	37	F v M	2.09	1.54	0.123
Ethnicity	Chinese (C)	387	38	I+Ma v C	1.25	0.42	0.675
	Indian (I)	7	2	Ma+C v I	2.67	1.35	0.176
	Malay (Ma)	45	2	C+I v M	0.46	−1.06	0.287
Age (years)	29–49 (A1)	99	7		1		
	50–59 (A2)	169	11	A1 v A2+A3	1.38	0.78	0.433
	60–69 (A3)	171	24	A1+A2 v A3	1.96	2.15	0.031
Tardive	Absent (Ab)	264	14		1		
dyskinesia	Mild (Mi)	35	3	Ab v Mi+De	2.74	3.08	0.0021
	Definitive (De)	**140**	**25**	**Ab+Mi v De**	**2.86**	**3.40**	**0.00067**
				Right Node ≥ 70 years			
Gender	Female (F)	31	5		1		
	Male (M)	63	25	F v M	2.00	1.41	0.160
Ethnicity	Chinese (C)	86	27	I+Ma v C	0.71	−0.56	0.578
	Indian (I)	3	2	M+C v I	2.37	1.18	0.239
	Malay (Ma)	5	1	C+I v M	0.75	−0.29	0.773
Tardive	Absent (Ab)	31	9		1		
dyskinesia	Mild (Mi)	7	2	Ab v Mi+De	1.07	0.17	0.864
	Definitive (De)	56	19	Ab+Mi v De	1.06	0.14	0.885

Figure 9.19 Gender, ethnicity, age and presence or otherwise of tardive dyskinesia in psychiatric patients in the Left and Right daughter nodes formed by a cut-point of 70 years and the associated hazard ratios (part data from Chong, Tay, Subramaniam, *et al.*, 2009)

TREE PRUNING

Purpose

As Zhang, Holford and Bracken (1996) indicate, the process of creating daughter nodes will sooner or later arrive at a situation in which further partitioning is no longer possible. This will arise, for example, if there is only one observation within the node, all node defining covariate values have, within the node, the same value, or all subjects within the node have the same outcome value. However, Zhang, Crowley, Sox and Olshen (1999) point out that, in general, the splitting process may end up with a very large tree, as does the final tree of 20 terminal nodes of Cohn, Pearson, London, *et al.* (2009) part of which is illustrated in Figure 1.13. In this particular study a very large number of patients were concerned and so many homogeneous subgroups might be anticipated. Nevertheless, a large tree may be too large to be useful and so methods are required by which such complexity may be reduced by 'pruning away' some of the nodes. These essentially examine each tree branch of the intermediate nodes leading to terminal nodes, and question whether or not these final nodes are required.

We use the regression tree of Figure 9.1, which is designed to identify those patients with low FFR in small coronary arteries, for illustration and which we reproduce again in structural form only in Figure 9.21(a).

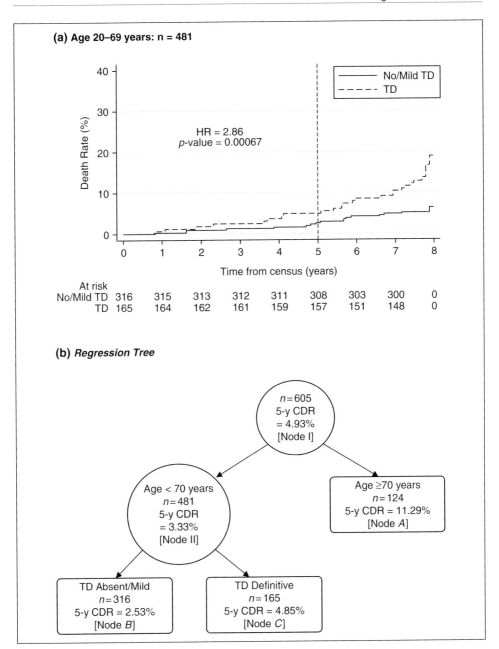

(a) Age 20–69 years: n = 481

HR = 2.86
p-value = 0.00067

At risk

No/Mild TD	316	315	313	312	311	308	303	300	0
TD	165	164	162	161	159	157	151	148	0

(b) Regression Tree

n=605
5-y CDR
= 4.93%
[Node I]

Age < 70 years
n=481
5-y CDR
= 3.33%
[Node II]

Age ≥70 years
n=124
5-y CDR = 11.29%
[Node A]

TD Absent/Mild
n=316
5-y CDR = 2.53%
[Node B]

TD Definitive
n=165
5-y CDR = 4.85%
[Node C]

Figure 9.20 (a) Cumulative death rates (CDR) by absence or presence of definitive TD in those aged 20–69 years at the census, and (b) the corresponding regression tree analysis in long-stay patients in a psychiatric hospital (part data from Chong, Tay, Subramaniam, et al., 2009)

Sub-trees, branches and complexity

The full tree, T_0, of Figure 9.21 has $N_{Terminal}=4$ terminal nodes and $N_{Intermediate}=3$ intermediate nodes. If nodes C and D are pruned from this tree, this leaves sub-tree T_1 with $N_{Terminal}=3$ (A, III and B) and $N_{Intermediate}=2$ (I and II). Pruning further, tree T_2 has $N_{Terminal}=2$ (A and II) and

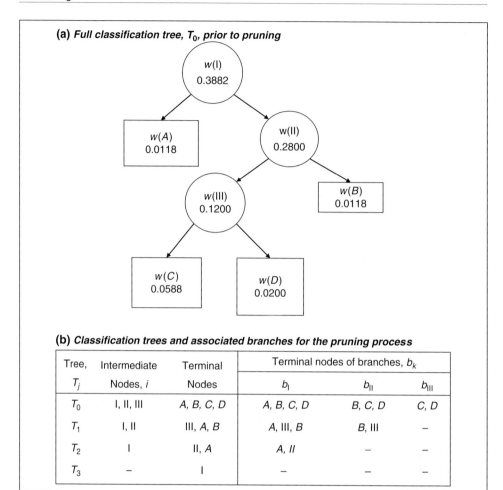

(a) Full classification tree, T_0, prior to pruning

(b) Classification trees and associated branches for the pruning process

Tree, T_j	Intermediate Nodes, i	Terminal Nodes	Terminal nodes of branches, b_k		
			b_I	b_{II}	b_{III}
T_0	I, II, III	A, B, C, D	A, B, C, D	B, C, D	C, D
T_1	I, II	III, A, B	A, III, B	B, III	–
T_2	I	II, A	A, II	–	–
T_3	–	I	–	–	–

Figure 9.21 (a) Schematic representation of the binary classification tree, T_0, of Figure 9.1 where I, II and III represent intermediate, and A, B, C and D terminal, nodes with their corresponding weighted misclassification costs, $w(Node)$, and (b) the potential sub-trees for the final choice of regression tree following pruning (part data from Lee, Tai, Soon, et al., 2010)

$N_{Intermediate} = 1$ (I), and the final possible prune leaves tree T_3 as the mother or root node with $N_{Terminal} = 1$ and $N_{Intermediate} = 0$. This process therefore identifies four possible classification trees, T_0, T_1, T_2 and T_3, of Figure 9.21(b) with associated branches from which the complexity parameter is determined. The root nodes of these branches are the associated intermediate nodes of the specific sub-tree. The size of a tree, or equivalently the total number of nodes, is defined as, $S_{Tree} = 2 N_{Terminal} - 1$. Thus for T_0, $S_0 = (2 \times 4) - 1 = 7$, whereas for the sub-tree T_2, $S_2 = (2 \times 2) - 1 = 3$. As the size of the tree is directly related to the number of terminal nodes, $N_{Terminal}$, this also defines the *complexity* of a given tree.

Tree quality

The objective of the regression tree-based method is to determine homogeneous subgroups of the subjects recruited to the study and whether this is achieved depends on the degree of homogeneity in the terminal nodes of the branches of the corresponding tree. One measure of homogeneity is

$$H(T) = \sum_{NTerminal} p(i)r(i) = \sum_{All\,Terminal\,Nodes} w(i) \qquad (9.8)$$

where $p(i)$ is the proportion of subjects in, and $r(i)$ the misclassification costs of, the terminal nodes, i, of a sub-tree or one of the branches of the sub-tree.

Misclassification costs

The purpose of the tree of Figure 9.21 is to distinguish those small coronary arteries with a LowFFR from those of HighFFR. However, if a patient is misclassified by the process then some 'cost' is attached to this. There are two possible misclassifications that can arise. The first is when the artery is thought to be LowFFR but is actually HighFFR, denoted *Cost*(L *but is* H), and the second when it is regarded as HighFFR but is actually LowFFR, *Cost*(H *but is* L). For medical reasons it is likely that the cost of missing the diagnosis of LowFFR is higher and so we presume *Cost*(H *but is* L)>*Cost*(L *but is* H). However, it is the relative costs that are important so we can assume *Cost*(L *but is* H)=1 and *Cost*(H *but is* L)=C with $C>1$.

The process of costing begins by listing all the nodes, distinguishing the intermediate from the terminal, identifying the number of subjects, $n(i)$, and calculating the proportion of individuals concerned at each node, $p(i)$, as in the first three columns of Figure 9.22. Columns (iv) and (vi) then list the number of cases of LowFFR and HighFFR respectively in the corresponding nodes. The cost associated with each node is then calculated as $c_{Low}(i)=1 \times n_{Low}(i)=n_{Low}(i)$ in column (v) and, in column (vii), $c_{High}(i)=C \times n_{High}(i)$. The designated class of column (viii) is then determined as that associated with the minimum of the $c_{Low}(i)$ and $c_{High}(i)$ values. Further,

$$r(i) = \frac{\min[c_{Low}(i), c_{High}(i)]}{n(i)} = \frac{c_{Minimum}(i)}{n(i)}, \qquad (9.9)$$

and this is calculated in column (ix).

To illustrate the process we assume $C=1.7$, the approximate ratio of High versus Low FFR, although this is quite arbitrary. We have deliberately chosen an 'odd and decimalized' number so its presence can be easily detected in the calculation process of Figure 9.22. However, in practical applications the value would be based on the experience of the clinical teams concerned. The weighted misclassification costs, $w(i)$, are included for each node of tree, T_0, in Figure 9.21(a).

Equation (9.8) is evaluated for each tree and the summation is made over the terminal nodes of the particular tree concerned. Thus, for tree T_0 the total weighted cost is the sum of costs of all terminal nodes or $H(T_0)=w(A)+w(B)+w(C)+w(D)=0.0118+0.0118+0.0200+0.0588=0.1024$. Similarly, $H(T_1)=w(A)+w(III)+w(B)=0.0118+0.1200+0.0118=0.1436$ and $H(T_2)=w(II)+w(A)=0.2800+0.0118=0.2918$. These, and the calculation of $H(T_3)$, are summarized in Figure 9.23, column (iii).

(i)	(ii)	(iii)	(iv)	(v)	(vi)	(vii)	(viii)	(ix)	(x)
		Node					Class	Cost	Weighted cost
Label	size $n(i)$	Proportion in node $p(i)$	Low $n_{Low}(i)$	$c_{Low}(i)=1$ $\times n_{Low}(i)$	High $n_{High}(i)$	$c_{High}(i)=1.7$ $\times n_{High}(i)$	Minimum of col (v) and (vii)	$r(i)=$ $c_{Minimum}(i)/n(i)$	$w(i)=$ $p(i) \times r(i)$
I	85	$85/85=1$	33	33	52	88.4	Low	33/85	$w(I)=$ 0.3882
II	46	$46/85=$ 0.5412	32	32	14	23.8	High	23.8/46	$w(II)=$ 0.2800
III	37	$37/85=$ 0.4353	31	31	6	10.2	High	10.2/37	$w(III)=$ 0.1200
A	39	$39/85=$ 0.4588	1	1	38	64.6	Low	1/39	$w(A)=$ 0.0118
B	9	$9/85=$ 0.1059	1	1	8	13.6	Low	1/9	$w(B)=$ 0.0118
C	27	$27/85=$ 0.3176	26	26	1	1.7	High	1.7/27	$w(C)-$ 0.0200
D	10	$10/85=$ 0.1176	5	5	5	8.5	Low	5/10	$w(D)=$ 0.0588

Figure 9.22   Estimation of the misclassification costs for the binary FFR75 classification tree, T_0, of Figure 9.21(a)

(i)	(ii)	(iii)	(iv)	(v)	(vi)	(vii)
	Terminal nodes	Misclassification cost	Tree quality $Qal(T_j, \alpha)$			Tree quality
Sub-tree	$N_{Terminal}$	$H(T_j)$	$H(T_j)+\alpha N_{Terminal}$	Range of α	Chosen α	$Qal(T_j, \alpha)$
T_0	4	0.1024	$0.1024+4\alpha$	$0-0.0412$	0.01	$0.1024+(4\times0.01)$ $=0.1424$
T_1	3	0.1436	$0.1436+3\alpha$	$0.0412-0.1223$	0.1	$0.1436+(30.1)$ $=0.4436$
T_2^*	2	0.2918				
T_3	1	0.3882	$0.3882+\alpha$	$0.1223+$	0.2	$0.3882+(1\times0.2)$ $=0.5882$

$^*T_2$ - this sub-tree is not part of the nested sequence but is included here for reference only

Figure 9.23   Tree quality for chosen CP of size α for the nested sequence of the binary FFR75 classification trees of Figure 9.21

Tree quality (Qal)

The tree homogeneity, as determined by the misclassification costs and the tree complexity, as defined by the number of terminal nodes, are combined to give an overall measure of tree quality as

$$Qal(T_j, \alpha) = H(T_j) + \alpha N_{Terminal} \tag{9.10}$$

where ($\alpha \geq 0$) is termed the complexity parameter (CP). We detail how α is chosen in the next section.

Pruning

According to Breiman, Freedman, Olshen and Stone (1984), there is a unique smallest sub-tree of T_0 that minimizes the cost complexity. This is termed the optimal sub-tree with respect to the cost complexity and is determined using a tree pruning process.

A tree is pruned of some of its terminal nodes only if the tree cost complexity, $Qal(T, \alpha)$, is thereby improved by the pruning. The decision depends on the choice of the CP. In the simplest situation, CP$=\alpha=0$ and so $Qal(T, 0)=H(T)$ and, if this is used to determine the *final* tree, then T_0 with a cost complexity $Qal(T_0, 0)=0.1024$ would be chosen as sub-trees T_1, T_2, and T_3 each have an associated greater cost. Thus, no terminal nodes are pruned in this case. However, in other examples, the sub-tree corresponding to $\alpha=0$ need not be the optimal sub-tree.

To determine the optimal sub-tree, the smallest CP which permits pruning is calculated for each sub-tree, starting with the full tree, T_0. This is defined by

$$\alpha(T_0) = \min_i \left[\frac{W_{Intermediate}(i) - H(b_i)}{[N_{Terminal}(i) - 1]} \right] \tag{9.11}$$

where $i=$I, II, and III are the intermediate nodes of T_0. They are similarly defined for T_1, T_2, and T_3.

From Figure 9.21 the branch b_1 of tree, T_0, has four terminal nodes, so $H(b_1)=w(A)+w(B)+w(C)+w(D)=0.0118+0.0118+0.0200+0.0588=0.1024$, $H(b_{II})=0.0906$, and $H(b_{III})=0.0788$. Thus,

$$\alpha(T_0) = \min \left[\frac{0.3882-0.1024}{[4-1]}, \frac{0.2800-0.0906}{[3-1]}, \frac{0.1200-0.0788}{[2-1]} \right]$$
$$= \min[0.0953, 0.0947, 0.0412] = 0.0412.$$

As $\alpha(T_0)=0.0412$ is associated with the branch, b_{III}, the terminal nodes C and D can be pruned without loss of cost complexity, leaving the sub-tree T_1 for potential pruning. Following the same procedures, we have

$$\alpha(T_1) = \min \left[\frac{0.3882-0.1436}{[3-1]}, \frac{0.2800-0.1318}{[2-1]} \right] = \min[0.1223, 0.1482] = 0.1223.$$

As $\alpha(T_1)=0.1223$ is associated with the branch, b_1 of sub-tree T_1, all nodes following Node I in this sub-tree, that is, A, B, II, and III can be pruned with little loss of cost complexity, leading to the single Node I of sub-tree T_3. Pruning stops as the root node is reached.

Following the pruning procedures, only T_0, T_1, and T_3 are found to be optimal sub-trees in the nested sequence, and any of these may be chosen depending on the choice of CP. As shown in column (v) of Figure 9.23, for α ranging from 0.0412 to 0.1223, the resultant optimal sub-tree is T_1. However, with CP$=0.0412$ in Figure 9.23 the penalty, or cost complexity at this threshold, is at a minimum for T_0 and T_1 with values of $(0.1024+4\times0.0412)$

and $(0.1436+3\times0.0412)$ both equal to 0.2672. The other sub-trees all have penalties higher than this with $Qal(T_2, 0.0412)=0.3742$ and $Qal(T_3, 0.0412)=0.4294$. As consequence the full classification tree T_0 is pruned to T_1 and this is presented in Figure 9.24(a) as the final tree selected for the study concerned.

If the R program is used in this situation, then the user may specify a value for CP directly rather than expressing this via the relative cost, C, of misclassification. Thus, the commands and output in Figure 9.24(b) set a default value of CP=0.1, but still result in the same pruned tree, T_1.

Finally, it should be noted that the regression tree of Figure 9.16(a), considering the continuous endpoint FFR, and the classification tree of Figure 9.24(a), considering binary FFR75, both comprise two Intermediate and three Terminal nodes. However, the characteristics of the patients within these two sets of nodes (although likely to be overlapping) will be different.

PRACTICAL CONSIDERATIONS

Classification Trees or Regression Trees

The Classification Tree methodology essentially deals with an endpoint variable that is binary or categorical in nature, whereas Regression Trees deal with other endpoints. The term Regression Trees is essentially generic. However, in the example of fractional flow reserve (FFR) we have used both a binary dichotomy at 75% to obtain a Classification Tree and the continuous form of the data to obtain a Regression Tree. In general terms, creating a binary variable from a continuous variable will be wasteful of information. However, in a medical decision making context, it may be more useful to think in binary terms. For example, a physician concerned with the diastolic blood pressure (DBP) of a patient, will record the actual DBP but will only be concerned if it exceeds a certain value. In which case, he may treat the patient for hypertension, otherwise not. Thus, with respect to any study, the design team needs to be clear as to the intended purpose of the regression tree that will be ultimately constructed.

Establishing the cut-points

Although in many circumstances a clear division in covariate values may be found to establish distinct daughter nodes, there will be situations where the choice may not be so evident. For example, Figure 9.12(b) suggests that the cut of MLA at 2.05 mm^2 is not firmly established as other MLA values in the vicinity give cut-criteria of very similar magnitude to Δ_{MLA} (2.05)=0.4708. In this circumstance, the choice of division may not be very robust, as the subsequent structure of the tree will depend critically on the selection of the daughters at this stage. The same difficulty arises in many applications whenever a continuous covariate is dichotomized, or an ordered categorical covariate is grouped into broad categories.

Graphical examination

In Chapter 7 describing model building, we warn against uncritical use of automatic variable selection methods when choosing a final regression model. The same warning equally applies when constructing classification and regression trees. As an illustration, the terminal Node A of

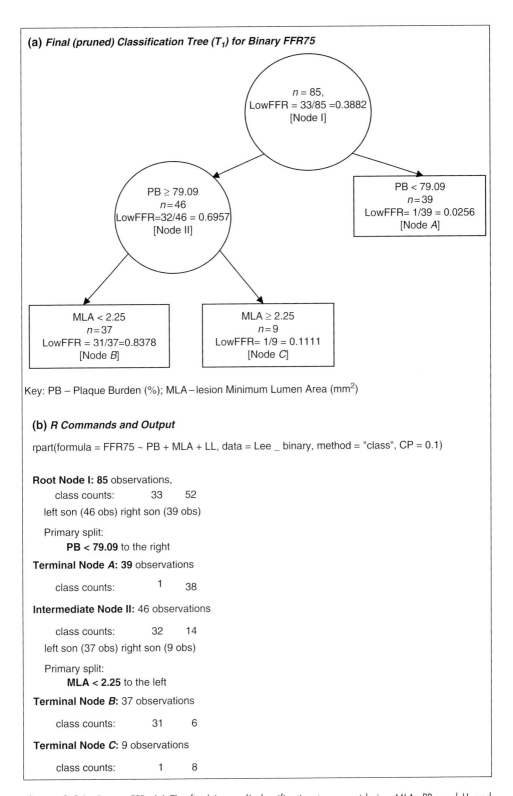

(a) *Final (pruned) Classification Tree (T₁) for Binary FFR75*

$n = 85$,
LowFFR $= 33/85 = 0.3882$
[Node I]

PB $\geq$ 79.09
$n = 46$
LowFFR $= 32/46 = 0.6957$
[Node II]

PB $<$ 79.09
$n = 39$
LowFFR $= 1/39 = 0.0256$
[Node A]

MLA $<$ 2.25
$n = 37$
LowFFR $= 31/37 = 0.8378$
[Node B]

MLA $\geq$ 2.25
$n = 9$
LowFFR $= 1/9 = 0.1111$
[Node C]

Key: PB – Plaque Burden (%); MLA – lesion Minimum Lumen Area (mm²)

(b) *R Commands and Output*

rpart(formula = FFR75 ~ PB + MLA + LL, data = Lee _ binary, method = "class", CP = 0.1)

Root Node I: 85 observations,
    class counts: 33   52
    left son (46 obs) right son (39 obs)

    Primary split:
        PB < 79.09 to the right
Terminal Node A: 39 observations

    class counts: 1   38

Intermediate Node II: 46 observations

    class counts: 32   14
    left son (37 obs) right son (9 obs)

    Primary split:
        MLA < 2.25 to the left
Terminal Node B: 37 observations

    class counts: 31   6

Terminal Node C: 9 observations

    class counts: 1   8

Figure 9.24 Binary FFR: (a) The final 'pruned' classification tree considering MLA, PB, and LL and (b) associated annotated R commands and output (part data from Lee, Tai, Soon, *et al.*, 2010)

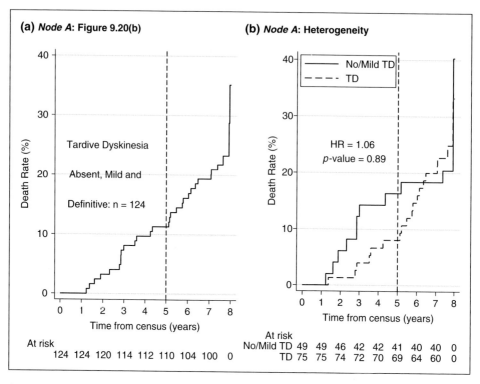

Figure 9.25 Evidence of some residual heterogeneity in the terminal Node A of Figure 9.20(b) (part data from Chong, Tay, Subramaniam, *et al.*, 2009)

Figure 9.20(b) comprised patients aged 70 or more years. Within this node, a comparison of the TD groups had been made resulting in a statistically non-significant $HR=1.06$ with p-value$=0.89$ and so is assumed to be relatively homogeneous. Thus, Node A is designated as terminal and the single K-M curve of Figure 9.25(a) summarizes their CDR. However, examination of the corresponding K-M curves in Figure 9.25(b) among those aged ≥ 70 years with respect to TD, suggests that Node A may not after all be truly homogeneous. This situation would have gone (possibly) unnoticed without graphical presentation. In such cases, if the graph reflects reality, the investigating team must ponder how to proceed. In such situations, should Node A be retained as terminal, the predictive value of the regression tree is likely to be low.

In a similar way, graphical examination of Figure 9.6(a) may help to resolve a situation issue where there are two or more local maxima in close proximity and with very similar reduction in impurity values, Δ. However, such problems may be resolved using a cross-validation process.

Cross-validation

In our examples, we have developed a single tree which, once pruned, is then in theory used for future diagnostic purposes. However, experience suggests that prospective use of trees often results in less satisfactory diagnostic value than that obtained by the development tree. Essentially this is because the tree is chosen as the 'best' or 'optimum' for the study sample. To avoid this difficulty, final tree selection can be determined following cross-validation (CV), which results in a more robust final tree and hence one with potentially more satisfactory diagnostic potential.

This CV process involves first splitting the data randomly into M mutually exclusive subsets of roughly equal size, organized in such a way that each subset contains a similar distribution for the outcome variable of concern. As Everitt (2003) describes, the results of these M models are then averaged to provide an indication of the performance of the tree. This complex process results in a set of fairly reliable estimates of the independent predictive accuracy of the tree, and provides information on how well the chosen tree will perform on completely fresh data even if we do not have an independent test sample.

For example, in developing the potential tree for the patients with schizophrenia, one might create $M=3$ groups or training sets (TS) labeled I, II and III each consisting of 200 patients in such a way that equal numbers of deaths, here 24, are in each group and that the diagnostic groups (Absent, Mild, and Definitive TD) are also in the ratio of about 6: 1: 4 as in the sample as a whole. Two of these three samples, say I and II, are then combined to form a training set and a full regression tree, T_0, is then constructed with the data from these (400) patients alone. The resulting training-tree is then tested on the validation data set (here set III of 200 patients) by allocating the validation data to the nodes defined by the cuts in the tree structure. The next step is to repeat this process but with the training set consisting of II and III and using I as the validation set. Finally, to repeat again with I and III comprising the training set and using II as the validation set. This generates three (in general k) training-trees T_{0I}, T_{0II} and T_{0III} each with corresponding CP of α_I, α_{II}, and α_{III} based on the procedures described in *Tree pruning*. From these $Qal(T_{0I})$, $Qal(T_{0II})$ and $Qal(T_{0III})$ are obtained, and the final cross-validation estimate, $Qal^{CV}(T_0)$, is obtained by averaging these. This process is repeated for each sub-tree of T_0, and the final tree chosen is that with the smallest Qal^{CV}.

For any tree, T, in the above process, each $Qal(T)$ calculated is only an estimate and so has an associated standard error, SE(T). Breiman, Freedman, Olshen and Stone (1984) pointed out that some of these SEs may be considerable, and therefore proposed a revised strategy to take the magnitude of the variability of each $Qal(T)$ into account when averaging to obtain the final Qal^{CV} and thereby identify the corresponding 'final' regression tree.

Missing covariate values

In most clinical studies, there will be several covariates that are possible candidates for splitting the mother (and subsequent daughters) into homogeneous groups and thereby constructing a classification or regression tree. If indeed there are missing data, then clearly when considering the primary cut there will be variable numbers of patients to consider depending on the covariate in question. Nevertheless, unlike standard regression procedures that omit incomplete observations during the modeling, the classification and regression tree methods will include any observation with values for the outcome and at least one independent variable in the tree construction (Therneau and Atkinson, 2011). When the variable chosen for the primary cut is missing, it may be imputed based on information of the other covariates. In Figure 9.1, if an individual has missing PB, surrogate variables will be defined to predict the split for 'PB < 79.09' versus 'PB ≥ 79.09' using available information on MLA and LL. As shown in Figure 9.26, the R package defines MLA < 2.35 as the first surrogate split and LL < 10.635 as the second. This suggests that an individual with missing PB will be assigned to node II based on the first surrogate split of MLA < 2.35. If the subject is also missing on MLA, then the next surrogate split LL < 10.635 will be considered. Nevertheless, in planning and conducting a study, every effort should be made to minimize the potential for missing

```
rpart(formula = FFR75 ~ PB + MLA + LL, data = Lee _ Binary, method = "class")
```

Root Node: 85 observations

class counts: 33   52
left son (46 obs) right son (39 obs)

Primary splits:
    PB   < **79.09** to the right
    MLA < 2.05
    LL   < 13.97

Surrogate splits:
    MLA < 2.35 to the left
    LL   < 10.635 to the right

Figure 9.26   Binary FFR75: Edited and annotated R commands and output illustrating surrogate splits of PB at the root node (part data from Lee, Tai, Soon, et al., 2010)

		TreeRisk		
PIRisk	Tree-Low	Tree-Med	Tree-High	Total
PI-Low	**36**	0	0	36
PI-Medium	12	**10**	0	22
PI-High	0	0	**27**	27
Total	48	10	27	85

Figure 9.27   Agreement between the Classification Tree and Prognostic Index in assigning patients having undergone non-urgent coronary angiography to risk groups (part data from Lee, Tai, Soon, et al., 2010)

data. If it is known in advance, that a particular covariate may be difficult to obtain from each patient, then it is probably best not to include such a covariate into the study.

Regression models or regression trees

We gave an example in Chapter 7 of how a prognostic index (PI) might be constructed to categorize patients reported by Lee, Tai, Soon, et al. (2010) into low, medium and high risk groups with respect to FFR. These same data were used to construct the classification tree of Figure 9.1 and so one might then compare these with the nodes A, B, C and D, identified. Both nodes A and B have low rates for LowFFR, node C has the highest whereas node D is intermediate. Figure 9.27 compares these risk groups with those derived using the PI and the diagonal terms show agreement between the two approaches in 36+10+27=73 or 86% of the cases. The intention here is not to argue which is the better of the two approaches, but only to illustrate that different conclusions can be drawn from the same data when alternative assumptions are made. Here both approaches have used binary covariates derived from continuous variables, and the PI does not include the possibility of interactions between them.

As we have just implied, the regression-tree process may more easily deal with interactions between covariates than a standard regression approach. This is because the regression-tree approach does not estimate parameters, whereas a regression model does Thus, with three covariates, LL, MLA and PB, the three first-level interactions add three more parameters to any regression model which then need to be estimated. Should the covariates be categorical in nature then more parameters would be necessary. This is avoided using the binary (covariate) splitting process, where any 'interaction' is accounted for by splitting on a particular covariate in (say) the left daughter node but not splitting by this same covariate in the right daughter. Nevertheless, Marshall (2001) refers to some of the problems associated with this strategy. In particular, he warns that '… clinicians may be misled into thinking the clusters [nodes] have biologic meaning …' and quotes Feinstein (1996, p. 566) who states the clusters may be composed of '… heterogeneous constituents with no apparent coherence', seemingly to imply that the resulting 'nodes' may have little clinical relevance.

STATISTICAL SOFTWARE

Throughout this text, we have used Stata to illustrate the type of commands that may be required to implement the regression techniques described. However, the regression tree methodology is not included within Stata so alternative packages have to be used. In particular, we have used the *rpart* library of *R* as described by Therneau and Atkinson (2011). This is a free software environment for statistical computing and graphics. Apart from modeling binary and continuous outcome variables, *rpart* may also be used for categorical, survival time and count data. Routines for analysis are also available as part of SAS Enterprise Miner (EM) 12.1 (SAS Institute, 2012). These routines provide pruning and CV procedures and graphical output of the regression trees. The programs also allow other options for creating classification and regression trees in addition to those described here. For example, the information function component of equations (9.1) and (9.2) may be replaced by $Q_{Root}(1 - Q_{Root})$. This is termed the Gini information index, after Corrado Gini 1884–1965, and the change in impurity calculated on this basis. Also there are options to curtail the node splitting in order to prevent the daughter nodes containing less than a pre-specified number of subjects.

10 Further Time-to-Event Models

SUMMARY

In this chapter we consider the situation where, rather than having a single outcome which defines the event of interest in a time-to-event study, there are several competing event types defined. Competing in the sense that once any one of these events has occurred within a study participant it may prevent, or at least influence, the times at which the remaining events can occur. Our purpose is to describe how such studies may be best summarized.

The chapter also discusses parametric models, which utilize the assumed distribution of the survival times under study, as alternatives to the semi-parametric Cox regression model.

In addition there are situations in which covariates, usually first determined at the commencement of a survival-time study, may themselves vary with time. We describe how such covariates may be incorporated into the modeling process and how they can help overcome difficulties associated with situations when the assumption of proportional hazards is violated.

COMPETING RISKS

Introduction

In cancer survival studies, the main outcome event with which to compare treatments is usually the time to death (D) post-diagnosis, although the times of local recurrence (LR) of the disease, development of distant metastasis (DM) and/or a second cancer (SC) are always of relevance. Although all patients will eventually die, before this they may (or may not) experience any one or more of the other events. Theoretically, the time to these respective events from diagnosis (or from the date of randomization in a clinical trial), t_{LR}, t_{DM}, t_{SC} and t_D can be recorded for each patient. However, if D occurs first, then only t_D will be recorded, and the times to the other competing events t_{LR}, t_{DM} and t_{SC} cannot be observed. Similarly, if LR occurs before the other events are observed, then this may potentially initiate a change in therapeutic strategy and hence change the course of the disease and thereby (hopefully) prevent the events DM and SC occurring and also postpone D. The different events are

Regression Methods for Medical Research, First Edition. Bee Choo Tai and David Machin.
© 2014 Bee Choo Tai and David Machin. Published 2014 by John Wiley & Sons, Ltd.

regarded as competing with each other to be the first to occur, hence the term competing risks (CR). In other contexts death may be the only endpoint but it is the cause of death, perhaps from cardiovascular failure, cancer, diabetes or other cause, that provides the competing risk. For example, Poole-Wilson, Uretsky, Thygesen, *et al.* (2003) conducted a randomized, double-blind clinical trial of lisinopril in patients with chronic heart failure in which other modes of death (sudden unexpected, other causes) were considered as competing risks for chronic heart failure death.

A specific example of where an appropriate analysis of CR is important is that of Grundy, Wilne, Weston, *et al.* (2007) in their trial designed to delay or avoid irradiation among children with malignant brain tumours. Here, although having to initiate radiotherapy (RT) following disease progression is the important event, competing events include declining RT following disease progression and initiating RT despite no evidence of disease progression.

Competing risks occur in many other areas of clinical medicine and they are particularly prominent in trials concerned with fertility regulation. Thus, a particular feature when using an Intra-Uterine Device (IUD) is the large number of possible causes of discontinuation of use (failure) including, for example, involuntary pregnancy, expulsion of the device itself, medical removals for pain and or bleeding, and non-medical removals such as the woman concerned having no further need for contraception. In trials of IUDs, such as those conducted by the World Health Organization and discussed by Tai, Peregoudov and Machin (2001), the objective is to quantify the different discontinuation rates and to compare the devices with respect to each of these.

Cause-specific rates (*CSR*)

One approach to regression modeling in the competing risks situation is to focus on one event type, say *LR*, and if this is the first of the competing events to occur, then t_{LR} is recorded. Should one of the other possible events occur first (say *DM* at t_{DM}), then the time to *LR* is censored and is recorded at that value as $T_{LR}^+ = t_{DM}$. Thus, the data of interest only concerns local recurrences and the Kaplan-Meier (K-M) survival curves and Cox regression models of Chapter 6 use such data. The focus of the analysis may then switch to a different event type, say *DM*, in which case the analysis will concern different values of t_{DM} and T_{DM}^+. To make the K-M calculations, equation (6.10) is modified to indicate which of the $k=1, 2, \ldots, K$ competing risks is being considered. Thus:

$$S_k(t_{ki}) = (1 - d_{ki}/n_{ki}) \times (1 - d_{ki-1}/n_{ki-1}) \times \ldots \times (1 - d_{k1}/n_{k1}) = S_k(t_{ki-1}) \times (1 - d_{ki}/n_{ki}) \quad (10.1)$$

From which the Cause-specific *failure* rate (CSR) for competing risk k is

$$CSR_k(t_{ki}) = 1 - S_k(t_{ki}) \quad (10.2)$$

and examples of which are the cumulative death rate (CDR) curves of Figure 6.7 for patients with schizophrenia, although in that study, $K=1$ as there are no CRs considered.

Wee, Tan, Tai, *et al.* (2005) conducted the SQNP01 trial in patients with locally advanced nasopharyngeal cancer to compare RT alone with CRT, which comprised concurrent radiochemotherapy followed by adjuvant chemotherapy using cisplatin and 5-fluorouracil. The primary outcome of the trial was event-free survival (EFS). For illustration, we consider the occurrence of local regional recurrence (*LR*), distant metastasis (*DM*) and death (*D*) as

(a) Reported events

tabulate CRisk treat

```
----------------------------------+----------------------------------------
                                  |        |      Treatment      |
              Event               | CRisk  |   RT        CRT     | Total
----------------------------------+--------+---------------------+----------
      Local Recurrence (LR)       |   1    |   10          9     |   19
      Distant Metastasis (DM)     |   2    |   38         18     |   56
                     Dead (D)     |   3    |    6          7     |   13
                        Alive     |   –    |   56         77     |  133
----------------------------------+--------+---------------------+----------
                                  | Total  |  110        111     |  221
----------------------------------+----------------------------------------
```

(b) Cause-Specific Rate for Local Recurrence for patients randomized to CRT

stset, clear
stset reltimed, fail(LR)
sts list if treat==1

```
-----------------------------------------------------------------------
 Time                                    Survivor
 to LR    Total    Fail    Lost          Function        CSR
-----------------------------------------------------------------------
   0       111       0       0              1             0
  153      109       1       0            0.9908        0.0092
  248      100       1       0            0.9809        0.0191
  274       95       1       0            0.9706        0.0294
  277       94       1       0            0.9603        0.0397
  295       93       1       0            0.9499        0.0501
  370       91       1       0            0.9395        0.0605
  399       86       1       0            0.9286        0.0714
  524       78       1       0            0.9167        0.0833
 1660       15       1       0            0.8556        0.1444
-----------------------------------------------------------------------
```

Figure 10.1 Results from the SQNP01 trial. (a) Number and type of events observed by randomized treatment, (b) times to local recurrence and associated Cause-specific rates (CSR) (counting local recurrence as the event and censoring times of any distant metastasis, death and alive free of disease) (part data from Wee, Tan, Tai, et al., 2005)

the competing risks. As shown in Figure 10.1(a), a total of 110 patients were randomized to receive RT alone, and 111 received CRT. Among these patients a total of 19 local recurrences, 56 distant metastases and 13 deaths, without either recurrence or distant metastases, were identified. The remaining 133 patients were alive free of disease when last examined.

The times at which the nine *LR* events occurred among the patients receiving CRT are given in Figure 10.1(b). For example, one subject experienced this event at Day 153 post-randomization to treatment, whereas for a second subject his recurrence occurred at Day 248. Tied times-to-recurrence of *LR* events were not reported, and so there is a single event at each recurrence time, in which case $d_{LRi} = 1$ at whatever time i.

The *CSR* for local recurrence, expressed as a cumulative failure rate, is shown for the CRT group in Figure 10.2(a) and indicates, for example, a 3-year CSR = 8.3%. However, the corresponding CSR for distant metastasis of Figure 10.2(b) is higher at 16.5%.

The results for the two IUDs described in Tai, Peregoudov and Machin (2001, Table II) with respect to *CSR* at 1-year are given in Figure 10.3. In this example, there are six reasons for discontinuation (the competing risks), among these the *CSR* for TCu380A for the event 'involuntary pregnancy' is 2.20% and for 'expulsion' is higher at 12.49%. It should be

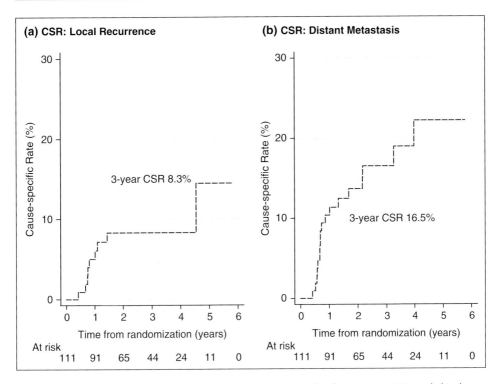

Figure 10.2 Cause-specific rates (CSR) with respect to (a) local recurrence (LR) and (b) distant metastasis (DM) among patients receiving concurrent radio-chemotherapy (CRT) (part data from Wee, Tan, Tai, *et al.*, 2005)

Competing risks	Cause Specific (*CSR*)	
	TCu380A	TCu220C
Involuntary pregnancy	2.20	5.79
Expulsion	12.49	12.79
Total medical removals	40.15	39.09
Total non-medical removals	53.92	53.95
Loss to follow-up	38.41	38.76
Other discontinuations	15.19	15.17
Arithmetic sum of each *CSR*	162.36	165.55

Figure 10.3 1-year post-insertion cause-specific discontinuation rates (%) comparing two IUDs, TCu380A and TCu220C, for fertility regulation (after Tai, Peregoudov and Machin, 2001, table II)

noted that, in contrast to most other clinical trial situations, 'loss to follow-up' is often regarded in contraceptive efficacy studies as an 'event' rather than treated as a 'censored' observation. In such one-year duration trials, only the women who complete 12 months of use with their IUD remaining in situ are regarded as truly censored. The sum of the *CSR*s for all six event types with TCu380A is $2.20+12.49+40.15+53.92+38.41+15.19=162.36$. The corresponding sum for TCu220C is 165.55. These both clearly exceed 100%. Thus, for either IUD it is difficult to ascertain the true contribution of each competing risk as each

CSR is inflated to an uncertain extent. This highlights a problem of using the *CSR* as a summary measure in competing risks studies. Nevertheless, the *CSR* enables the different event types to be ranked in terms of their relative contribution to device failure.

CuMulative Incidence Rates (CMIR)

In contrast to the CSR which deals with a single risk and regards all the others as censored, the CuMulative Incidence Rate (CMIR) takes full account of all the competing risks present. There are two component parts to the calculation of the CMIR. The first component is the cause-specific hazard of the primary risk of interest, denoted k, at event time t_i. This is defined by:

$$h_k(t_{ki}) = \frac{d_{ki}}{n_i} \qquad (10.3)$$

where n_i is the number of subjects event-free just before t_{ki} and d_{ki} is the number who fail from competing risk k at t_{ki}. Thus, if we are considering *LR* as the event of interest in those receiving CRT in Figure 10.1(b), then there are nine event times $t_{LR1} = 153$, $t_{LR2} = 248$, ... , $t_{LR9} = 1660$.

The second component considers the 'first of *any* one of the several, K, competing events to occur' as 'the event of interest'. Thus, in Figure 10.1(a), $K = 3$ as there are three failure types in all and, as *any* one of these occurs, this provides the corresponding survival time. In total, there are now $9 + 18 + 7 = 34$ events to consider among those receiving CRT, each with individual failure time denoted t_j. These survival times are then used as the outcome variable for equation (6.10) to obtain the Kaplan-Meier estimates:

$$KM_j = S_{Any}(t_j) \qquad (10.4)$$

However, although these have a specific value whenever an event of any type occurs, we only need to note their value immediately before the times, t_{ki}, when each event of type k occurs, and we denote these by $KM_{Any}(t_{ki} - 1)$.

The two components, (10.3) and (10.4), are then combined to give at event time t_{ki}:

$$KM_{Any}(t_{ki} - 1) \times \frac{d_{ki}}{n_i} = S_{Any}(t_{ki} - 1) \times h_k(t_{ki}) \qquad (10.5)$$

from which the cumulative incidence rate is obtained as

$$CMIR_k(t_{ki}) = CMIR_k(t_{ki-1}) + S_{Any}(t_{ki} - 1) h_k(t_{ki}) \qquad (10.6)$$

The calculation begins by setting $CMIR_k(0) = 0$ at the beginning of follow-up, when time is zero, and this remains zero until t_{k1}; the time when the first event of type k occurs. Similarly, $S_{Any}(0) = 1$ from time zero and remains so until the time of occurrence of the first event of *any* type.

Once the first event (of type k) has occurred, the calculation then proceeds by continually updating (10.6) on every subsequent occasion of time when a further event of type k occurs.

Note that t_{ki-1} means the time when the previous event of type k has occurred prior to that at t_{ki}. For example, in Figure 10.4 the seventh local recurrence occurs on Day 399, so $k = LR$, $i = 7$ and $t_{LR7} = 399$ so $t_{ki-1} = t_{LR6} = 370$ of column (ii). In contrast, $S_{Any}(t_{ki} - 1)$ indicates the

i	t_{LRi} Day(Year)	d_{LRi}	n_i	$S_{Any}(t_{LRi}-1)$	$h_{LR}(t_{LRi})$	$CMIR_{LR}(t_{LRi})$
(i)	(ii)	(iii)	(iv)	(v)	(vi)	(vii)
0	0	0	111	1	–	0
1	153 (0.42)	1	109	0.9820	0.0092	0.0090
2	248 (0.68)	1	100	0.9094	0.0100	0.0181
3	274 (0.75)	1	95	0.8639	0.0105	0.0272
4	277 (0.76)	1	94	0.8548	0.0106	0.0363
5	295 (0.81)	1	93	0.8457	0.0108	0.0454
6	370 (1.01)	1	91	0.8276	0.0110	0.0545
7	399 (1.09)	1	86	0.8094	0.0116	0.0639
8	524 (1.43)	1	78	0.7807	0.0128	0.0739
9	1660 (4.54)	1	15	0.6169	0.0667	0.1150

Figure 10.4 Times to recurrence, t_{LRi}, number of recurrences, d_{LRi}, number of patients at risk, n_i, any event-free survival (counting the first of LR, DM or D as the event), $S_{Any}(t_{LRi} - 1)$, cause-specific hazard, $h_{LR}(t_{LRi})$, and the cumulative incidence rate for event LR, $CMIR_{LR}(t_{LRi})$, of treatment CRT of the SQNP01 trial (part data from Wee, Tan, Tai, et al., 2005)

calculation at any of the competing events, including type *LR*, that immediately precede that at t_{LRi}, the time of the *i*th local recurrence. Thus, for $i=7$, this implies that $(t_{LR7}-1)=398$ and the entry in column (v) is the *K-M* estimate of survival obtained from all events, *LR*, *DM* or *D*, preceding event *LR* at 399 days; thus, $S_{Any}(398)=0.8094$. Some extra clarity with respect to the notation is given in Figure 10.25 of *Technical details*.

The cause-specific hazard, $h_{LR}(t_{LRi})$, of equation (10.3) is calculated for the data from Wee, Tan, Tai, *et al.* (2005) by dividing the number of local recurrences, d_{LRi}, by the number of patients n_i, remaining at risk at t_{LRi} of column (iv) in Figure 10.4 to obtain column (vi). Although S_{Any} is calculated whenever an event occurs, whether *LR*, *DM* or *D*, column (v) only gives the estimated value of S_{Any} for the day prior to each *LR* occurring. Finally multiplying columns (v) and (vi) gives the *CMIR* of column (vii).

The calculation begins with $CMIR_{LR}(0)=0$, as this corresponds to having $n_0=111$ patients just randomized with no follow-up time to permit any event to occur as shown in Figure 10.1(b). Prior to the first *LR* event at 153 days, 2 patients are censored for this analysis. Thus, $n_1=(111-2)=109$ at $t_{LR1}=153$, $CMIR_{LR}(153)=CMIR_{LR}(0)+S_{Any}(152)\times h_{LR}(153)=0+(0.9820 \times 0.0092)=0.0090$. In fact, prior to the *LR* at 153 days, there were deaths at 29 and 43 days. These gave $S_{Any}(29)=0.9910$ then $S_{Any}(43)=0.9820$. However, as there were no further events after Day 43 until Day 153, the K-M estimate remains at this value up to and including Day 152 and so $S_{Any}(152)=0.9820$. Following the first local recurrence, the next *LR* occurs at $t_{LR2}=248$, hence $CMIR_{LR}(248)=CMIR_{LR}(153)+S_{Any}(247)\times h_{LR}(248)=0.0090+(0.9094\times0.0100)$ $=0.0181$. This process continues until the final *LR* event at $t_{LR9}=1660$, and so $CMIR_{LR}(1660)=$ $CMIR_{LR}(524)+S_{Any}(1659)\times h_{LR}(1660)=0.0739+(0.6169 \times 0.0667)=0.1150$.

The CMIR can be calculated directly by use of the command (**stcompet CMIR=ci, compet1(2) compet2(3)**). Here (**ci**) is an acronym for cumulative incidence and (2) and (3) refer to the competing risks (*CRisk*) of *DM* and *D* of Figure 10.1(a). The results are summarized in Figure 10.5(a).

Similar calculations can be made for the *DM* events in the CRT group of patients, and these are summarized graphically in Figure 10.5(b). As was the case for *CSR*, it is clear from Figure 10.5

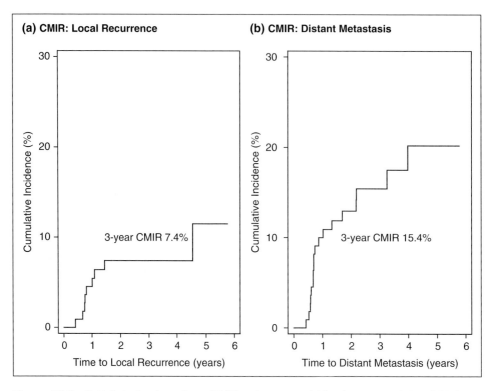

Figure 10.5 CuMulative Incidence Rates (CMIR) with respect to (a) local recurrence (LR) and (b) distant metastasis (DM) among patients receiving CRT (part data from Wee, Tan, Tai, *et al.*, 2005)

Competing risks	Cumulative Incidence Rate (*CMIR*) (%)	
	TCu380A	TCu220C
Involuntary pregnancy	1.29	3.51
Expulsion	8.09	8.74
Total medical removals	23.29	21.20
Total non-medical removals	30.80	29.94
Loss to follow-up	19.13	19.48
Other discontinuations	5.09	5.16
Any discontinuation	87.69	88.03
Also equals the arithmetic sum of each *CMIR*		

Figure 10.6 1-year post-insertion cumulative incidence discontinuation rates (*CMIR%*) comparing two IUDs, TCu380A and TCu220C, for fertility regulation (after Tai, Peregoudov and Machin, 2001, table II)

that the estimated *CMIR* for local recurrence is much less than that for distant metastasis. In addition, the *CMIR*s are numerically smaller than the corresponding *CSR*s of Figure 10.2.

Applying this methodology to the comparison of the two IUDs considered by Tai, Peregoudov and Machin (2001) gives the *CMIR* estimates at 1-year of Figure 10.6, which are all less than the corresponding *CSR* for each discontinuation reason of Figure 10.3. Thus, for example, for 'expulsion of the IUD' with TCu380A, $CSR=12.49\%$, whereas $CMIR=8.09\%$. These are quite substantial differences and are likely to have an important influence on how these data are interpreted. Further, the six individual $CMIRs$ now sum to give the estimated 1-year failure rates of 87.69% and 88.03% for TCu380A and TCu220C, respectively. These correspond exactly to calculations made when *any* of the six discontinuation reasons is counted as the 'event'. The corresponding censored rates for those completing the one-year trial without an event occurring are very similar at $100-87.69=12.31$ and $100-88.03=11.97\%$.

Adjusting for covariates

There are no new principles involved when adjusting for covariates when estimating the $CSRs$, as the Cox regression model described in Chapter 6 is immediately applicable. Thus, for local recurrence, LR, in the SQNP01 randomized trial, a comparison of the alternative treatments is made by fitting the model

$$\lambda_{LR}(t) = \lambda_{0LR}(t)\exp(\beta_{LR,Treat}Treat) \tag{10.7}$$

from which

$$CSR:HR_{LR} = \exp(\beta_{LR,Treat}Treat) \tag{10.8}$$

is the hazard ratio for comparing treatments with respect to local recurrence. Here $Treat=0$ when RT is given and $Treat=1$ for CRT. These have exactly the same form as equations (6.2) and (6.3). The essential command structure uses (`stcox Treat`) preceded by (`stset reltime, fail(CRisk==1)`) and estimates $CSR:HR_{LR}=0.84$ in favor of CRT. The corresponding cumulative event curves for local recurrence for each treatment group are shown in Figure 10.7(a). A similar analysis for distant metastasis, DM, is summarized in Figure 10.7(b) and gives $CSR:HR_{DM}=0.43$. In summary, these calculations suggest low LR rates with little difference between treatments, whereas DM rates are higher and much greater with RT.

The same algebraic format for the Cox proportional hazards model is also used in competing risks regression so that we have

$$\lambda_{LR}^{sub}(t) = \lambda_{0LR}^{sub}(t)\exp(\beta_{LR,Treat}Treat) \tag{10.9}$$

Although this describes the key features of the model, the detailed calculation process of Fine and Gray (1999) is explained further by Tai, Grundy and Machin (2011). This model takes better account of the other competing risks when making comparisons between groups. The 'sub' is therefore attached to emphasize that, although the expression looks similar to equation (10.7), the basis of the calculation is the *sub-distribution* variant of the CMIR. It is named sub-distribution as the method is dealing with the distributions of *each* of several competing risks. This leads to the sub-distribution hazard ratio:

$$Sub:HR_{LR} = \frac{\lambda_{LR}^{sub}(t)}{\lambda_{0LR}^{sub}(t)} = \exp(\beta_{LR,Treat}Treat) \tag{10.10}$$

The corresponding command now utilizes a competing risks option of the form (`stcrreg Treat, compete(CRisk==2, 3)`). Here the variable, $CRisk$ now indicates that distant metastasis ($CRisk=2$) and death ($CRisk=3$) are the competing risks for a local recurrence

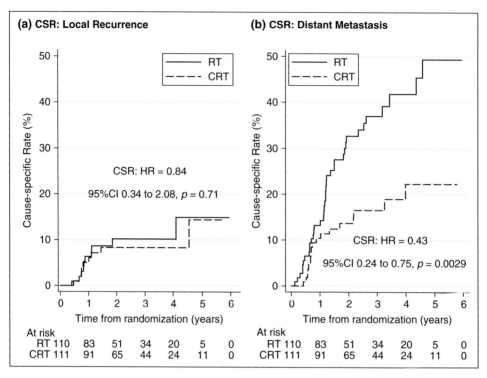

Figure 10.7 Cause-specific hazard ratio (CSR:HR) to compare RT and CRT for the treatment of patients with nasopharyngeal cancer with respect to (a) local recurrence (LR) and (b) distant metastasis (DM) (part data from Wee, Tan, Tai, et al., 2005)

($CRisk=1$). The corresponding output in Figure 10.8(a) gives a $Sub{:}HR_{LR}=0.91$ indicating less difference, that is the estimate is closer to the null hypothesis value of $HR_0=1$, between the treatment groups than indicated by $CSR{:}HR_{LR}=0.84$.

There is little to choose between, for example, the $CSR{:}HR_{DM}$ and that of $Sub{:}HR_{DM}$ for comparing treatments RT and CRT with respect to distant metastasis in the SQNP01 trial. However, quoting these, and the associated confidence intervals, in more detail than those presented as captions in Figures 10.7(b) and 10.8(b) gives $CSR{:}HR_{DM}=0.4263$, 95% CI 0.2432 to 0.7472 and $Sub{:}HR_{DM}=0.4343$, 95% CI 0.2476 to 0.7617, respectively. Thus, there are differences between them but, as they are so small, they will not affect the interpretation that fewer distant metastasis develop with CRT.

The competing risks version of the Cox model of (10.9) can be extended to include more than a single covariate. We noted in Chapter 7, *Practical considerations*, that nodal status, in two groups (N_0, N_1, N_2) and (N_3), was used to stratify the patients before randomization to RT and CRT in the SQNP01 trial. Fuller details of the numbers in each component nodal group are given in Figure 10.9(a). For illustrative purposes (we ignore the fact that the design was stratified on nodal status) if we add the categorical covariate *Node* to *Treat* then the corresponding CR model for LR takes the form:

$$\lambda_{LR}^{sub}(t) = \lambda_{0LR}^{sub}(t)\exp(\beta_{LR,Treat}Treat + \beta_{LR,Node}Node) \tag{10.11}$$

from which $Sub{:}HR_{LR}(Treat, Node) = \exp(\beta_{LR,Treat}Treat + \beta_{LR,Node}Node)$ is obtained.

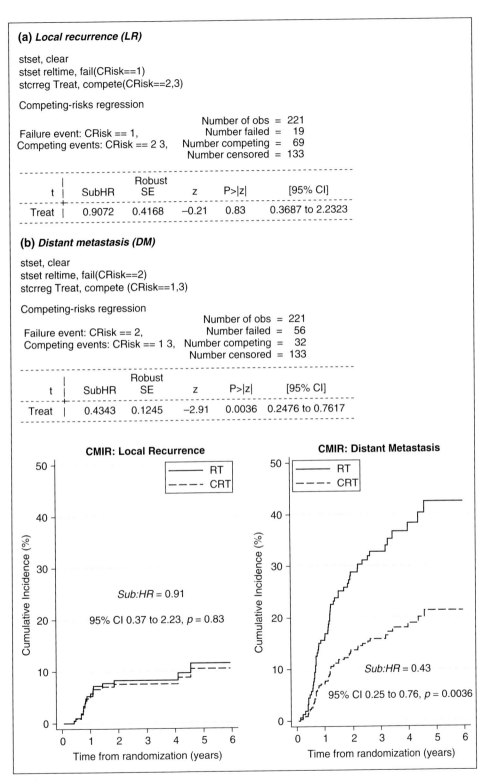

(a) *Local recurrence (LR)*

stset, clear
stset reltime, fail(CRisk==1)
stcrreg Treat, compete(CRisk==2,3)

Competing-risks regression

	Number of obs = 221
Failure event: CRisk == 1,	Number failed = 19
Competing events: CRisk == 2 3,	Number competing = 69
	Number censored = 133

t	SubHR	Robust SE	z	P>|z|	[95% CI]
Treat	0.9072	0.4168	−0.21	0.83	0.3687 to 2.2323

(b) *Distant metastasis (DM)*

stset, clear
stset reltime, fail(CRisk==2)
stcrreg Treat, compete (CRisk==1,3)

Competing-risks regression

	Number of obs = 221
Failure event: CRisk == 2,	Number failed = 56
Competing events: CRisk == 1 3,	Number competing = 32
	Number censored = 133

t	SubHR	Robust SE	z	P>|z|	[95% CI]
Treat	0.4343	0.1245	−2.91	0.0036	0.2476 to 0.7617

CMIR: Local Recurrence

Sub:HR = 0.91

95% CI 0.37 to 2.23, p = 0.83

CMIR: Distant Metastasis

Sub:HR = 0.43

95% CI 0.25 to 0.76, p = 0.0036

Figure 10.8 Commands and corresponding output for calculating the sub-distribution hazard ratio (*Sub:HR*) to compare RT and CRT with respect to (a) local recurrence (LR) and (b) distant metastasis (DM) (part data from Wee, Tan, Tai, et al., 2005)

(a) *Local Recurrence*

table Node LR Treat

```
----------------------------------------------------
         |        Treatment and LR       |       |
         |  ----- RT ---   ---- CRT - |       |
  Node   |   0      1       0      1  |  All  |
---------+-----------------------------+-------|
  N0  |   10      2       10      1 |   23  |
  N1  |   11      1       15      1 |   28  |
  N2  |   49      4       50      5 |  108  |
  N3  |   30      3       27      2 |   62  |
----------------------------------------------------
```

stset, clear
stset reltime, fail(CRisk==1)
xi: stcrreg Treat i.Node, compete(CRisk==2,3)

```
-------------------------------------------------------------------
        |                 Robust
      t |    SubHR         SE        z      P>|z|        [95% CI]
--------+----------------------------------------------------------
  Treat |   0.9147       0.4214    -0.19     0.85     0.3708 to 2.2564
  N0  |   1
  N1  |   0.5252       0.4585
  N2  |   0.6762       0.4460
  N3  |   0.6468       0.4689
-------------------------------------------------------------------
```

(b) *Distant Metastasis*

table Node DM Treat

```
----------------------------------------------------
         |        Treatment and DM       |       |
         |  ---- RT ---   ---- CRT -- |       |
  Node   |   0      1       0      1  |  All  |
---------+-----------------------------+-------|
  N0  |   10      2       10      1 |   23  |
  N1  |    7      5       14      2 |   28  |
  N2  |   35     18       50      5 |  108  |
  N3  |   20     13       19     10 |   62  |
----------------------------------------------------
```

stset, clear
stset reltime, fail(CRisk==2)
xi: stcrreg Treat i.Node, compete(CRisk==1,3)

```
-------------------------------------------------------------------
        |                 Robust
      t |    SubHR         SE        z      P>|z|        [95% CI]
--------+----------------------------------------------------------
  Treat |   0.4494       0.1312    -2.74    0.0061    0.2535 to 0.7965
  N0  |   1
  N1  |   2.2178       1.5033
  N2  |   1.9822       1.1993
  N3  |   3.6545       2.2215
-------------------------------------------------------------------
```

Figure 10.9 Commands and corresponding output for calculating the sub-distribution hazard ratio (*Sub:HR*) to compare RT and CRT for patients with nasopharyngeal cancer adjusted for nodal status with respect to (a) local recurrence (LR) and (b) distant metastasis (DM) (part data from Wee, Tan, Tai, *et al.*, 2005)

	Randomized Treatment		Cause-specific	Sub-distribution
	RT	CRT	*CSR:HR* (95% CI)	*Sub:HR* (95% CI)
Local Recurrence (*n*)	10	9		
Treat (Unadjusted)			0.8435 (0.3426 to 2.0766)	0.9072 (0.3687 to 2.2323)
Treat (Adjusted for *Node*)			0.8631 (0.3492 to 2.1332)	0.9147 (0.3708 to 2.2564)
Distant metastasis (*n*)	38	18		
Treat (Unadjusted)			0.4263 (0.2432 to 0.7472)	0.4343 (0.2476 to 0.7617)
Treat (Adjusted for *Node*)			0.4462 (0.2538 to 0.7843)	0.4494 (0.2535 to 0.7965)

Figure 10.10 Cox type regression estimates of the hazard ratio for comparing RT and CRT using the cause-specific and sub-distribution estimates (part data from Wee, Tan, Tai, *et al.*, 2005)

Fitting this model to the trial data of Wee, Tan, Tai, *et al.* (2005) using the command structure (**xi: stcrreg Treat i.Node, compete(CRisk==2,3)**) gives for local recurrence the results of Figure 10.9(a) and for distant metastases those of Figure 10.9(b). Use of (**xi:**) and hence (**i.Node**) are necessitated as *Node* is regarded as a covariate of four unordered categories.

Figure 10.10 compares the CSR and CMIR estimates of the hazard ratios for the SQNP01 trial for local recurrence and distant metastasis. Although general conclusions should not be drawn from this, the *Sub:HR*s are closer to the null hypothesis value, $HR_0 = 1$, than the corresponding *CSR:HR*. Differences are greater between the values for local recurrence where there are fewer events, 19 in all, compared with distant metastasis with 56. Adjusting for nodal status also move the estimated HRs closer to the null, but the small sizes of these changes would not affect interpretation with respect to the magnitude of the treatment differences. As Beyersmann, Dettenkofer, Bertz and Schumacher (2007) emphasize, when treatment has no effect on the relative hazard rates of the competing risks concerned, the results from both the CSR and CMIR regression models will concur well. Nevertheless, there may be appreciable differences between *CSR:HR* and *Sub:HR* if the main and competing events are influenced in opposite directions by an intervention.

PARAMETRIC MODELS

Introduction

Regression models are not only an integral part of the (non-parametric) Cox approach of Chapter 6, but they are also relevant to situations where the time-to-event is assumed to have an Exponential or Weibull distribution form. The shape of these distributions depends on values of one and two parameters, respectively, and these have to be estimated using model fitting procedures.

Single group – no covariate

The simplest time-to-event distribution arises when the hazard rate, $\lambda(t)$, does not depend on t but remains constant over time. A constant value of the hazard rate, here denoted η (Greek eta), implies that the probability of an event occurring for each individual concerned remains constant as successive days go by. This idea extends to saying that the probability of an event in any time interval depends only on the width of that interval. Thus, the wider the time interval, the greater the probability of an event in that interval, but where the interval begins (and ends) has no influence on the event rate.

In this case the time-to-event follows the Exponential distribution, which has a survival function of the form:

$$S_{Exponential}(t) = \exp(-\eta t) \tag{10.12}$$

The unchanging hazard rate, $\lambda_{Exponential}(t) = \eta$ is a unique property of the Exponential distribution and it is estimated by

$$\eta = \frac{e}{f + F} \tag{10.13}$$

where e is the total number of events observed, f is the total follow-up time of the e patients experiencing an event, and F is the total follow-up time of the remaining $(n - e)$ censored observation times obtained from those not yet experiencing an event.

In the example of Sridhar, Gore, Boiangiu, *et al.* (2009), there were $e = 30$ deaths with $f = 25.6564$ years and for the $(35 - 30) = 5$ alive patients, $F = 12.7830$ years. The command (**strate**) in Figure 10.11(a) gives the estimated hazard rate as $\eta = 0.78$ per year. However, this command must be preceded by (**stset survy, fail(dead)**), which defines the events and the corresponding survival times. Alternatively, this can be calculated using the regression command (**streg, distribution(exponential)**) of Figure 10.11(b).

The shape of the Exponential survival function of equation (10.12) is shown as the hatched curve in Figure 10.11(c) following the commands (**predict**), which calculates the curve, and (**sts graph**), which produces the plot. The Exponential function provides a close, but smoothed, summary of the K-M survival curve. Hence, we can conclude that patients with this disease are therefore dying at an approximately constant rate.

It follows from the fitted line that about $\exp(-0.7804 \times 1) = 0.46$ or 46% of the patients remain alive at one year, and at two years $\exp(-0.7804 \times 2) = 0.21$ or 21%. For a value of the hazard rate $\eta < 0.7804$, the corresponding exponential survival function lies above that of Figure 10.11(c) as the death rate is lower, whereas for $\eta > 0.7804$ it will fall below as, in this case, the death rate is higher.

The Weibull distribution of event times has two parameters η and κ (kappa) and takes the form

$$S_{Weibull}(t) = \exp\left[-(\eta t)^{\kappa}\right], \kappa > 0 \tag{10.14}$$

The parameter η is referred to as the scale parameter and κ the shape. It can be shown that this model corresponds to a hazard rate described by

$$\lambda_{Weibull}(t) = \eta \kappa (\eta t)^{\kappa - 1} \tag{10.15}$$

Thus, in contrast to the Exponential distribution, the hazard rate of the Weibull distribution does change with time, t. In fact, as time increases when $\kappa > 1$ the value of $\lambda(t)$ also increases, whereas if $\kappa < 1$ it decreases. However, when $\kappa = 1$, equation (10.15) becomes

(a) *Estimating the constant death rate*

stset survy, fail(dead)
strate

Estimated rates and lower/upper bounds of 95% confidence intervals
(35 records included in the analysis)

```
+---------------------------------------------+
|  D    Y        Rate      Lower     Upper   |
|--------------------------------------------|
|  30   38.4394  0.7805    0.5457 to 1.1162  |
+---------------------------------------------+
```

(b) *Estimating the constant death rate using an Exponential model*

streg, distribution(exponential)

Exponential regression -- log relative-hazard form

No. of subjects = 35, No. of failures = 30, Time at risk = 38.4394
Log-likelihood = –51.7487

```
---------------------------------------------------------------
     t |  ExpRate    SE        z    P>|z|      [95% CI]
-------+-------------------------------------------------------
  cons |  0.7804    0.1425   -1.36   0.17   0.5457 to 1.1162
---------------------------------------------------------------
```

(c) *Plotting the survival curve*

predict SExp, surv
sts graph, addplot(line SExp_t, sort)

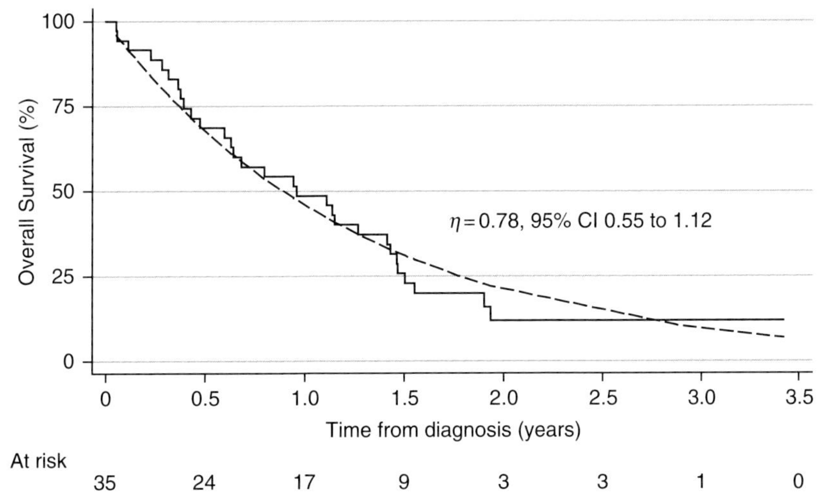

$\eta = 0.78$, 95% CI 0.55 to 1.12

At risk
```
            35        24        17       9       3        3        1       0
```

Figure 10.11 Exponential regression model fitted to overall survival of 35 patients with glioblastoma treated with temozolomide and radiation (data from Sridhar, Gore, Boiangiu, *et al.*, 2009)

$\lambda(t) = \eta \times 1 \times (\eta t)^{1-1} = \eta \times (\eta t)^0 = \eta$, and this is now the unchanging hazard of the Exponential distribution. Thus, the Exponential distribution is nested within the Weibull distribution.

The corresponding fit of the Weibull distribution to the survival data of those with glioblastoma using the command (**streg, nohr distribution(weibull)**) is shown

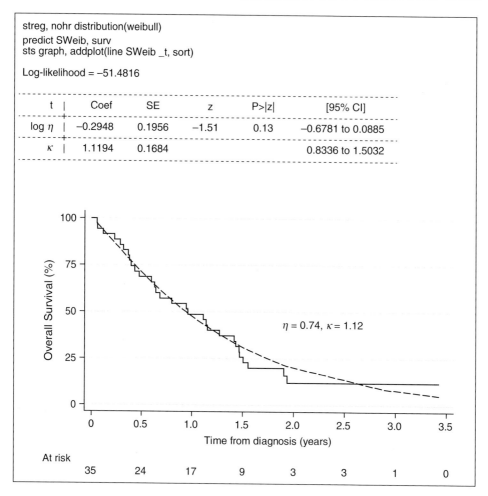

```
streg, nohr distribution(weibull)
predict SWeib, surv
sts graph, addplot(line SWeib _t, sort)
```

Log-likelihood = –51.4816

t	Coef	SE	z	P>|z|	[95% CI]
log η	–0.2948	0.1956	–1.51	0.13	–0.6781 to 0.0885
κ	1.1194	0.1684			0.8336 to 1.5032

$\eta = 0.74$, $\kappa = 1.12$

At risk

| | 35 | 24 | 17 | 9 | 3 | 3 | 1 | 0 |

Figure 10.12 Weibull regression model fitted to overall survival of 35 patients with glioblastoma treated with temozolomide and radiation (data from Sridhar, Gore, Boiangiu, *et al.*, 2009)

in Figure 10.12, and this also provides close agreement with the K-M curve. Here (cons) corresponds to log $\eta = -0.2948$, hence $\eta = \exp(-0.2948) = 0.7447$ while $\kappa = 1.1194$. These are the maximum likelihood estimates which are obtained by solving equations (10.23) and (10.24) described in *Technical details*.

The fact that $\kappa > 1$ means that the hazard of failure increases with time, although not dramatically here so that if we were to compare $\lambda(0.5) = \eta\kappa(\eta \times 0.5)^{\kappa-1}$ with one year later when $\lambda(1.5) = \eta\kappa(\eta \times 1.5)^{\kappa-1}$, their ratio is $(1.5/0.5)^{1.1194-1} = 3^{0.1194} = 1.14$ or a 14% increase in failure rate.

The Weibull estimates of the parameters are both close to those of the corresponding Exponential model: namely $\eta = 0.7804$ and $\kappa = 1$. As the Exponential model is nested within the Weibull model, the 'extra' fit provided by the latter can be tested using the likelihood ratio statistic (LR). In this example $\log L_{Exponential} = -51.7487$ from Figure 10.11(b), and $\log L_{Weibull} = -51.4816$ from Figure 10.12, hence the $LR = 2 \times [-51.7487 - (-51.4816)] = 0.534$. As the Weibull distribution has two parameters, one more than the Exponential distribution, the comparison has $df = 1$ so Table T5 of the χ^2 distribution gives the corresponding p-value > 0.2. More precise tabulations give a p-value $= 0.47$, which is far from statistically significant. Hence the extra complexity of the Weibull distribution does not seem justified to describe these data.

Further, it is clear that the estimated survival values at one and two years of $S_{Weibull}(1)=$ $\exp[-(0.7447 \times 1)^{1.1194}]=0.49$ or 49% and $S_{Weibull}(2)=\exp[-(0.7447 \times 2)^{1.1194}]=0.21$ or 21% are very similar to the 46% and 21% estimated by the Exponential distribution.

Models with covariates

When comparing two groups, say A and B, each with constant but possibly different hazards, and hence each have a corresponding Exponential distribution of survival times, the hazard for group A can be specified by $\eta_A=\eta$, whereas for group B, $\eta_B=\eta \times \exp(\beta_1)$ neither of which depend on t. These two hazards can be combined into one regression model as:

$$\lambda_{Exponential}(t,x_1) = \eta \times \exp(\beta_1 x_1) \tag{10.16}$$

where $x_1=0$ for group A and $x_1=1$ for group B. The right-hand side of this equation does not include t, as the hazard is constant regardless of time. Consequently, we replace $\lambda_{Exponential}$ (t, x_1) by $\lambda_{Exponential}(\,.\,, x_1)$ to make it clear it does not depend on t, but only on the value of the associated covariate, x_1. In this case the $HR=\lambda_{Exponential}(\,.\,,1)/ \lambda_{Exponential}(\,.\,,0)=[\eta \times \exp(\beta_1)]/ [\eta \times \exp(0)]=\exp(\beta_1)$. Thus, the Exponential distribution provides a proportional hazards (PH) model as the (now unchanging) baseline hazard rate divides out when calculating the HR.

In the study reported by Sridhar, Gore, Boiangiu, *et al.* (2009), two types of patients with glioblastoma were recruited: those with very extensive (*Extent*=0) and those with less extensive (*Extent*=1) disease; the latter with the better anticipated prognosis as is evident from Figure 6.6. As we noted earlier, and repeated in Figure 10.13(a), using a Cox regression model comparing the *Extent* groups gives $HR_{Cox}=0.1378$, indicating a greater mortality in those with very extensive disease.

However, assuming an Exponential distribution of survival times, and using the command (**streg Extent, distribution(exponential)**) of Figure 10.13(b), gives the estimated hazard ratio directly as $HR_{Exponential}=0.2303$. This is larger (closer to the null hypothesis value of 1) than the estimate provided by the Cox model. Adding (**nohr**) to the previous command provides estimates of $\log\eta$ and β_1 so that from Figure 10.13(b) $\log \eta=0.8523$ giving $\eta=\exp(0.8523)=2.3450$. The estimate of β_1 is $b_1=-1.4682$ from which $HR_{Exponential}=\exp(-1.4682)=0.2303$ once more.

In a similar way a covariate model can be derived for the situation where the Weibull distribution of survival times is appropriate. However, in this case the corresponding hazard is anticipated to change with time, t, as well as with the covariate, x_1, and the expression corresponding to (10.16) takes the form:

$$\lambda_{Weibull}(t,x_1) = \eta\kappa(\eta t)^{\kappa-1} \times \exp(\beta_1 x_1) \tag{10.17}$$

It is clear from this that the value of $\lambda_{Weibull}(t, x_1)$ depends on both t and x_1. The hazard ratio for comparing groups $x_1=1$ with $x_1=0$ is

$$HR = \frac{\lambda_{Weibull}(t,1)}{\lambda_{Weibull}(t,0)} = \frac{\left[\eta\kappa(\eta t)^{\kappa-1} \times \exp(\beta_1)\right]}{\left[\eta\kappa(\eta t)^{\kappa-1} \times \exp(0)\right]} = \exp(\beta_1) \tag{10.18}$$

Thus, the Weibull distribution also provides a PH model as the baseline hazard rate divides out when calculating the HR.

(a) *Cox regression model*

tabulate status Extent

```
----------+--------------------+--------
          |        Extent      |
status    |   Very      Less   | Total
----------+--------------------+--------
  Alive   |     0         5    |    5
  Dead    |    12        18    |   30
----------+--------------------+--------
  Total   |    12        23    |   35
----------+--------------------+--------
```

stcox Extent

No. of subjects = 35, No. of failures = 30, Time at risk = 38.4394
Log likelihood = −77.859693

```
----------------------------------------------------------------
   t  |  HRCox      SE       z      P>|z|        [95% CI]
------+---------------------------------------------------------
Extent|  0.1378   0.0644   −4.24   0.00002   0.0551 to 0.3444
----------------------------------------------------------------
```

(b) *Exponential regression*

streg Extent, distribution(exponential)

Log likelihood = −45.169571

```
----------------------------------------------------------------
   t  |  HRExp      SE       z      P>|z|        [95% CI]
------+---------------------------------------------------------
Extent|  0.2303   0.0858   −3.94   0.00008   0.1110 to 0.4782
----------------------------------------------------------------
```

streg Extent, nohr distribution (exponential)

```
----------------------------------------------------------------
   t    |  Coef      SE       z      P>|z|        [95% CI]
--------+-------------------------------------------------------
 logη   |  0.8523   0.2887   2.95   0.0032    0.2865 to  1.4181
 Extent | −1.4682   0.3727  −3.94   0.00008  −2.1986 to −0.7378
----------------------------------------------------------------
```

(c) *Weibull regression*

streg Extent, distribution(weibull)

Log likelihood = −42.421906

```
----------------------------------------------------------------
   t  | HRWeibull   SE       z      P>|z|        [95%CI]
------+---------------------------------------------------------
Extent|  0.1417   0.0616   −4.50   0.00001   0.0605 to 0.3321
------+---------------------------------------------------------
  κ   |  1.4599   0.2160    2.56   0.011     1.0925 to 1.9508
----------------------------------------------------------------
```

streg Extent, nohr distribution (weibull)

```
----------------------------------------------------------------
    t    |  Coef      SE       z      P>|z|        [95% CI]
---------+------------------------------------------------------
log(ηκ)  |  1.0763   0.3021   3.56   0.00037   0.4843 to  1.6683
 Extent  | −1.9537   0.4343  −4.50   0.00001  −2.8050 to −1.1025
---------+------------------------------------------------------
   κ     |  1.4599   0.2160   2.56   0.011     1.0925 to  1.9508
----------------------------------------------------------------
```

Figure 10.13 A comparison of the Cox, Exponential and Weibull regression models in patients with glioblastoma having very and less extensive disease at diagnosis (data from Sridhar, Gore, Boiangiu, *et al.*, 2009)

Assuming a Weibull distribution of survival times for the patients with glioblastoma using the command (**streg Extent, distribution(weibull)**) of Figure 10.13(c), gives $HR_{Weibull} = 0.1417$. Further, if the previous command is modified to include (**nohr**) then $\kappa = 1.4599$, while $\log(\eta\kappa) = 1.0763$. From the latter $\eta\kappa = \exp(1.0763) = 2.9338$, and so $\eta = 2.9338/\kappa = 2.9338/1.4599 = 2.0096$. This contrasts with the greater estimated hazard rate of $\eta = 2.3450$ when assuming the Exponential distribution, which, as we have stated previously, implicitly has $\kappa = 1$. Finally, $HR_{Weibull} = \exp(-1.9537) = 0.1417$ as before.

The latter estimate is close to that given by use of the Cox model. However, as the Weibull is also a PH model and both allow the hazard rates to change over time, these may explain why the two approaches produce similar estimates of the HR. In contrast, the Exponential model, although also PH, makes the restrictive assumption that the hazard rates do not fluctuate over time. This firm requirement may explain the large difference from the corresponding estimated HRs from the other models.

The format of equations (10.16) and (10.17) can be extended to a multiple regression situation including several covariates by adding, for example, $\beta_2 x_2 + \beta_3 x_3$, to the model.

One way to check the validity of the constant hazard assumption underlying the Exponential distribution is by plotting the smoothed hazard function of the two groups against time as in Figure 10.14 using the command (**sts graph, hazard by(Extent)**). Superimposed on these graphs are the estimated (constant) hazards of the disease groups provided by the model of Figure 10.13(b) where $\log[\lambda_{Exponential}] = 0.8523 - 1.4682 \times Extent$. This gives for $Extent = 0$, $\log[\lambda_{Exponential,Very}] = 0.8523$ or $\lambda_{Exponential,Very} = \exp(0.8523) = 2.35$, whereas for $Extent = 1$, $\log[\lambda_{Exponential,Less}] = 0.8523 - 1.4682 \times 1 = -0.6159$ or $\lambda_{Exponential,Less} = \exp(-0.6159) = 0.54$. These (constant) values, which could have been directly calculated using equation (10.16), are indicated in Figure 10.14 (which is a repeat of Figure 6.5 with some extra details added), and do not provide a reasonable description of each of the respective increasing hazard profiles. Further, it appears that $\kappa \neq 1$ as the 95% CI of 1.09 to 1.95 does not include 1 and the associated p-value $= 0.011$. Hence both reasons suggest that assuming that the survival distributions are Exponential is untenable in this instance.

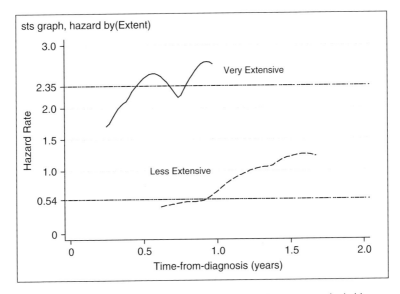

Figure 10.14 Graph of smoothed hazard estimate against time for patients with glioblastoma with very and less extensive disease at diagnosis (data from Sridhar, Gore, Boiangiu, et al., 2009)

Assuming a Weibull distribution of survival times gives $HR=0.1417$, which is quite close to that obtained from the Cox model with $HR=0.1378$. The plot of Figure 10.14 indicates that the hazards in the two disease groups are both increasing as time-from-diagnosis increases in an approximately parallel way. Nevertheless, there is a suggestion of a somewhat steeper rise in those with very extensive disease, although the departure from 'parallelism' is not great. This suggests that, although there is some evidence to suggest that PH does not hold, it may not be a serious violation.

When the hazards are clearly proportional, then a choice between the Cox and, for example, Exponential or Weibull models might be made in terms of ease of interpretation of the final model. Preference would be given to the Exponential model if the hazards plots, such as those of Figure 10.14, each took an approximately constant but possibly different value about straight lines parallel to the 'Time-from-diagnosis' axis. When the evidence for or against PH is unclear, then Cox and a Weibull model (although there is a range of other possibilities) may both be used and the results compared to guide the ultimate choice.

TIME-VARYING COVARIATES

Introduction

In some circumstances in a survival-time study for which death is the primary endpoint, an incident may occur in the life-time of an individual which may precipitate a sudden change in the underlying death rate of the person concerned. Thus, in following a cohort of individuals over time, Korenman, Goldman and Fu (1997) recognized that widowhood may be one such factor. Thus, the discrete covariate (actually binary taking values No or Yes) widowhood potentially varies over time. One aim of their study was to examine whether becoming a widow/widower precipitated an earlier death. In order to capture any change in status in this respect, the study participants were interviewed every two years and their current widowhood status noted. Consequently, the covariate 'widowhood' is time-varying or time-dependent in nature.

In other situations there may be time-varying covariates (TVC) that are continuous in nature. These covariates may correspond to a series of measures made over time in a group of individuals, such as their body mass index, serum triglyceride level, serum HDL cholesterol, and systolic or diastolic blood pressure. Such measures are likely to take different values when recorded at different follow-up visits and so are time-varying. It is important to distinguish TVCs from the repeated observations on the primary endpoint (y-variable) of a study.

In some instances, the analyst may create TVCs to deal with regression model situations in which the assumption of PH does not hold.

Single time-varying covariate

In order to retain a distinction between a fixed covariate (denoted by x) recorded at the start of the study and a TVC assessed at time t post-commencement of the study, we denote the latter by $z(t)$ and use τ for the corresponding regression coefficients. In the presence of a single fixed covariate, x_1, with parameter β_1, and a single time-varying covariate, $z_1(t)$ with parameter τ_1, the Cox regression model of equation (6.2) becomes:

$$\lambda(t) = \lambda_0(t)\exp\left[\beta_1 x_1 + \tau_1 z_1(t)\right]$$

(10.19)

From this the, now time-varying, hazard ratio, is obtained as

$$HR(t) = \lambda(t)/\lambda_0(t) = \exp\left[\beta_1 x_1 + \tau_1 z_1(t)\right] \qquad (10.20)$$

This model can be extended by adding more fixed and/or time-varying covariates as the design of the study to be analyzed requires.

Discrete time-varying covariate

A trabeculectomy is a surgical procedure designed to relieve intraocular pressure (IOP) by removing part of the eye's trabecular meshwork. Husain, Liang, Foster, *et al.* (2012) investigated whether the timing of any succeeding cataract surgery adversely influences the time-to-trabecular-failure in patients who had received a trabeculectomy for their glaucoma. Failure was defined as an IOP>21 mmHg and the post-operative time-to-failure, t_{Fail}, was recorded. In addition, the time to any cataract surgery prior to this failure, $t_{Cataract}$, was also recorded.

Cataract surgery post-trabeculectomy is a binary TVC as, at any time point during follow-up, a patient will or will not have had subsequent cataract surgery. Thus, the covariate $z(t) = TVCCat(t)$ takes the value of 0 after the trabeculectomy and remains 0 until cataract surgery is performed at $t_{Cataract}$. Thereafter it becomes 1 until t_{Fail}. In summary:

$$TVCCat(t) = \begin{bmatrix} 0 & if\ t < t_{Cataract} \\ 1 & if\ t \geq t_{Cataract} \end{bmatrix} \qquad (10.21)$$

Thus, for each patient the date of trabeculectomy, the date of any later cataract surgery, and the date of failure were each recorded. For example, Patient id = 1 of Figure 10.15(a) with fixed-covariates of age of 71 years and Open glaucoma, had cataract surgery (*Cat* = 1) at $t_{Cataract}$ = 43.5 months post trabeculectomy and then failed (*Fail* = 1) some 24.2 months later at t_{Fail} = 43.5 + 24.2 = 67.7 months. In contrast, Patient id=2, aged 43 years with Closed glaucoma, did not have cataract surgery (*Cat* = 0) and after 84 months observation post-trabulectomy had not failed (*Fail*=0). In this case time-to-cataract-surgery and time-to-fail-ure are censored observations both taking the same (censored) value, that is $T^+_{Cataract} = T^+_{Fail} = $ 84 months. Of the 235 patients in the study, 97 (41.3%) had cataract surgery and there were a total of 79 (33.6%) trabeculectomy failures.

However, if the fact that a patient has had a cataract operation and at a specific time post-trabeculectomy is to be regarded as a TVC, then the additional covariate *TVCCat(t)* of equation (10.21) has to be created. For patient id = 1, *TVCCat* = 0 (No) from the time of trabeculectomy until $t_{Cataract}$, thereafter it takes the value *TVCCat* = 1 (Yes). In contrast, for patient id = 2, *TVCCatTV* = 0 for the whole 84 months. Thus, the first patient has two distinct values of *TVCCat*, whereas the second has only one.

The data as presented in Figure 10.15(a) are of the 'wide' format, whereas, in order to accommodate the possible change in status of *TVCCat* at subsequent follow-up, the 'long format' (as discussed in Chapter 8) of Figure 10.15(b) has to be created. In this latter format Patient id = 1 now has two rows (each containing repeats of the fixed-covariate values of *Age* and *Glaucoma*): Row 1 containing *Cat* = 0 (No) and Row 2 containing *Cat* = 1 (Yes). These are now relabeled as the single time-varying covariate *TVCCat* with values 0 and 1.

(a) *Wide file*

list id Age Glaucoma Cat tCat Fail tFail

```
+------------------------------------------------------------------+
| id   Age   Glaucoma      Cat      tCat      Fail      tFail  |
|------------------------------------------------------------------|
| 1    71    Open          Yes      43.5      Yes       67.7   |
| 2    43    Closed        No       84.0      No        84.0   |
| 3    41    Open          No       60.0      No        60.0   |
| 5    70    Open          No       84.0      No        84.0   |
| 6    57    Open          No       59.8      Yes       59.8   |
|------------------------------------------------------------------|
| 8    70    Closed        Yes      23.7      Yes       49.9   |
| 9    75    Open          Yes      20.7      No        84.0   |
| 12   71    Open          Yes      41.9      No        84.0   |
| 14   68    Closed        Yes      32.7      Yes       47.2   |
| 16   69    Closed        Yes      58.9      No        84.0   |
+------------------------------------------------------------------+
```

tabulate Cat Fail

```
--------+-----------------+--------
        |      Fail       |
 Cat    |   No      Yes   |  Total
--------+-----------------+--------
 No     |   79      59    |   138
 Yes    |   77      20    |    97
--------+-----------------+--------
 Total  |  156      79    |   235
--------+-----------------+--------
```

(b) *Long file*

reshape long Age Glaucoma Cat Fail tFail, i(id) j(number)

list id Age Glaucoma TVCCat TVCFail tTVCFail

```
+------------------------------------------------------------+
| id   Age   Glaucoma   TVCCat   TVCFail   tTVCFail |
|------------------------------------------------------------|
| 1    71    Open        No       No        43.5    |
| 1    71    Open        Yes      Yes       67.7    |
| 2    43    Closed      No       No        84.0    |
| 3    41    Open        No       No        60.0    |
| 5    70    Open        No       No        84.0    |
|------------------------------------------------------------|
| 6    57    Open        No       Yes       59.8    |
| 8    70    Closed      No       No        23.7    |
| 8    70    Closed      Yes      Yes       49.9    |
| 9    75    Open        No       No        20.7    |
| 9    75    Open        Yes      No        84.0    |
|------------------------------------------------------------|
| 12   71    Open        No       No        41.9    |
| 12   71    Open        Yes      No        84.0    |
| 14   68    Closed      No       No        32.7    |
| 14   68    Closed      Yes      Yes       47.2    |
| 16   69    Closed      No       No        58.9    |
|------------------------------------------------------------|
| 16   69    Closed      Yes      No        84.0    |
+------------------------------------------------------------+
```

Figure 10.15 Type of glaucoma and age at trabeculectomy and time to subsequent failure as defined by an intra-ocular pressure > 21 mmHg. (a) Wide file format also including time from trabeculectomy to any cataract surgery and time-to trabeculectomy-failure. (b) Long file format to assess the influence of the time-varying covariate cataract surgery on time-to-failure (part data from Husain, Liang, Foster, et al., 2012)

The corresponding times $tCat = 43.5$ and $tFail = 67.7$ are now both in the single column of variable $tTVCFail$, whereas the binary $TVCFail$ records whether (Yes) or not (No) a failure had occurred.

Once the associated data are in the format as required by the specific statistical program to be used, the commands for fitting the corresponding survival time model are usually straightforward. Thus, to test the effect of the discrete TVC cataract surgery ($TVCCat$) in this setting using Cox regression, the associated command will be of the form (`stcox TVCCat, vce(cluster id)`). The purpose of 'cluster' is to take into account the possible within-subject correlation when a participant contributes two rows of data. This component is identified by using (`id`) to link, as necessary, the two rows of information (the cluster) contributed by those patients who experience cataract surgery. The term (`vce(.)`) refers to variance-component estimates which take account of the clusters when calculating the standard errors. The results of the calculations are summarized in Figure 10.16(a), and give a $HR = 1.40$ suggesting an increased risk of trabeculectomy failure once cataract surgery had been performed. However, the associated 95% CI of 0.80

(a) *Influence of cataract surgery (time-varying covariate) on trabeculectomy failure*

stset tTVCFail, id(id) failure(TVCFail==1)

stcox TVCCat, vce(cluster id) nohr
stcox TVCCat, vce(cluster id)

No. of subjects = 235, Number of obs = 332, No. of failures = 79

(SE adjusted for 235 clusters in id)

t	Coef	Robust SE	z	P>|z|	[95% CI]
TVCCat	0.3391	0.2888	1.17	0.24	−0.2269 to 0.9051

t	HR	Robust SE	z	P>|z|	[95% CI]
TVCCat	1.4037	0.4053	1.17	0.24	0.7970 to 2.4721

(b) *Influence of cataract surgery (time-varying covariate) on trabeculectomy failure adjusted for type of glaucoma (fixed covariate)*

stcox TVCCat Glaucoma, vce(cluster id)

(SE adjusted for 235 clusters in id)

t	HR	Robust SE	z	P>|z|	[95% CI]
TVCCat	1.5029	0.4294	1.43	0.15	0.8585 to 2.6312
Glaucoma	1.7758	0.4316	2.36	0.018	1.1029 to 2.8592

Figure 10.16 Estimated hazard ratio for estimating the influence of the time-varying covariate cataract surgery (a) alone and (b) also taking account of the fixed covariate—type of glaucoma (part data from Husain, Liang, Foster, et al., 2012)

to 2.47 is wide and includes the null hypothesis value of $HR_0 = 1$. This, and the associated p-value $= 0.24$, indicate a lack of statistical significance.

As indicated in equation (10.19), the Cox model including a TVC can also include one or more covariates of the more usual (fixed) format. Thus if the influence of the initial type of glaucoma (*Glaucoma*) on subsequent trabeculectomy failure is to be investigated, while taking account of possible cataract surgery, the model command is extended to (`stcox TVCCat Glaucoma, vce(cluster id)`) with the corresponding output of Figure 10.16(b). This suggests that adjusting for the type of glaucoma increases the estimated risk associated with cataract surgery from $HR = 1.4037$ to $HR = 1.5029$. However, the relative change $C = 1.5029/1.4037 = 1.07$ or 7% is not likely to be regarded as clinically important, and so it may be reasonable to omit *Glaucoma* from the model. However, as we caution in the Preface, no clinical conclusions should be drawn from this illustrative analysis.

Continuous time-varying covariate

In the study of Grundy, Wilne, Robinson, *et al.* (2010), some of the children with cancer received chemotherapy and immediately prior to each cycle of treatment their weight was recorded. For illustration purposes only, there might be a primary concern of the study to know if gender was prognostic for outcome within the first three years from commencement of treatment, and whether weight changes over the active treatment period or metastatic status at diagnosis influenced the magnitude of this effect. The gender, metastatic status at initial diagnosis, and successive recorded weights (kg) of 10 children with a cancer together with their subsequent survival time in years (OSy) censored at three years from the date treatment began are given in a wide file format in Figure 10.17(a). Of the children listed, two remain alive at three years. Potentially each child has seven weight recordings made, but there may be occasional missing documentation within the series such as patient id $= 4$ or the series may be curtailed as with patient id $= 1$. The corresponding date on which the weights are taken is also recorded. The weight change over time for one patient is shown in Figure 10.17(b). In this example, the weight of the child increases from 8.2 kg at the start of treatment to 10.7 kg at 8.7 months, thereafter there is a small decrease to 10.6 kg and the child remains at that weight when weighed again at 12.6 months. The child then dies 2.6 months later. Thus, weight is a continuous TVC, albeit assessed at discrete time intervals, and is one which may affect the ultimate outcome in terms of patient survival time.

If the sole interest with these data is to investigate whether the (fixed) covariate gender (*Gender*) was influential on ultimate outcome, then standard K-M curves, with a Cox regression model to obtain the HR, would be calculated with the results shown in Figure 10.18(a). Thus, the risk is marginally less for the females with $HR_{Gender} = 0.9726$, but is far from statistically significant, p-value $= 0.93$. Using the weight assessment ($w0$), recorded as treatment was about to commence, as a *fixed* covariate suggested that adding this to the model with *Gender* alone had little influence. Thus, the weight-adjusted value in Figure 10.18(b) of $HR_{Gender} = 0.9957$ is close to that unadjusted value, and very near to $HR_0 = 1$ of the null hypothesis. The associated p-value $= 0.99$.

However, if weight is to be regarded as a TVC then some adjustment needs to be made to the format of the wide database. In particular, the 'gaps' in the database may need to be filled. The method of filling these gaps will depend on the functionality of the particular type of database in which the data is stored. But, by whatever means this is established,

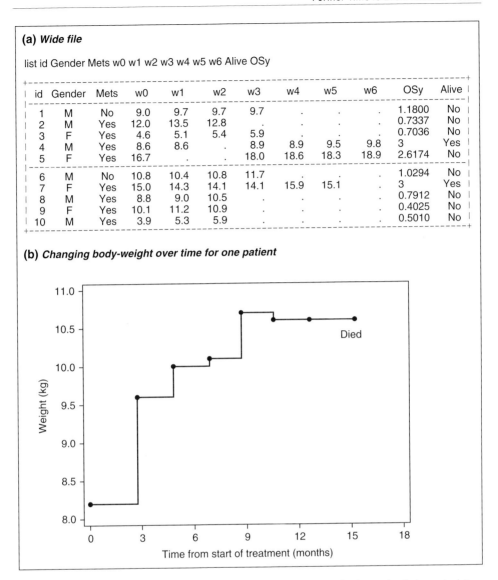

(a) Wide file

list id Gender Mets w0 w1 w2 w3 w4 w5 w6 Alive OSy

id	Gender	Mets	w0	w1	w2	w3	w4	w5	w6	OSy	Alive
1	M	No	9.0	9.7	9.7	9.7	.	.	.	1.1800	No
2	M	Yes	12.0	13.5	12.8	.	.	.	.	0.7337	No
3	F	Yes	4.6	5.1	5.4	5.9	.	.	.	0.7036	No
4	M	Yes	8.6	8.6	.	8.9	8.9	9.5	9.8	3	Yes
5	F	Yes	16.7	.	.	18.0	18.6	18.3	18.9	2.6174	No
6	M	No	10.8	10.4	10.8	11.7	.	.	.	1.0294	No
7	F	Yes	15.0	14.3	14.1	14.1	15.9	15.1	.	3	Yes
8	M	Yes	8.8	9.0	10.5	.	.	.	.	0.7912	No
9	F	Yes	10.1	11.2	10.9	.	.	.	.	0.4025	No
10	M	Yes	3.9	5.3	5.9	.	.	.	.	0.5010	No

(b) Changing body-weight over time for one patient

Figure 10.17 Gender and metastatic status at diagnosis, successive body-weights (kg), survival times and survival status of children with cancer: (a) wide data file format, (b) profile of weight change over time of one patient (part data from Grundy, Wilne, Robinson, et al., 2010)

the compact form of the database for the weights shown in Figure 10.19(a) is what is required. This is formed by filling the 'gaps' by moving the next recorded weight to the left. For clarity, the variable names are now denoted by (wght*), where the * denotes possible values from 0 to 6. By this means, the gaps are eliminated but the weight section of the file remains 'ragged'; that is, different rows in the database may have different numbers of entries.

In fact the situation is even more complex, as each weight has to be attached to the cumulative survival time, t*, until the next weighing and their survival status, d*, and finally

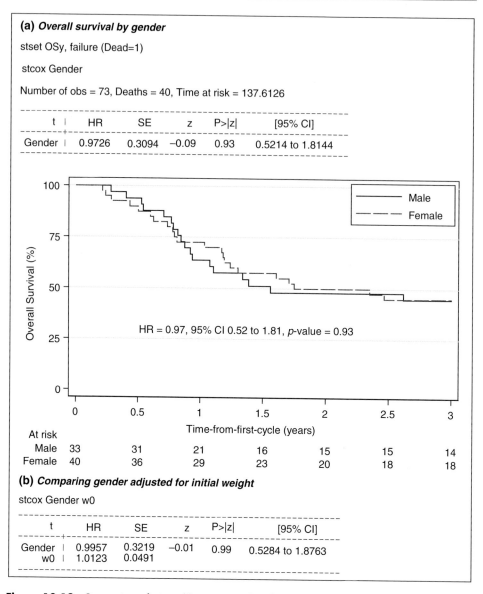

Figure 10.18   Comparison of survival between gender of children with a cancer: (a) estimated hazard ratio and K-M survival curves and (b) estimated hazard ratio after adjustment for body-weight immediately prior to commencing chemotherapy (part data from Grundy, Wilne, Robinson, *et al.*, 2010)

(for the last weight recorded) the cumulative survival time to death or last follow-up and final survival status also. The complexity of the information required suggests considerable care needs to be taken with the data collection, storage and processing of continuous TVC data. A point that has been stressed in the context of clinical trials by Little, Cohen, Dickersin, *et al.* (2012), but equally applies to all longitudinal studies including repeated assessments of whatever type.

(a) *Compacted wide file*

id	Gender	Mets	wght0	wght1	wght2	wght3	wght4	wght5	wght6	OSy	Alive
1	M	No	9.0	9.7	9.7	9.7	.	.	.	**1.1800**	**No**
2	M	Yes	12.0	13.5	12.8	.	.	.	.	**0.7337**	**No**
3	F	Yes	4.6	5.1	5.4	5.9	.	.	.	0.7036	No
4	M	Yes	8.6	8.6	8.9	8.9	9.5	9.8	.	3	Yes
5	F	Yes	16.7	18.0	18.6	18.3	18.9	.	.	2.6174	No
6	M	No	10.8	10.4	10.8	11.7	.	.	.	1.0294	No
7	F	Yes	15.0	14.3	14.1	14.1	15.9	15.1	.	3	Yes
8	M	Yes	8.8	9.0	10.5	.	.	.	.	0.7912	No
9	F	Yes	10.1	11.2	10.9	.	.	.	.	0.4025	No
10	M	Yes	3.9	5.3	5.9	.	.	.	.	0.5010	No

(b) *More detail of compacted wide file*

list id Gender Mets wght0 t0 d0 wght1 t1 d1 wght2 t2 d2 wght3 t3 d3 if id<3

id	Gen	Mets	wght0	t0	d0	wght1	t1	d1	wght2	t2	d2	wght3	t3	d3
1	M	No	9.0	0.1780	0	9.7	0.3313	0	9.7	0.5120	0	9.7	**1.1800**	1
2	M	Yes	12.0	0.1862	0	13.5	0.3614	0	12.8	**0.7337**	1	.	.	.

Figure 10.19 Gender and metastatic status at diagnosis, successive body-weights, survival time and survival status of children with cancer. (a) Compacted form of the wide data file, and (b) expanded detail of the wide file (part data from Grundy, Wilne, Robinson, *et al.*, 2010)

Thus, Figure 10.19(b) shows that for patient id = 1: wght0 = 9.0, t0 =0.1780, d0 = 0, wght1 = 9.7, t1 = 0.3313, d1 = 0, and so on until finally wght3 = 9.7, t3 = 1.1800, d3=1. Up to and including the final weighing d* = 0 (as they must be alive to be weighed) in all cases, whereas following the period after the last weighing, the patient may or may not have died, hence d*(*Last*) can take values 0 or 1. The values given in bold are the final survival status and corresponding survival time (OSy) of Figure 10.17(a).

As with repeated measures studies discussed in Chapter 8, the next step is to convert the file from wide to long format using a command such as (**reshape long wght t d, i(id) j(cycle)**) as in Figure 10.20.

The associated command to assess the influence of changing weight takes the same format as for a discrete time-varying covariate apart from the **tvc** option. Thus (**stcox, tvc(wght) vce(cluster id)**) provides the output of Figure 10.21(a). As survival is expressed in years in the database, then the output gives $HR(1) = 0.9892$ (95% CI 0.9658 to 1.0131, p-value =0.37) and this indicates the estimated magnitude of the decreasing risk for every 1 kg increase in body-weight one year post commencement of treatment. However, if we need the time-varying hazard ratios at (say) 0.5 and 1.5 years, then these are $HR(0.5)=0.9892^{0.5}=0.9946$ and $HR(2.0)=0.9892^{2.0}=0.9785$, respectively. These suggest that with increasing time from commencement of therapy, increasing weight implies contin- uously improving prognosis.

However, the object of the illustration is to see if a comparison between the genders is affected by the TVC weight. Thus, adjusting the analysis for *Gender* by means of the

```
reshape long wght t d, i(id) j(cycle)

list id cycle Gender Mets wght t d
+-----------------------------------------------+
|  id   cycle   Gender   Mets   wght    t      d |
|-----------------------------------------------|
|  1     0       M       No      9     0.1780   0 |
|  1     1       M       No      9.7   0.3313   0 |
|  1     2       M       No      9.7   0.5120   0 |
|  1     3       M       No      9.7   1.1800   1 |
|  2     0       M       Yes    12     0.1862   0 |
|-----------------------------------------------|
|  2     1       M       Yes    13.5   0.3614   0 |
|  2     2       M       Yes    12.8   0.7337   1 |
|  3     0       F       Yes     4.6   0.1506   0 |
|  3     1       F       Yes     5.1   0.3231   0 |
|  3     2       F       Yes     5.4   0.4764   0 |
|-----------------------------------------------|
|  3     3       F       Yes     5.9   0.7036   1 |
|  4     0       M       Yes     8.6   0.1506   0 |
|  4     1       M       Yes     8.6   0.4764   0 |
|  4     2       M       Yes     8.9   0.6297   0 |
|  4     3       M       Yes     8.9   0.7830   0 |
|-----------------------------------------------|
|  4     4       M       Yes     9.5   0.9665   0 |
|                                                 |
|  4     5       M       Yes     9.8   3        0 |
+-----------------------------------------------+
```

Figure 10.20   Long file format for gender and metastatic status at diagnosis, successive body-weights, survival time and survival status of children with cancer (part data from Grundy, Wilne, Robinson, et al., 2010)

changing weight of the children over time using the command (**stcox   Gender, tvc(wght) vce(cluster id)**) gives the results of Figure 10.21(b). Now the adjusted $HR_{Gender} = 0.9920$, which is very close to 0.9957 of Figure 10.18(b) when adjusting the gender comparison by the (fixed) covariate *wght0*. Further, Figure 10.21(c) adds the fixed covariate *Mets* to the model and suggests also that this has little influence on the gender comparison. Consequently, in this illustrative example, we would conclude that gender had little influence on survival up to three years post commencement of treatment. In other contexts, the fixed covariate and/or the TVC could influence the magnitude of the hazard ratio of primary concern.

Non-proportional hazards

In Chapter 6, *Verifying proportional hazards*, we described some methods of verifying whether or not the assumption of proportional hazards (PH) holds for a particular situation where survival time from two or more groups is to be compared. If the data do not appear to satisfy the PH assumption, the creation of a TVC may be useful in tracking changing differences between groups over time. Figure 10.22(a) shows the overall survival curves of patients with advanced nasopharyngeal cancer from the SQNP01 trial undertaken by Wee, Tan, Tai, *et al.* (2005).

It is evident from examining the K-M curves for CRT and RT that there is a difference between the treatments, but the hazards do not appear proportional over the whole 6-year

(a) *Influence of changing weight on survival time*

stset t, id(id) failure(d=1)

stcox, tvc(wght) vce(cluster id) nohr
stcox, tvc(wght) vce(cluster id)

No. of subjects = 73, Number of obs = 325, No. of failures = 40
Time at risk = 145.2533

(SE adjusted for 73 clusters in id)

		Coef	Robust SE	z	P>|z|	[95% CI]
TVC	wght	−0.01085	0.01220	−0.89	0.37	−0.0348 to 0.0131

		HR	Robust SE	z	P>|z|	[95% CI]
TVC	wght	0.9892	0.0121	−0.89	0.37	0.9658 to 1.0131

(b) *Influence of gender adjusted for time-varying weight*

stcox Gender, tvc(wght) vce(cluster id) nohr
stcox Gender, tvc(wght) vce(cluster id)

(SE adjusted for 73 clusters in id)

		Coef	Robust SE	z	P>|z|	[95% CI]
Main	Gender	−0.0081	0.3185	−0.03	0.98	−0.6322 to 0.6161
TVC	wght	−0.01083	0.01222			

		HR	Robust SE	z	P>|z|	[95% CI]
Main	Gender	0.9920	0.3159	−0.03	0.98	0.5314 to 1.8517
TVC	wght	0.9892	0.0121			

(c) *Influence of gender, adjusted for metastatic status at diagnosis and time-varying weight*

stcox Gender Mets, tvc(wght) vce(cluster id) nohr
stcox Gender Mets, tvc(wght) vce(cluster id)

(SE adjusted for 73 clusters in id)

		Coef	Robust SE	z	P>|z|	[95% CI]
Main	Gender	−0.0086	0.3205	−0.03	0.98	−0.6368 to 0.6196
Main	Mets	0.0094	0.3224			
TVC	wght	−0.01083	0.01224			

		HR	Robust SE	z	P>|z|	[95% CI]
Main	Gender	0.9914	0.3178	−0.03	0.98	0.5290 to 1.8581
Main	Mets	0.9907	0.3193			
TVC	wght	0.9892	0.01211			

Figure 10.21 Cox regression analysis with (a) weight as a time-varying covariate, (b) adjusted for gender and (c) adjusted for gender and metastatic status at diagnosis (part data from Grundy, Wilne, Robinson, *et al.*, 2010)

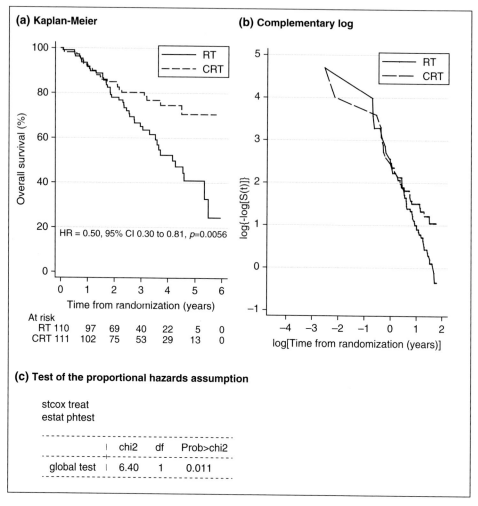

Figure 10.22 (a) Overall survival of patients with nasopharyngeal cancer by treatment received, (b) the complementary log plot to check for proportional hazards and (c) the corresponding test of the proportional hazards assumption (part data from Wee, Tan, Tai, et al., 2005)

span of the survival time. For example, the two curves overlap until 1-year post randomization and thereafter diverge. The lack of PH is also suggested by the complementary log plot of Figure 10.22(b), which also suggests divergence in the later stages. This is confirmed by the associated global test for PH of Figure 10.22(c), which is statistically significant, p-value$=0.011$.

In order to account for the situation where the effect of treatment possibly changes over time, the Cox regression model for *Treat* alone is modified to include an additional term, *TVCTrtSurvy*. Here *TVCTrtSurvy* is calculated as the product of the treatment (*Treat*=0 or 1) and the actual survival time (*Survy*) of each patient (whether censored or not). Its inclusion in the model allows the assessment of possible interaction between the treatment received and the corresponding survival time to be quantified. If statistically significant, the difference

---

(a) *Estimating the time-varying hazard model*

xi: stcox i.Treat, tvc(Treat) nohr
xi: stcox i.Treat, tvc(Treat)

No. of subjects = 221, No. of failures = 68

```
------------------------------------------------------------------------
         Time  |    Coef     SE       z     P>|z|        [95% CI]
---------------+--------------------------------------------------------
Main  ITreat_0 |   0
      ITreat_1 |   0.3555   0.4874   0.73   0.47     -0.5998 to  1.3109
---------------+--------------------------------------------------------
TVC      Treat |  -0.5468   0.2295  -2.38   0.017    -0.9967 to -0.0970
------------------------------------------------------------------------
         Time  |    HR       SE       z     P>|z|        [95% CI]
---------------+--------------------------------------------------------
Main  ITreat_0 |   1
      ITreat_1 |   1.4269   0.6955   0.73   0.47      0.5489 to  3.7095
---------------+--------------------------------------------------------
TVC      Treat |   0.5788   0.1328  -2.38   0.017     0.3691 to  0.9076
------------------------------------------------------------------------
```

(b) *Estimating the hazard ratio at 3 years*

lincom _ITreat_1 + Treat*3, hr

```
---------------------------------------------------------------------
   Time  |  HR(3)    SE(3)     z     P>|z|          [95% CI]
---------+-----------------------------------------------------------
3 years  |  0.2767   0.1059  -3.36   0.00078    0.1307 to 0.5858
---------------------------------------------------------------------
```

Figure 10.23 Time-varying differences in the hazard ratio comparing treatments with respect to overall survival in patients with nasopharyngeal cancer estimated at one and three years from randomization (part data from Wee, Tan, Tai, *et al.*, 2005)

between treatments is no longer regarded as constant and its magnitude will change as *Survy* changes. The corresponding Cox regression model now leads to a time-varying hazard ratio to compare treatments of the form:

$$TV : HR(Survy) = \exp[(\beta_{Treat} \times Treat) + (\beta_{TVCTrtSurvy} \times TVCTrtSurvy)] \qquad (10.22)$$

Here, once the regression coefficients β_{Treat} and $\beta_{TVCTrtSurvy}$ are estimated, they determine the magnitude of any time-varying changes in the main effect (the treatment group difference).

The need to generate the extra covariate, *TVCTrTSurvy*, directly is not essential as the following command (`xi:stcox i.Treat, tvc(Treat)`) does this automatically by making use of the TVC subcommand (`tvc(.)`). This generates the dummy variables (`Itreat_0`) and (`Itreat_1`) associated with the binary (design) covariate *Treat*. These dummy variables are then used to establish the necessary interaction terms.

The results of fitting the time-varying Cox model to compare RT with CRT in Figure 10.23(a) give $HR(Survy) = \exp[0.3555 + (-0.5468 \times Survy)]$. Thus, for $Survy = 3$ years, $HR(3) = \exp[0.3555 + (-0.5468 \times 3)] = \exp[-1.2849] = 0.2767$ in favour of CRT.

This latter calculation can be made directly using the command (`lincom Itreat_1+Treat* 3, hr`) as in Figure 10.23(b). The output gives $HR(3) = 0.2767$ as

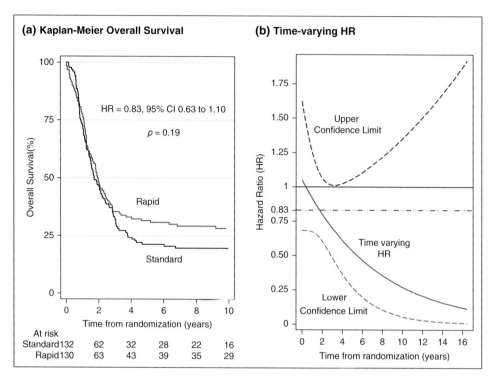

Figure 10.24 (a) Overall survival (OS) of patients with neuroblastoma randomized to either COJEC (Rapid) or OPEC/OJEC (Standard) chemotherapy and (b) estimated change with time in the corresponding hazard ratio with associated upper (UCL) and lower (LCL) 95% confidence limits (HR=0.83 estimated assuming no change with time) (adapted from Pearson, Pinkerton, Lewis, et al., 2008)

we have calculated, but it also includes the estimated 95% CI of 0.13 to 0.59. In a similar way, $HR(1)=0.8259$ while $HR(5)=0.0927$. Thus, the *declining* hazard ratios at one, three and five years indicate the *increasing* advantage of CRT over RT as survival time increases. However, the associated confidence intervals become wider as the time from randomization increases. By these means, although PH assumptions do not appear justified, a sensible and time-independent interpretation of these data may be obtained using a standard Cox regression model.

A further example, on similar lines to that we have just described, is provided by the analysis of a randomized trial conducted by Pearson, Pinkerton, Lewis, et al. (2008) in patients over one year of age with Stage 4 neuroblastoma. The overall survival curves of Figure 10.24(a) plateau in both treatment groups with a more favorable long-term outcome for those receiving the *Rapid* chemotherapy. These plateaux indicate the presence of non-PHs. The authors conclude: '… the underlying assumption that the HR remains constant over time is not supported beyond about 3 years with … OS. Fitting the Cox model, … suggests a far from constant HR gradually decreasing in favour of *Rapid* treatment [our Figure 10.24(b)]. However, the upper 95% CI always exceeds $HR=1$'.

Any of $k=1, 2$ or 3			Local Recurrence $k=1$			Distant Metastasis $k=2$			Death $k=3$		
j	t_j	Any	i	t_{LRi}	LR	i	t_{DMi}	DM	i	t_{Di}	D
1	29	1			+			+	1	29	1
2	43	1			+			+	2	43	1
3	153	1	1	153	1			+			+
4	154	1			+	1	154	1			+
	185+	0+			0+			0+			0+
5	189	1			+	2	189	1			+
6	210	1			+	3	210	1			+
7	214	1			+	4	214	1			+
8	219	1			+	5	219	1			+
9	246	2			+	6	246	2			+
10	248	1	2	248	1			+			+
11	249	1			+			+	3	249	1
12	252	1			+	7	252	1			+
13	255	1			+	8	255	1			+
14	270	1			+	9	270	1			+
15	274	1	3	274	1			+			+
16	277	1	4	277	1			+			+
17	295	1	5	295	1			+			+
18	315	1			+	10	315	1			+
19	370	1	6	370	1			+			+
20	371	1			+	11	371	1			+
											+

Figure 10.25 Event times for a Competing Risks assessment of times to Local Recurrence, Distant Metastasis or Death in patients with nasopharyngeal cancer (part data from Wee, Tan, Tai, et al., 2005)

TECHNICAL DETAILS

Event times for Competing Risk data

Figure 10.25 gives the lowest 21 ranked survival times from the 111 patients randomized to CRT in the SQNP01 clinical trial of Wee, Tan, Tai, et al. (2005). In this trial there were $K = 3$ competing risks: Local Recurrence (LR, $k = 1$), Distant Metastasis (DM, $k = 2$) and Death (D, $k = 3$). All but one of the patients experienced a first event. The one patient who did not has an associated survival time of 185+ days, which is therefore censored whichever of the competing risks is considered. This is indicated by the '0+' entries within the table indicating that no event has yet occurred for this patient. The remaining patients listed are numbered by $j = 1$ to 20 with corresponding event times: $t_1 = 29$, $t_2 = 43$, ... , $t_{20} = 371$. Each of these has a '**1**', indicating an event has occurred at that time, except for $t_9 = 246$, which has a '**2**' indicating that there are two patients who experienced an event (both DM) with the same survival time post-randomization when they occurred.

Among these, six patients had a LR ($k = 1$), at $t_{LR1} = 153$, $t_{LR2} = 248$, ... , $t_{LR6} = 370$, as listed in Figure 10.1(b), and each has a '1' indicating that a LR has occurred, the remaining survival times are all regarded as censored for this risk. These are indicated by a '+'. Similarly, 12 patients developed DM ($k = 2$), at $t_{DM1} = 154$, $t_{DM2} = 189$, ... , $t_{DM12} = 371$, with all others giving censored observations for this second competing risk. Finally, three patients died, D ($k = 3$), at $t_{D1} = 29$, $t_{D2} = 43$ and $t_{D3} = 249$, with all others giving censored observations for this third competing risk.

Estimating the parameters of the Weibull distribution

To obtain the maximum likelihood estimates of the parameters η and κ of the Weibull distribution, it is necessary to solve quite complicated equations. These equations are

$$W(\kappa) = \frac{\Sigma t^{\kappa} \log t + \Sigma (T^{+})^{\kappa} \log T^{+}}{\Sigma t^{\kappa} + \Sigma (T^{+})^{\kappa}} - \frac{\Sigma \log t}{d} - \frac{1}{\kappa} = 0 \qquad (10.23)$$

and

$$\eta = \left[e / \{ \Sigma t^{\kappa} + \Sigma (T^{+})^{\kappa} \} \right]^{1/\kappa} \qquad (10.24)$$

where e is the total number of events among n subjects recruited to the study, t are their corresponding survival times and T^{+} are the $(n - e)$ censored survival times. This takes the same form as equation (10.13) when $\kappa = 1$.

To solve equation (10.23) for κ involves finding a particular κ which makes $W(\kappa) = 0$. Once κ is obtained, η is calculated using equation (10.24). One method of solving equation (10.23) is by 'trial-and-error'. For example, we could start by assuming $\kappa = \kappa_0 = 1$ which corresponds to the situation of the nested Exponential distribution. We then substitute κ_0 in equation (10.23) to obtain $W(\kappa_0) = W(1)$. If $W(1) = 0$, then this initial estimate itself is indeed the solution to the equation. More usually, $W(\kappa_0) \neq 0$ and we need to choose a second value of $\kappa = \kappa_1$ perhaps a little smaller (or larger) than κ_0 and calculate $W(\kappa_1)$. If this is nearer to zero, or perhaps of the opposite sign to the previous value, $W(\kappa_0)$, this may indicate the next value of κ to choose and the calculations are repeated once more. For example if $W(\kappa_0) > 0$ but $W(\kappa_1) < 0$, then a suitable choice for the next value might be $\kappa_2 = (\kappa_0 + \kappa_1)/2$. The process is repeated as necessary with differing values until κ_{Final} gives $W(\kappa_{Final}) = 0$. This final value of κ is then the maximum likelihood solution, κ_{ML}, of equation (10.23). Substituting κ_{ML} in equation (10.24) then gives the maximum likelihood estimate of η, or η_{ML}.

In practice an appropriate statistical package will, for a given data set, usually perform these calculations automatically.

11   Further Topics

SUMMARY

The topics discussed in previous chapters are concerned with describing the basics for regression modeling but, as is common in most areas of investigation, there are issues beyond the 'basics' which may be relevant in the context of the clinical study that is the main focus for the use of such models. However, we first stress, although in a different sense from our earlier emphasis, that simple models are to be preferred.

In certain situations, individuals recruited to a study may belong to specific groups, perhaps patients with a particular condition but treated in different hospitals or by different clinical teams. The data from within the same group are termed clustered, and it might be anticipated that there is some association between them with respect to the study outcome measures. The concept of clusters can be extended to various levels, for example, one level of clustering may be the hospitals involved, and a second level would be the wards within the hospitals concerned. Methods for taking into account this multi-level clustering in the regression modeling process are described.

Finally, we include situations where we may wish to depart from the 'simple' model approach in order to describe more complex profiles. In this context, we describe some applications of fractional polynomials, which allow more flexible regression models to be considered.

MODEL STRUCTURE

Introduction

In Chapter 8 we discussed repeated measures designs in which the endpoint variable of concern is measured on successive occasions over time. One type of repeated measures design is that of a clinical trial in which a number of pre-randomization observations are taken at different times in addition to a number of post-randomization observations on each participant. In such a design, the post-randomization observations are, in our terminology, the repeated and therefore auto-correlated observations, y, whereas the pre-randomization observations are repeated measures of a covariate, x. In this section we consider circumstances in which y, the endpoint variable, itself is also assessed before randomization. For example, if there is a single measure of y pre-randomization to give values (say) y_0 for each patient, then these values are used as the covariate $x = y_0$.

Modeling change

Adjusting for baseline

The simplest case of the pre- and post-repeated measures design is when one is comparing two treatments (*Treat*), interventions or groups and there is a single baseline measure of y itself, which we term y_0, followed by a single post-intervention assessment of the same variable, say y_1. This is often termed a before-and-after design. In this situation, the simple linear model involving this single-covariate can be expressed as

$$y_1 = \beta_0 + \beta_{Treat}Treat + \beta_{y_0}y_0 + \varepsilon \tag{11.1}$$

As well as the self-assessed Physical Component Summary (PCS) score of Figure 8.2 recorded in the trial conducted by Nejadnik, Hui, Choong, *et al.* (2010), several other measures were also used to compare the two implants. In particular, Physical Function (PF) was also noted at the same times that PCS was recorded. Thus, if we consider the baseline y_0 as PF0 and y_1 as the first assessment measure PF1, then an analysis of these data, with *Treat* replaced by *Implant*, corresponds to fitting a model of the form (11.1). Even so, we would generally precede this analysis by one which assumes no covariate is involved, that is using a model with the covariate term absent implying, in this example, that $\beta_{y_0} = \beta_{PF0} = 0$. So if PF is can be regarded as a continuous variable, the necessary command omitting the covariate is (**regress PF1 Implant**). The results of this calculation are given in Figure 11.1(a). The estimated $b_{Implant} = 4.6970$ units, but with a wide

---

(a) *Ignoring baseline PF0*

regress PF1 Implant

Diff	Coef	SE	z	p-value	[95% CI]
cons	53.9394	3.5954			
Implant	4.6970	5.0847	0.92	0.36	−5.4608 to 14.8547

(b) *Adjusting for baseline PF0*

regress PF1 Implant PF0

Diff	Coef	SE	z	p-value	[95% CI]
cons	46.2105	6.7625			
Implant	4.8786	5.0545	0.97	0.34	−5.2220 to 14.9792
PF0	0.1332	0.0989	1.35	0.18	−0.0645 to 0.3309

Figure 11.1 Alternative models when assessing the effect of the type of implant for cartilage repair on the first post-treatment assessment, PF1 (a) ignoring baseline PF0, and (b) adjusting for baseline PF0 (part data from Nejadnik, Hui, Choong, *et al.*, 2010)

95% CI from −5.4608 to 14.8547 covering the null hypothesis value of $\beta_{Implant}=0$. The associated p-value$=0.36$. These suggest a non-significant difference between the two implants with respect to PF1.

As we have indicated, this analysis takes no note of the baseline values, PF0. Nevertheless, it seems prudent to verify whether or not, after adjusting for PF0, it is indeed reasonable to conclude $\beta_{Implant}=0$. In which case, the command (**regress PF1 Implant PF0**) is required to fit the extended model of equation (11.1). The results given in Figure 11.1(b) show that the adjusted estimate $b_{Implant}=4.8786$ (95% CI: −5.2220 to 14.9792, p-value$=0.34$) is slightly larger than the 4.6970 obtained previously. This marginal change in the estimated regression coefficient of $C=4.8786/4.6970=1.04$ or 4%, suggests that the baseline PF0 has little influence on the estimated difference between implants in terms of PF1. As a consequence, it seems reasonable to revert back to the unadjusted model PF1$=53.9394+4.6970$*Implant*, where *Implant*$=0$, for the ACC implant and *Implant*$=1$ for BMSC. Thus, when presenting the results of this trial, the data summary is essentially provided by a simple comparison of the two respective means, of $\overline{PF1}_{BMSC}-\overline{PF1}_{ACC}=58.6364-53.9394=4.6970$ units.

Modeling a difference

However, in the situation of a single post- and a single pre-measure of the same variable, it is common practice for investigators to directly model the difference, $d=y_1-y_0$, between the post- and pre-randomization observations rather than y_1 itself. In which case the model, omitting the residual element, takes the form

$$d = y_1 - y_0 = \beta_0 + \beta_{Treat}Treat \qquad (11.2)$$

This model has two parameters, β_0 and β_{Treat}, one fewer than model (11.1) as the term with β_{y_0} is no longer included.

However, if the analysis for the study of Nejadnik, Hui, Choong, *et al.* (2010) is conducted in the form of equation (11.2), the regression coefficient corresponding to $\beta_{Implant}$ now represents a difference of differences. In fact, $b_{Implant}=(\overline{d}_{BMSC}-\overline{d}_{ACC})=\left[\overline{PF1}_{BMSC}-\overline{PF0}_{BMSC}\right]-\left[\overline{PF1}_{ACC}-\overline{PF0}_{ACC}\right]=(58.6364-56.6667)-(53.9394-58.0303)$ $=1.9697-(-4.0909)=6.0606$. If we denote the population differences by δ_{BMSC} and δ_{ACC}, then their difference is $\Delta=\delta_{BMSC}-\delta_{ACC}$ and the comparison of the implants is made by testing the hypothesis, $\Delta=0$. This hypothesis is tested by the command (**regress Diff Implant**), where the variable *Diff*=PF1 − PF0. Figure 11.2(a) confirms our calculation that $b_{Implant}=6.0606$, and also indicates a non-statistically significant 'difference' between the implants measured on this basis with p-value$=0.42$. However, this latter measure of the difference between implants is not directly comparable with either of the estimates obtained previously in Figure 11.1(a) and (b), which were 4.6970 and 4.8786, respectively. This is because the models concerned are not estimating the same quantity.

It should be noted that the p-value$=0.42$ using the *Diff* variable is larger than both the p-values of 0.36 and 0.34 obtained for the models of Figure 11.1. This is suggestive that the approach of Figure 11.2(a) is less statistically efficient in comparing the implants. This arises, at least in part, from the auto-correlation that is present between PF1 and PF0, which is shown graphically in Figure 11.2(b) and has an estimated value of $r=0.1630$.

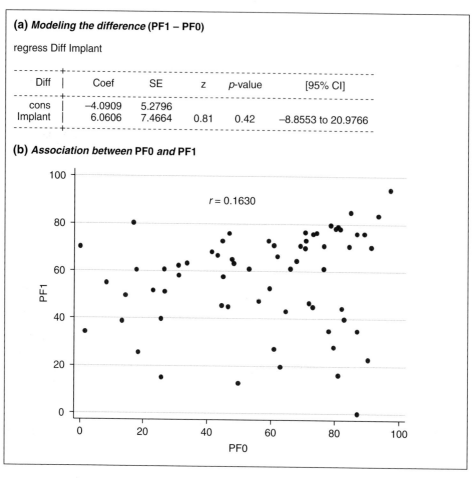

(a) *Modeling the difference* (PF1 – PF0)

regress Diff Implant

Diff	Coef	SE	z	p-value	[95% CI]
cons	−4.0909	5.2796			
Implant	6.0606	7.4664	0.81	0.42	−8.8553 to 20.9766

(b) *Association between* **PF0** *and* **PF1**

$r = 0.1630$

Figure 11.2 (a) Modeling the difference between implants based on the difference between pre- and post-randomization assessments of PF and (b) scatter plot of the association between the two assessments PF1 and PF0 with the estimated auto-correlation coefficient (part data from Nejadnik, Hui, Chong, et al., 2010)

In general, it can be shown that the variance of a difference between two auto-correlated measures Y_0 and Y_1 on the same individual is

$$Var(Y_1 - Y_0) = Var(Y_1) - 2\rho\sqrt{Var(Y_1)Var(Y_0)} + Var(Y_0) \qquad (11.3)$$

Here ρ is the auto-correlation between the two measures and $Var(.)$ is the variance of the term within the braces.

Figure 11.3(a) gives estimates of the standard deviation (SD) of PF0 and PF1 from which $Var(PF1) = 20.631^2$ and $Var(PF0) = 25.739^2$. Substituting these values, and the estimated $\rho = 0.1630$ in equation (11.3), gives $Var(PF1 - PF0) = 20.631^2 - (2 \times 0.1630 \times 20.631 \times 25.739) + 25.739^2 = 915.02 = 30.25^2$. Thus, the SD is estimated $s = 30.25$. This result can be obtained by first finding the actual differences PF1 − PF0 and then calculating their SD, which gives $s = 30.249$ as is also shown in Figure 11.3(a).

(a) Summary statistics

stats	PF0	PF1	PF1-PF0	PF1/PF0
n	66	66	66	64
median	62.5	60	0	1
mean	57.348	56.288	−1.061	1.242
sd	25.739	20.631	30.249	0.996
CV	0.45	0.37	--	0.80

(b) Regression model utilizing a ratio

regress Ratio Implant   [Ratio = PF1/PF0]

PCS1	Coef	SE	z	p-value	[95% CI]
cons	1.1211	0.1761			
Implant	0.2424	0.2491	0.97	0.33	−0.2555 to 0.7402

(c) Regression model utilizing a percentage

regress Percent Implant   [Percent = (PF1-PF0)/PF0]

cons	0.1211	0.1761			
Implant	0.2424	0.2491	0.97	0.33	−0.2555 to 0.7402

Figure 11.3 Comparative standard deviations of PF0, PF1, their difference (PF1 − PF0), and their ratio PF1/PF0 (part data from Nejadnik, Hui, Choong, *et al.*, 2010)

Now the SD of the difference, $d = y_1 - y_0$, is actually greater than $s = 20.631$ of $y_1 = $ PF1 alone, which implies that the amount of variation to be explained by the model is greater if a model is chosen based on (11.2) rather than (11.1). Thus, model (11.1) is intrinsically more efficient than (11.2), and so is preferred.

In the situation where $Var(Y_0)$ and $Var(Y_1)$ are both equal to (say) σ^2, equation (11.3) simplifies to become $Var(Y_1 - Y_0) = \sigma^2 - 2\rho\sigma^2 + \sigma^2 = 2\sigma^2(1-\rho)$. The auto-correlation coefficient, ρ, usually takes positive values so this expression suggests that if it is less than 0.5 then $Var(Y_1 - Y_0) > \sigma^2$. This leads to the general recommendation that model (11.1) is likely to be preferred if $\rho < 0.5$, and (11.2) if it is larger.

However, Frison and Pocock (1992) point out that model (11.2) is actually the same model as (11.1) but with the presumption that $\beta_{y_0} = 1$. The advantage of (11.1) is that it allows alternative values for the (covariate) parameter, including the possibility that $\beta_{y_0} = 0$. Thus, by ignoring equation (11.1) and using (11.2), one precludes the possibility of the simplest model, $y_1 = \beta_0 + \beta_{Treat}Treat$, being considered as possibly the 'best' and most parsimonious for the situation.

Modeling a ratio

In *Example 1.1*, Busse, Lemanske Jr and Gern (2010) use the dependent variable $y = $ [Reduction in FEV$_1$ from baseline value (%)] and the covariate $x = $ [Generation of interferon-λ (pg/ml)] to derive a fitted linear model of the simple form of $y = \beta_0 + \beta_x x$. Here, for brevity and in what follows in this section, we omit the error terms.

What the investigators have done in this study is to measure on each subject $f=\text{FEV}_1$ at baseline (giving f_0), then at some time later record FEV_1 again (f_1) and the interferon-λ covariate measure, x. Their scatter plot therefore graphs $y=(f_1 - f_0)/f_0$ (expressed as a percentage) against x, and the fitted model is used to summarize this relationship. In essence, the proposed model for subject i is

$$\left(f_{1i} - f_{0i}\right)/f_{0i} = \beta_0 + \beta_1 x_i \tag{11.4}$$

After some algebra, this can be rewritten as $f_{1i}=[f_{0i}+\beta_0 f_{0i}]+\beta_1[f_{0i}] x_i$. Further, if we write $B_{0i}=[f_{0i}+\beta_0 f_{0i}]$ and $B_{1i}=\beta_1[f_{0i}]$, then $f_{1i}=B_{0i}+B_{1i}x_i$ and the right-hand side of this expression looks superficially like a linear regression equation. However, the regression parameters, here B_{0i} and B_{1i}, now potentially differ from patient-to-patient. In essence, therefore, this is a far more complex model than the standard linear regression model and hence is one that is very difficult to interpret. A better choice of model is $f_1=\beta_0+\beta_1 x+\beta_2 f_0$, which is of the form of (11.1) and so has the advantages we have previously described.

In the example of Busse, Lemanske Jr and Gern (2010) there is a further aspect of their analysis which is important to note, as equation (11.4) can be rewritten as

$$\frac{f_{1i}}{f_{0i}}-1 = \beta_0 + \beta_1 x_i \tag{11.5}$$

In which case the endpoint variable is now the ratio, $y_i=f_{1i}/f_{0i}$, of the two auto-correlated variables.

It can be shown that the variance of the ratio of two auto-correlated variables Y_1 and Y_0 is approximately:

$$Var\left(\frac{Y_1}{Y_0}\right) = \left(\frac{Y_1}{Y_0}\right)^2 \left[\frac{Var(Y_1)}{Y_1^2} - \frac{2\rho\sqrt{Var(Y_1)Var(Y_0)}}{Y_1 Y_0} + \frac{Var(Y_0)}{Y_0^2}\right] \tag{11.6}$$

In the situation where $Var(Y_1)=Var(Y_0)=\sigma^2$, this simplifies to

$$Var\left(\frac{Y_1}{Y_0}\right) = \sigma^2 \left(\frac{Y_1}{Y_0}\right)^2 \left[\frac{1}{Y_1^2} - \frac{2\rho}{Y_1 Y_0} + \frac{1}{Y_0^2}\right] \tag{11.7}$$

but nevertheless remains a complicated expression. As a consequence it is difficult to know what effect this will have on the corresponding regression analysis, but it is likely that $Var(Y_1/Y_0)>Var(Y_1)$. It follows that by using the ratio there may be some unnecessary loss of statistical efficiency.

Returning to the trial of Nejadnik, Hui, Choong, et al. (2010), if the ratio approach, which essentially removes the covariate from the right-hand side of the model, is used then the model to fit is

$$Ratio_i = \frac{\text{PF1}_i}{\text{PF0}_i} = \beta_0 + \beta_{Implant}Implant_i \tag{11.8}$$

This is fitted by the command (**regress Ratio Implant**), and the results are shown in Figure 11.3(b). The corresponding $b_{Implant}=0.2424$ cannot be compared directly with those obtained from the earlier models fitted but, nevertheless, the associated confidence interval and p-value also indicate a non-statistically significant difference between implants.

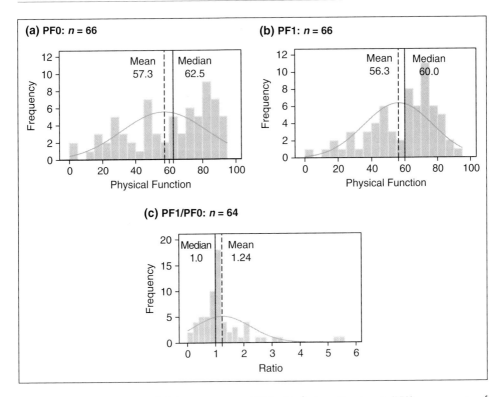

Figure 11.4 Histograms of (a) pre-treatment (PF0), (b) first post-treatment (PF1) assessments of performance status, and (c) their ratio with the corresponding median and mean values indicated (part data from Nejadnik, Hui, Choong, *et al.*, 2010)

In some circumstances the outcome is expressed with the left-hand side of equation (11.8) replaced (omitting the multiple of 100) by $Percent_i = \dfrac{PF1_i - PF0_i}{PF0_i}$. In this case, it is important to note from Figure 11.3(b) and (c) that whether *Ratio* or *Percent* are used, the estimate for the parameter $\beta_{Implant}$ remains the same. However, the constant term differs by unity as $b_{0,Percent} = b_{0,Ratio} - 1 = 1.1211 - 1 = 0.1211$.

Coefficient of variation (CV)

A relative measure of the variation in a single sample is provided by the coefficient of variation, defined by $CV = \dfrac{s}{\bar{x}}$, provided the variable concerned only takes non-negative values and $\bar{x} > 0$. Thus, for PF0, $CV_0 = 25.74/57.35 = 0.45$ and for PF1, $CV_1 = 20.63/56.29 = 0.37$, which are quite similar. The *CV* measure is not appropriate for the difference PF1 − PF0 as this can take negative values. However, for the ratio, *Ratio*=PF1/PF0, $\bar{x} = 1.242$, $s = 0.996$, hence $CV_R = 0.996/1.242 = 0.80$ and, as Figure 11.3(a) indicates, this is clearly the largest *CV*. Thus, in relative terms there is much more variation if the ratio scale is used for analysis. This in turn results in a loss of statistical efficiency, and may result in a 'non-statistically significant' model when a simpler model may indicate the contrary. Further, for two patients PF0=0 and so the ratio could not be calculated even though zero is a valid score. Figure 11.4(c) also illustrates how the skewness of a distribution based on the ratio tends to be greater than those of their

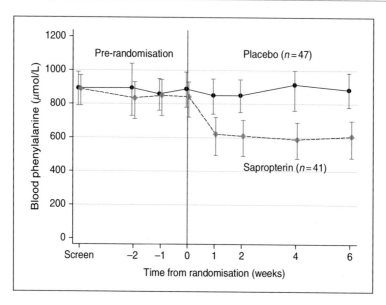

Figure 11.5 Mean blood phenylalanine concentration over time – bars indicate 95% confidence intervals (based on Levy, Milanowski, Chakrapani, et al., 2007, Figure 3)

component parts as shown in Figures 11.4(a) and (b): in this illustrative case caused by one outlier observation, corresponding to a patient with a low PF0 but high PF1 giving the *Ratio*=80/15=5.33.

Several pre-intervention assessments

In some situations, the intended endpoint variable, y_1, may also be monitored several times before the intervention is introduced. In which case, a summary of the profile of these initial values may be required to convert these to a single covariate. In certain circumstances, this summary may be provided by their mean, which would then imply that the values in an individual study participant are fluctuating about a constant value. In such a case the model to adopt for analysis would take the form:

$$y_1 = \beta_0 + \beta_{Treat} Treat + \beta_{\bar{y}_0} \bar{y}_0 \qquad (11.9)$$

Here again we assume the comparison is of two treatments, with *Treat* taking the values 0 or 1. The main focus of the analysis is to estimate β_{Treat} and to check if this estimate is materially affected by the covariate $\bar{y}_0$ by testing the null hypothesis: $\beta_{\bar{y}_0} = 0$.

An example of such a design is the randomized trial conducted by Levy, Milanowski, Chakrapani, *et al.* (2007), who compare sapropterin dihydrochloride with (double-blind) placebo in patients with phenylketonuria to assess its role in reducing blood phenylalanine concentration and therefore its potential for preventing mental retardation in these patients. As illustrated in Figure 11.5, their design consisted of 4 pre-treatment initiation and 4 post-randomization measures, taken at first screen then at weeks −2, −1, 0 (baseline), 1, 2, 4 and 6 weeks. However, their stated primary endpoint was the *change* in blood phenylalaline concentration from baseline to week 6. As we have pointed out, using change as an endpoint is not usually optimal so an analysis using equation (11.9) with $y_1 = y_{Week6}$ and $\bar{y}_0 = (y_{Screen} + y_{-2} + y_{-1} + y_0)/4$ may be more optimal. In addition, the analysis may be further improved if a repeated measures approach making use of y_{Week1}, y_{Week2} and y_{Week4} has also been adopted.

MULTI-LEVEL MODELS

Introduction

In certain situations, the method of delivery of the intervention prevents it being given on an individual participant basis, rather it can only be delivered to collections of individuals. For example, if a public health campaign conducted through the local media is to be tested, it may be possible to randomize locations, which are then termed clusters, to either receive or not the planned campaign. It would not be possible to randomize individuals.

In a 2-group cluster-randomized trial, several (usually half) of the clusters will receive one intervention and the remainder the other. Thus, a whole cluster, consisting of a number of individuals who then become the trial participants, is assigned to the intervention en-bloc.

Sackley, van den Berg, Lett, *et al.* (2009) used a cluster randomized controlled trial in which 24 nursing and residential homes from Birmingham, UK were randomly assigned to intervention or control groups, with the object to compare the clinical effectiveness of a programme of physiotherapy and occupational therapy with standard care in residents who have mobility limitations. The intervention was assigned to 12 homes, encompassing 128 eligible residents and the control to 12 homes with a total of 121 residents. The primary outcome measures were scores on the Barthel index and the Rivermead mobility index at 6-months post randomization. After adjustment for baseline characteristics, no significant differences were found in either the Barthel index or the Rivermead mobility index between the intervention groups.

Intra-class correlation

In a cluster design randomized trial despite the lack of individualized randomization and the receipt of a more group-based intervention, the assessment of the relative effect of the interventions is made at the level of the individual participant receiving the respective interventions. This is also the case in any type of observational study in which participants may be clustered on similar lines. As a consequence, the observations on the subjects within a single cluster are positively correlated as they are not completely independent of each other. Thus, patients treated by one health care professional team will tend to be more similar among themselves with respect to the outcome measure concerned than those treated by a different health care team. So if we know which team is involved with a particular patient, we can predict to some degree the outcome for that patient by reference to experience with similar patients treated by the same team.

The strength of this dependence among observations is measured by the intra-cluster correlation (ICC), or $\rho_{Cluster}$, which is defined as

$$\rho_{Cluster} = \frac{\sigma^2_{Between}}{\sigma^2_{Within} + \sigma^2_{Between}} = \frac{1}{1 + \dfrac{\sigma^2_{Within}}{\sigma^2_{Between}}} \qquad (11.10)$$

Here $\sigma_{Between}$ is the between clusters standard deviation and σ_{Within} that within clusters. In general, the more heterogeneity there is between the clusters, the greater $\sigma_{Between}$ is likely to be relative to σ_{Within}. As this increases, it brings their ratio, in the denominator of the right-hand expression in equation (11.10), closer to zero, and hence brings the value of $\rho_{Cluster}$ closer and closer to the maximum possible value of 1.

In general, however, values of the ICC tend to be small. For example, Bellary, O'Hare, Raymond, *et al.* (2008) quote the sizes for the ICC derived from primary care studies as 0.035 for systolic blood pressure, 0.05 for total cholesterol and 0.05 for haemoglobin type A_k, whereas Richards, Bankhead, Peters, *et al.* (2001) quote an even lower figure of 0.023 for breast screening uptake.

There are parallels here with the repeated measures designs of Figure 11.5 and Chapter 8 in which the auto-correlation between repeated measures within an individual is accounted. In these designs the associated auto-correlation implies that the next recorded observation from an individual can be predicted to some extent by previous values.

Multi-level models

In the model for a cluster design comparing two groups, the simple linear regression equation (1.1) has to be modified to take note of the different clusters involved. The model for subject i in cluster j is

$$y_{ij} = \beta_0 + \beta_{Group}Group_i + \varphi_j + \varepsilon_{ij} \tag{11.11}$$

Here the coefficients β_0 and β_{Group} have the same interpretation as the parameters of equation (1.7). In addition, φ_j is the effect for cluster j and is assumed random with mean $\bar{\varphi} = 0$ over all clusters with a *between*-clusters standard deviation of $\sigma_{Between}$. The term ε_{ij} is assumed to be random within the cluster j, with mean of $\bar{\varepsilon}_i = 0$ and a *within*-clusters standard deviation, σ_{Within}.

In the model fitting process, the structure of the residuals, $\varphi_j + \varepsilon_{ij}$, has to be specified in relation to the actual numbers of clusters involved. Thus, each subject is categorized by the cluster in which he or she belongs, the particular *Group* concerned, and their individual end-point value. For example, in-patients staying for treatment in a hospital may be residents in a certain ward of a particular section (or block) within the hospital. This leads to the concept of what are termed multi-level models, with the block as the highest level, the ward intermediate and the patient the lowest level unit. Thus, as illustrated in Figure 11.6, the blocks form the (so-called) Level-3 cluster, whereas the allocated ward within the block is the patients' Level-2 cluster. The patients themselves are termed as Level-1.

Again, there are parallels with the repeated measures designs of Chapter 8 in which the different individuals are regarded as the Level-2 units, whereas the repeated measures within an individual are regarded as the Level-1 units.

The majority of patients included in the study of Chong, Tay, Subramaniam, *et al.* (2009) were long-term residents living in the wards of one hospital. At the time of the study, those residents had their current cholinergic medication dose recorded. From the individual information of 403 residents, the mean of the logarithm of their current dose for each tardive dyskinesia (TD) diagnostic group (*TarDy*: No TD, Mild TD, Def TD) was calculated as shown in Figure 11.7(a). For all residents the mean logarithm was 2.1741 from which the geometric mean is $GM = \exp(2.1741) = 8.8$ units of medication.

To investigate if the levels of the medication differ between the three diagnostic groups (regarded as an unordered categorical variable), one might use the ordinary least squares command (**xi:regress LCHOL i.TarDy**). In which case Figure 11.7(b) suggests that there is little to choose between the diagnostic groups. For example, the change of +0.0826 in those with Mild-TD over the mean log(cholinergic medication) = 2.1836 of the No-TD group is very small and not statistically significant (p-value = 0.55). This can also be calculated from the difference in mean log(cholinergic medication) values between these groups

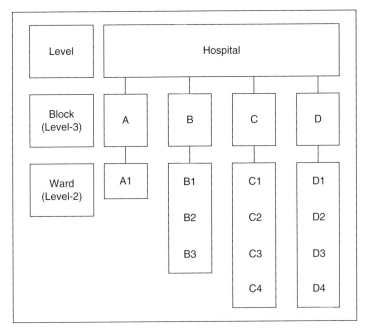

Figure 11.6   Schematic representation of cluster design of three levels: Block (Level-3) and Ward (Level-2) within a hospital. Design structure for a cluster based study in which the dosage of current medication is recorded for each patient (Level-1)

given in Figure 11.7(a). As this difference, and that for Def-TD compared with No-TD of −0.0419, are not statistically significant, we conclude that levels of cholinergic medication in the respective *TarDy* groups do not differ. The level of medication given is therefore summarized by the $GM=8.8$ units calculated from all 403 patients.

However, the above regression command ignores the clustering nature of the study design and the consequential ICC. The required command to take account of the effect of *BLOCK* is of the form(`xi:xtmixed LCHOL i.TarDy || BLOCK: covariance(exchangeable)`). This gives the output of Figure 11.7(c), which duplicates the estimates for the regression coefficients for *TarDy* of Figure 11.7(b). However, the corresponding *SEs* are marginally reduced from 0.1377 to 0.1372 for Mild-TD and from 0.0774 to 0.0771 for Def-TD. These lower values result in narrower confidence intervals but, in this example, will have little impact on the interpretation of the study. The hospital block mean is constrained to $\bar{\varphi}=0$, whereas the estimate of $\sigma_{BLOCK}=1.09 \times 10^{-9}$ is very small indeed, indicating that taking note of the effect of clustering has only marginal influence.

However, within each block there are different wards (*WARD*) and each of these too, as we have previously indicated, may be regarded as a cluster. Thus, in this situation if we were to investigate whether a continuous variable, y, varies with respect to a particular covariate, *Group*, then model (11.11) is extended to the 3-Level hierarchical model

$$y_{ijk} = \beta_0 + \beta_{Group}Group_i + \varphi_j + \omega_{jk} + \varepsilon_{ijk} \tag{11.12}$$

where φ_j describes the between blocks cluster variation as in equation (11.11), and ω_{jk} that between wards within a block j is constrained to have mean $\bar{\omega}_j = 0$. This in turn implies that

(a) *GM levels of medication by TarDy and Block*

tabulate BLOCK TarDy

BLOCK	WARDS	Tardive Dyskinesia			Total	Mean (log)	GM
		No TD	Mild TD	TD			
A	1	8	6	4	18	2.4334	11.3976
B	3	84	13	58	155	2.1023	8.8150
C	4	99	11	53	163	2.1741	8.7943
D	4	22	3	42	67	2.2704	9.6833
Total	12	213	33	157	403	2.1741	8.7943
mean(log)		2.1836	2.2662	2.1418	2.1741	8.7943	
GM		8.8782	9.6427	8.5148			

(b) *Regression model for TarDy ignoring any clustering*

xi:regress LCHOL i.TarDy

Number of obs = 403

LCHOL	Coef	SE	t	P>|t|	[95% CI]
cons	2.1836	0.0504			
No TD	0				
Mild TD	0.0826	0.1377	0.60	0.55	−0.1881 to 0.3533
Def TD	−0.0419	0.0774	−0.54	0.59	−0.1941 to 0.1104

(c) *Regression model for TarDy accounting for clustering within Blocks*

xi: xtmixed LCHOL i.TarDy, || BLOCK:, covariance(exchangeable)

Mixed-effects REML regression

Number of obs = 403, Group variable: BLOCK, Number of groups = 4
Obs per group: min = 18, avg = 100.8, max = 163

LCHOL	Coef	SE	z	P>|z|	[95% CI]
cons	2.1836	0.0502			
No TD	0				
Mild TD	0.0826	0.1372	0.60	0.55	−0,1863 to 0.3515
Def TD	−0.0419	0.0771	−0.54	0.59	−0.1930 to 0.1093

Random-effects Parameters	Estimate
BLOCK: Identity σ_{BLOCK}	1.09×10^{-9}
$\sigma_{RESIDUAL}$	0.7333

Figure 11.7 (a) Geometric mean (GM) dose of cholinergic medication received by diagnostic group according to clustering by Block and Ward accommodating the residential patients (b) regression analysis ignoring clusters, (c) regression analysis accounting for Block and (d) regression analysis accounting for Block and Ward (part data from Chong, Tay, Subramaniam, et al., 2009)

(d) *Regression model for TarDy accounting for clustering within Blocks and Wards*

xi:xtmixed LCHOL i.TarDy, || BLOCK:, covariance(exchangeable) ||
WARD:, covariance(exchangeable)

Group Variable	No. of Groups	Observations per Group		
		Minimum	Average	Maximum
BLOCK	4	18	100.8	163
WARD	12	10	33.6	57

LCHOL	Coef	SE	z	P>|z|	[95% CI]
cons	2.2339	0.0743			
No-TD	0				
Mild-TD	0.0186	0.1370	0.14	0.89	−0.2499 to 0.2871
Def-TD	−0.0554	0.0776	−0.71	0.48	−0.2076 to 0.0967

Random–effects Parameters		Estimate
BLOCK: Identity	σ_{BLOCK}	5.12×10^{-11}
WARD: Identity	σ_{WARD}	0.1792
	$\sigma_{RESIDUAL}$	0.7168

Figure 11.7   (Continued)

the mean of these means is $\bar{\bar{\omega}} = 0$. As previously, the residual terms, now ε_{ijk}, describe the unexplained or residual variation.

The output from fitting this model to the data on cholinergic medication is summarized in Figure 11.7(d). This shows that the estimated regression coefficients are further reduced over the previous analysis accounting for clustering within blocks only. In a relative sense, the reductions in size of 0.0186/0.0826=0.23 or 23% and −0.0554/(−0.0419)=1.32 or 32% are considerable but, despite this, the general conclusion of no difference in levels of cholinergic medication received among the three diagnostic groups is unaltered.

However, in contrast to the clustering within blocks which appears to be of little consequence as the corresponding estimated σ_{BLOCK} is so small, that for wards is quite considerable with estimated $\sigma_{WARD}=0.1792$. The latter measures the random effects variation among the ward components assumed to have an overall mean of zero.

Although we have used a continuous measure as the endpoint in our illustration of multi-level modeling, the methods can be adapted to settings with binary, ordered categorical, count or survival time endpoints. Further, they can also be extended to situations where repeated measures are concerned, implying that models of the random or mixed type of, for example, equation (8.10) can be incorporated within the 3-Level cluster model (11.12). In which case, this becomes a 4-level hierarchical design with Blocks that become Level-4, Wards Level-3, Patient Level-2 and the repeated measures within each patient the Level-1 units.

FRACTIONAL POLYNOMIALS

Introduction

In general we have tried to develop regression models with linear terms with respect to the various covariates concerned. Nevertheless, it is recognized that this constrains the manner in which we summarize the changing endpoint values as the covariates concerned change. Thus, we have described the possibility of adding a quadratic term, for example, in equation (3.5) where this is introduced to better investigate changes in HDL with weight. Further, equation (3.7) complicates the basic linear model of the two covariates gender and weight by adding an interaction term of gender by weight. In some situations the patterns to investigate may not be sufficiently well described by either formulation and even more complex models are required.

One example in which a more complex model is chosen is the change in self-reported pain levels of patients with oral lichen planus (OLP) recruited to the randomized trial of Poon, Goh, Kim, *et al.* (2006). In this case 'parallel', but non-linear profiles, were fitted to the repeated measures of each randomized treatment group as was shown in Figure 1.12.

Fractional polynomials

The linear regression model is termed a polynomial of order or degree-1, and that of a quadratic of order-2. In general, a polynomial may have order-q where q is an integer, and so models could be fitted such as:

$$y = \beta_0 + \beta_1 x + \beta_2 x^2 + \beta_3 x^3 + \ldots + \beta_q x^q. \tag{11.13}$$

Experience indicates that polynomials of order 3 and more often produce models which provide an unrealistic summary. In contrast, the linear and quadratic models are very restricted in their shapes. However, fractional polynomials (FP) increase the flexibility of the polynomial models by allowing the powers to which x can be raised to take non-integer values. Thus, FP take the form

$$y = \beta_0 + \beta_1 x^{(p1)} + \beta_2 x^{(p2)} + \beta_3 x^{(p3)} + \ldots + \beta_q x^{(pq)} \tag{11.14}$$

where x must be positive and

$$x^{(p)} = \begin{cases} x^p & \text{if } p \neq 0 \\ \log x & \text{if } p = 0 \end{cases} \tag{11.15}$$

In addition, each $x^{(p)}$ can imply terms involving both x^p and $x^p \log x$ are in the model, in which case, for $p=0.5$, the model choices become: $y = \beta_0 + \beta_1 x^{0.5}$; $y = \beta_0 + \beta_1 x^{0.5} \log x$ and $y = \beta_0 + \beta_1 x^{0.5} + \beta_2 x^{0.5} \log x$. The FP models can be fitted in Stata using the command (`fracpoly`) but which confines the possible options for the potential models to the powers $(-2, -1, -0.5, 0, 0.5, 1, 2, 3)$ because, as Stata (2007a, Volume A-H, p. 461) states, 'our experience ... including extra powers ... is not often worthwhile'. The implementation command selects the best choice of model from a range of potential alternatives.

In Figure 1.4(b) we summarized the relationship between HDL cholesterol levels and weight from data collected from the Singapore Cardiovascular Cohort Study 2 program, whereas in Figure 11.8(a) the relationship of HDL with subject age is illustrated. The

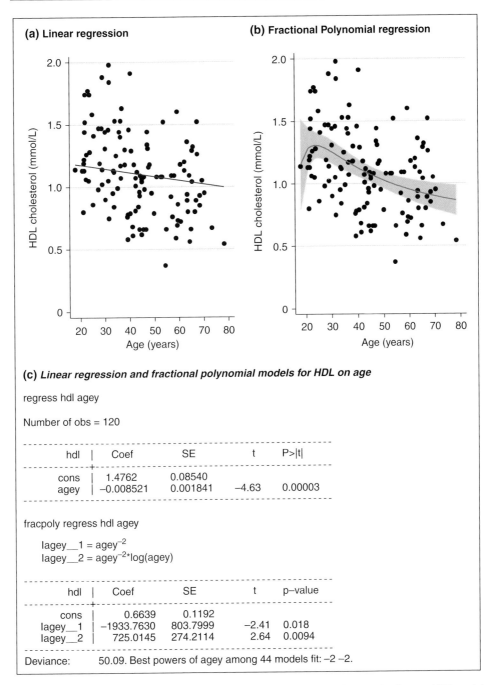

(a) Linear regression

(b) Fractional Polynomial regression

(c) *Linear regression and fractional polynomial models for HDL on age*

regress hdl agey

Number of obs = 120

hdl	Coef	SE	t	P>|t|
cons	1.4762	0.08540		
agey	−0.008521	0.001841	−4.63	0.00003

fracpoly regress hdl agey

lagey__1 = agey^{-2}
lagey__2 = agey^{-2}*log(agey)

hdl	Coef	SE	t	p–value
cons	0.6639	0.1192		
lagey__1	−1933.7630	803.7999	−2.41	0.018
lagey__2	725.0145	274.2114	2.64	0.0094

Deviance: 50.09. Best powers of agey among 44 models fit: −2 −2.

Figure 11.8 Contrast between a simple linear regression model and a fractional polynomial (FP) model to describe the changes in HDL with increasing age (part data from the Singapore Cardiovascular Cohort Study 2) corresponding linear regression model fitted to these data estimates a gradual decline of 0.08521 mmol/L for every 10 years of age in this group of 120 individuals. This is highly statistically significant (p-value$=0.00003$). However, using the model fitted using the command (**fracpoly regress hdl agey**) followed by (**fracplot agey**) gives a rather different profile in Figure 11.8(b).

The corresponding output is given in Figure 11.8(c) and the model chosen by the program takes the form $y=\beta_0+\beta_1x^{-2}+\beta_2x^{-2}\log x$. This is estimated by HDL$=0.6639-\{1933.7630\times Agey^{-2}\}+\{725.0145\times Agey^{-2}\times\log Agey\}$. Thus, for someone aged 49 years the predicted value is HDL$_{49}=0.6639-\{1933.7630/(49\times49)\}+\{(725.0154\times\log 49)/(49\times49)\}=0.6639-\{0.8054\}+\{1.1752\}=1.0337$. This is quite close to 1.0587 predicted from the fitted linear model HDL$=1.4762-0.008521Agey$ of Figure 11.8(a), but a greater disparity would be anticipated for those aged close to 20 years and for the oldest individuals concerned.

Which of the two model approaches is chosen to describe the study findings will depend critically on the specific objectives of the investigation concerned. If the main focus is to investigate the changing patterns of HDL with increasing age in detail, then the FP approach is likely to be more informative, whereas if age is only one of several covariates potentially influencing HDL, then adopting a linear model component for age may be the more likely choice.

Royston, Reitz, and Atzpodien (2006) use FPs to help determine prognosis in metastatic renal cancer, provide references to other applications and give a more complete description of the methodology.

Statistical Tables

Table T1 The probability density function of a standardized Normal distribution.

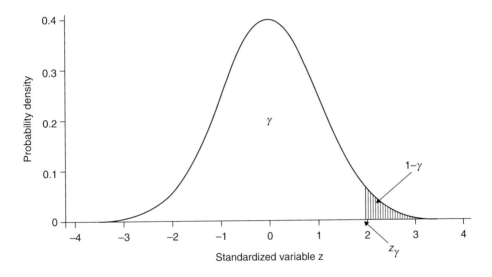

Regression Methods for Medical Research, First Edition. Bee Choo Tai and David Machin.
© 2014 Bee Choo Tai and David Machin. Published 2014 by John Wiley & Sons, Ltd.

Table T1 The Normal distribution function: probability that a Normally distributed variable is less than $z\gamma$ (some frequently used entries are highlighted).

z	0.00	0.01	0.02	0.03	0.04	0.05	0.06	0.07	0.08	0.09
0.0	0.50000	0.50399	0.50798	0.51197	0.51595	0.51994	0.52392	0.52790	0.53188	0.53586
0.1	0.53983	0.54380	0.54776	0.55172	0.55567	0.55962	0.56356	0.56749	0.57142	0.57535
0.2	0.57926	0.58317	0.58706	0.59095	0.59483	0.59871	0.60257	0.60642	0.61026	0.61409
0.3	0.61791	0.62172	0.62552	0.62930	0.63307	0.63683	0.64058	0.64431	0.64803	0.65173
0.4	0.65542	0.65910	0.66276	0.66640	0.67003	0.67364	0.67724	0.68082	0.68439	0.68793
0.5	0.69146	0.69497	0.69847	0.70194	0.70540	0.70884	0.71226	0.71566	0.71904	0.72240
0.6	0.72575	0.72907	0.73237	0.73565	0.73891	0.74215	0.74537	0.74857	0.75175	0.75490
0.7	0.75804	0.76115	0.76424	0.76730	0.77035	0.77337	0.77637	0.77935	0.78230	0.78524
0.8	0.78814	0.79103	0.79389	0.79673	0.79955	0.80234	0.80511	0.80785	0.81057	0.81327
0.9	0.81594	0.81859	0.82121	0.82381	0.82639	0.82894	0.83147	0.83398	0.83646	0.83891
1.0	0.84134	0.84375	0.84614	0.84849	0.85083	0.85314	0.85543	0.85769	0.85993	0.86214
1.1	0.86433	0.86650	0.86864	0.87076	0.87286	0.87493	0.87698	0.87900	0.88100	0.88298
1.2	0.88493	0.88686	0.88877	0.89065	0.89251	0.89435	0.89617	0.89796	0.89973	0.90147
1.3	0.90320	0.90490	0.90658	0.90824	0.90988	0.91149	0.91308	0.91466	0.91621	0.91774
1.4	0.91924	0.92073	0.92220	0.92364	0.92507	0.92647	0.92785	0.92922	0.93056	0.93189
1.5	0.93319	0.93448	0.93574	0.93699	0.93822	0.93943	0.94062	0.94179	0.94295	0.94408
1.6	0.94520	0.94630	0.94738	0.94845	0.94950	0.95053	0.95154	0.95254	0.95352	0.95449
1.7	0.95543	0.95637	0.95728	0.95818	0.95907	0.95994	0.96080	0.96164	0.96246	0.96327
1.8	0.96407	0.96485	0.96562	0.96638	0.96712	0.96784	0.96856	0.96926	0.96995	0.97062
1.9	0.97128	0.97193	0.97257	0.97320	0.97381	0.97441	**0.97500**	0.97558	0.97615	0.97670
2.0	0.97725	0.97778	0.97831	0.97882	0.97932	0.97982	0.98030	0.98077	0.98124	0.98169
2.1	0.98214	0.98257	0.98300	0.98341	0.98382	0.98422	0.98461	0.98500	0.98537	0.98574
2.2	0.98610	0.98645	0.98679	0.98713	0.98745	0.98778	0.98809	0.98840	0.98870	0.98899
2.3	0.98928	0.98956	0.98983	0.99010	0.99036	0.99061	0.99086	0.99111	0.99134	0.99158
2.4	0.99180	0.99202	0.99224	0.99245	0.99266	0.99286	0.99305	0.99324	0.99343	0.99361

z	0.00	0.01	0.02	0.03	0.04	0.05	0.06	0.07	0.08	0.09
2.5	0.99379	0.99396	0.99413	0.99430	0.99446	0.99461	0.99477	0.99492	**0.99506**	0.99520
2.6	0.99534	0.99547	0.99560	0.99573	0.99585	0.99598	0.99609	0.99621	0.99632	0.99643
2.7	0.99653	0.99664	0.99674	0.99683	0.99693	0.99702	0.99711	0.99720	0.99728	0.99736
2.8	0.99744	0.99752	0.99760	0.99767	0.99774	0.99781	0.99788	0.99795	0.99801	0.99807
2.9	0.99813	0.99819	0.99825	0.99831	0.99836	0.99841	0.99846	0.99851	0.99856	0.99861
3.0	0.99865	0.99869	0.99874	0.99878	0.99882	0.99886	0.99889	0.99893	0.99896	0.99900
3.1	0.99903	0.99906	0.99910	0.99913	0.99916	0.99918	0.99921	0.99924	0.99926	0.99929
3.2	0.99931	0.99934	0.99936	0.99938	0.99940	0.99942	0.99944	0.99946	0.99948	0.99950
3.3	0.99952	0.99953	0.99955	0.99957	0.99958	0.99960	0.99961	0.99962	0.99964	0.99965
3.4	0.99966	0.99968	0.99969	0.99970	0.99971	0.99972	0.99973	0.99974	**0.99975**	0.99976
3.5	0.99977	0.99978	0.99978	0.99979	0.99980	0.99981	0.99981	0.99982	0.99983	0.99983
3.6	0.99984	0.99985	0.99985	0.99986	0.99986	0.99987	0.99987	0.99988	0.99988	0.99989
3.7	0.99989	0.99990	0.99990	0.99990	0.99991	0.99991	0.99992	0.99992	0.99992	0.99992
3.8	0.99993	0.99993	0.99993	0.99994	0.99994	0.99994	0.99994	0.99995	0.99995	0.99995
3.9	0.99995	0.99996	0.99996	0.99996	0.99996	0.99996	0.99996	0.99996	0.99997	0.99997

Table T2 Percentage points of the Normal distribution (some frequently used entries are highlighted).

α		
2-sided	**1-sided**	**z**
0.001	0.0005	3.2905
0.005	0.0025	2.8070
0.010	0.0050	**2.5758**
0.020	0.0100	2.3263
0.025	0.0125	2.2414
0.050	0.0250	**1.9600**
0.100	0.0500	1.6449
0.200	**0.1000**	**1.2816**
0.300	0.1500	1.0364
0.400	**0.2000**	**0.8416**
0.500	0.2500	0.6745
0.600	0.3000	0.5244
0.700	0.3500	0.3853
0.800	0.4000	0.2533

Table T3 Percentage points of the Normal distribution for given α and 1 − β (some frequently used entries are highlighted).

α		1 − β	
1-sided	**2-sided**	**1-sided**	**z**
0.0005	0.001	0.9995	3.2905
0.0025	0.005	0.9975	2.8070
0.005	**0.01**	0.995	**2.5758**
0.01	0.02	0.99	2.3263
0.0125	0.025	0.9875	2.2414
0.025	**0.05**	0.975	**1.9600**
0.05	0.1	0.95	1.6449
0.1	0.2	**0.9**	**1.2816**
0.15	0.3	0.85	1.0364
0.2	0.4	**0.8**	**0.8416**
0.25	0.5	0.75	0.6745
0.3	0.6	0.7	0.5244
0.35	0.7	0.65	0.3853
0.4	0.8	0.6	0.2533

Table T4   Students t-distribution. The value tabulated is $t_{\alpha/2}$, such that if X is distributed as Student's t-distribution with f degrees of freedom, then α is the probability that $X \leq -t_{\alpha/2}$ or $X \geq t_{\alpha/2}$.

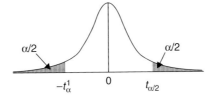

If following a Student t-test with $df = 10$, a value of the test statistic $X = 2.764$ is obtained, then this implies that probability that $X \leq -2.764$ or ≥ 2.764 is $\alpha = 0.02$.

df	α							
	0.20	**0.10**	**0.05**	**0.04**	**0.03**	**0.02**	**0.01**	**0.001**
1	3.078	6.314	12.706	15.895	21.205	31.821	63.657	636.6
2	1.886	2.920	4.303	4.849	5.643	6.965	9.925	31.60
3	1.634	2.353	3.182	3.482	3.896	4.541	5.842	12.92
4	1.530	2.132	2.776	2.999	3.298	3.747	4.604	8.610
5	1.474	2.015	2.571	2.757	3.003	3.365	4.032	6.869
6	1.439	1.943	2.447	2.612	2.829	3.143	3.707	5.959
7	1.414	1.895	2.365	2.517	2.715	2.998	3.499	5.408
8	1.397	1.860	2.306	2.449	2.634	2.896	3.355	5.041
9	1.383	1.833	2.262	2.398	2.574	2.821	3.250	4.781
10	1.372	1.812	2.228	2.359	2.528	2.764	3.169	4.587
11	1.363	1.796	2.201	2.328	2.491	2.718	3.106	4.437
12	1.356	1.782	2.179	2.303	2.461	2.681	3.055	4.318
13	1.350	1.771	2.160	2.282	2.436	2.650	3.012	4.221
14	1.345	1.761	2.145	2.264	2.415	2.624	2.977	4.140
15	1.340	1.753	2.131	2.249	2.397	2.602	2.947	4.073
16	1.337	1.746	2.120	2.235	2.382	2.583	2.921	4.015
17	1.333	1.740	2.110	2.224	2.368	2.567	2.898	3.965
18	1.330	1.734	2.101	2.214	2.356	2.552	2.878	3.922
19	1.328	1.729	2.093	2.205	2.346	2.539	2.861	3.883
20	1.325	1.725	2.086	2.196	2.336	2.528	2.845	3.850
21	1.323	1.721	2.079	2.189	2.327	2.517	2.830	3.819
22	1.321	1.717	2.074	2.183	2.320	2.508	2.818	3.790
23	1.319	1.714	2.069	2.178	2.313	2.499	2.806	3.763
24	1.318	1.711	2.064	2.172	2.307	2.492	2.797	3.744
25	1.316	1.708	2.059	2.166	2.301	2.485	2.787	3.722
26	1.315	1.706	2.056	2.162	2.396	2.479	2.779	3.706
27	1.314	1.703	2.052	2.158	2.291	2.472	2.770	3.687
28	1.313	1.701	2.048	2.154	2.286	2.467	2.763	3.673
29	1.311	1.699	2.045	2.150	2.282	2.462	2.756	3.657
30	1.310	1.697	2.042	2.147	2.278	2.457	2.750	3.646
∞	1.282	1.645	1.960	2.054	2.170	2.326	2.576	3.291

Table T5 The χ^2 distribution. The value tabulated is $\chi^2(\alpha)$, such that if X is distributed as χ^2 with degrees of freedom, df, then α is the probability that $X \geq \chi^2$.

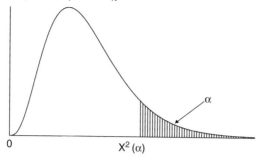

df	0.2	0.1	0.05	0.04	0.03	0.02	0.01	0.001
1	1.64	2.71	3.84	4.22	4.71	5.41	6.63	10.83
2	3.22	4.61	5.99	6.44	7.01	7.82	9.21	13.82
3	4.64	6.25	7.81	8.31	8.95	9.84	11.34	16.27
4	5.99	7.78	9.49	10.03	10.71	11.67	13.28	18.47
5	7.29	9.24	11.07	11.64	12.37	13.39	15.09	20.51
6	8.56	10.64	12.59	13.20	13.97	15.03	16.81	22.46
7	9.80	12.02	14.07	14.70	15.51	16.62	18.48	24.32
8	11.03	13.36	15.51	16.17	17.01	18.17	20.09	26.12
9	12.24	14.68	16.92	17.61	18.48	19.68	21.67	27.88
10	13.44	15.99	18.31	19.02	19.92	21.16	23.21	29.59
11	14.63	17.28	19.68	20.41	21.34	22.62	24.73	31.26
12	15.81	18.55	21.03	21.79	22.74	24.05	26.22	32.91
13	16.98	19.81	22.36	23.14	24.12	25.47	27.69	34.53
14	18.15	21.06	23.68	24.49	25.49	26.87	29.14	36.12
15	19.31	22.31	25.00	25.82	26.85	28.26	30.58	37.70
16	20.47	23.54	26.30	27.14	28.19	29.63	32.00	39.25
17	21.61	24.77	27.59	28.44	29.52	31.00	33.41	40.79
18	22.76	25.99	28.87	29.75	30.84	32.35	34.81	42.31
19	23.90	27.20	30.14	31.04	32.16	33.69	36.19	43.82
20	25.04	28.41	31.41	32.32	33.46	35.02	37.57	45.31
21	26.17	29.62	32.67	33.60	34.76	36.34	38.93	46.80
22	27.30	30.81	33.92	34.87	36.05	37.66	40.29	48.27
23	28.43	32.01	35.17	36.13	37.33	38.97	41.64	49.73
24	29.55	33.20	36.42	37.39	38.61	40.27	42.98	51.18
25	30.68	34.38	37.65	38.64	39.88	41.57	44.31	52.62
26	31.79	35.56	38.89	39.89	41.15	42.86	45.64	54.05
27	32.91	36.74	40.11	41.13	42.41	44.14	46.96	55.48
28	34.03	37.92	41.34	42.37	43.66	45.42	48.28	56.89
29	35.14	39.09	42.56	43.60	44.91	46.69	49.59	58.30
30	36.25	40.26	43.77	44.83	46.16	47.96	50.89	59.70

Example. For an observed test statistic of $X = 9.7$ with 3 degrees of freedom, the tabular entries for α equal to 0.03 and 0.02 are 8.95 and 9.84, respectively. Hence $X = 9.7$ suggests a p-value between 0.03 and 0.02, or more precisely close to 0.021.

Table T6 The F-distribution. The value tabulated is $F(\alpha, df_1, df_2)$, such that if X has an F-distribution with df_1 and df_2 degrees of freedom, then α is the probability that $X \geq F(\alpha, df_1, df_2)$.

df_2	α	df_1 1	2	3	4	5	6	7	8	9	10	20	∞
1	0.10	39.86	49.50	53.59	55.83	57.24	58.20	58.91	59.44	59.86	60.19	61.74	63.30
1	0.05	161.45	199.50	215.71	224.58	230.16	233.99	236.77	238.88	240.54	241.88	248.02	254.19
1	0.01	4052.18	4999.34	5403.53	5624.26	5763.96	5858.95	5928.33	5980.95	6022.40	6055.93	6208.66	6362.80
2	0.10	8.53	9.00	9.16	9.24	9.29	9.33	9.35	9.37	9.38	9.39	9.44	9.49
2	0.05	18.51	19.00	19.16	19.25	19.30	19.33	19.35	19.37	19.38	19.40	19.45	19.49
2	0.01	98.50	99.00	99.16	99.25	99.30	99.33	99.36	99.38	99.39	99.40	99.45	99.50
3	0.10	5.54	5.46	5.39	5.34	5.31	5.28	5.27	5.25	5.24	5.23	5.18	5.13
3	0.05	10.13	9.55	9.28	9.12	9.01	8.94	8.89	8.85	8.81	8.79	8.66	8.53
3	0.01	34.12	30.82	29.46	28.71	28.24	27.91	27.67	27.49	27.34	27.23	26.69	26.14
4	0.10	4.54	4.32	4.19	4.11	4.05	4.01	3.98	3.95	3.94	3.92	3.84	3.76
4	0.05	7.71	6.94	6.59	6.39	6.26	6.16	6.09	6.04	6.00	5.96	5.80	5.63
4	0.01	21.20	18.00	16.69	15.98	15.52	15.21	14.98	14.80	14.66	14.55	14.02	13.47
5	0.10	4.06	3.78	3.62	3.52	3.45	3.40	3.37	3.34	3.32	3.30	3.21	3.11
5	0.05	6.61	5.79	5.41	5.19	5.05	4.95	4.88	4.82	4.77	4.74	4.56	4.37
5	0.01	16.26	13.27	12.06	11.39	10.97	10.67	10.46	10.29	10.16	10.05	9.55	9.03
6	0.10	3.78	3.46	3.29	3.18	3.11	3.05	3.01	2.98	2.96	2.94	2.84	2.72
6	0.05	5.99	5.14	4.76	4.53	4.39	4.28	4.21	4.15	4.10	4.06	3.87	3.67
6	0.01	13.75	10.92	9.78	9.15	8.75	8.47	8.26	8.10	7.98	7.87	7.40	6.89
7	0.10	3.59	3.26	3.07	2.96	2.88	2.83	2.78	2.75	2.72	2.70	2.59	2.47
7	0.05	5.59	4.74	4.35	4.12	3.97	3.87	3.79	3.73	3.68	3.64	3.44	3.23
7	0.01	12.25	9.55	8.45	7.85	7.46	7.19	6.99	6.84	6.72	6.62	6.16	5.66
8	0.10	3.46	3.11	2.92	2.81	2.73	2.67	2.62	2.59	2.56	2.54	2.42	2.30
8	0.05	5.32	4.46	4.07	3.84	3.69	3.58	3.50	3.44	3.39	3.35	3.15	2.93
8	0.01	11.26	8.65	7.59	7.01	6.63	6.37	6.18	6.03	5.91	5.81	5.36	4.87

(Continued)

Table T6 (cont'd)

df_2	α	1	2	3	4	5	6	7	8	9	10	20	∞
								df_1					
9	0.10	3.36	3.01	2.81	2.69	2.61	2.55	2.51	2.47	2.44	2.42	2.30	2.16
9	0.05	5.12	4.26	3.86	3.63	3.48	3.37	3.29	3.23	3.18	3.14	2.94	2.71
9	0.01	10.56	8.02	6.99	6.42	6.06	5.80	5.61	5.47	5.35	5.26	4.81	4.32
10	0.10	3.29	2.92	2.73	2.61	2.52	2.46	2.41	2.38	2.35	2.32	2.20	2.06
10	0.05	4.96	4.10	3.71	3.48	3.33	3.22	3.14	3.07	3.02	2.98	2.77	2.54
10	0.01	10.04	7.56	6.55	5.99	5.64	5.39	5.20	5.06	4.94	4.85	4.41	3.92
20	0.10	2.97	2.59	2.38	2.25	2.16	2.09	2.04	2.00	1.96	1.94	1.79	1.61
20	0.05	4.35	3.49	3.10	2.87	2.71	2.60	2.51	2.45	2.39	2.35	2.12	1.85
20	0.01	8.10	5.85	4.94	4.43	4.10	3.87	3.70	3.56	3.46	3.37	2.94	2.43
30	0.10	2.88	2.49	2.28	2.14	2.05	1.98	1.93	1.88	1.85	1.82	1.67	1.46
30	0.05	4.17	3.32	2.92	2.69	2.53	2.42	2.33	2.27	2.21	2.16	1.93	1.63
30	0.01	7.56	5.39	4.51	4.02	3.70	3.47	3.30	3.17	3.07	2.98	2.55	2.02
40	0.10	2.84	2.44	2.23	2.09	2.00	1.93	1.87	1.83	1.79	1.76	1.61	1.38
40	0.05	4.08	3.23	2.84	2.61	2.45	2.34	2.25	2.18	2.12	2.08	1.84	1.52
40	0.01	7.31	5.18	4.31	3.83	3.51	3.29	3.12	2.99	2.89	2.80	2.37	1.82
50	0.10	2.81	2.41	2.20	2.06	1.97	1.90	1.84	1.80	1.76	1.73	1.57	1.33
50	0.05	4.03	3.18	2.79	2.56	2.40	2.29	2.20	2.13	2.07	2.03	1.78	1.45
50	0.01	7.17	5.06	4.20	3.72	3.41	3.19	3.02	2.89	2.78	2.70	2.27	1.70
100	0.10	2.76	2.36	2.14	2.00	1.91	1.83	1.78	1.73	1.69	1.66	1.49	1.22
100	0.05	3.94	3.09	2.70	2.46	2.31	2.19	2.10	2.03	1.97	1.93	1.68	1.30
100	0.01	6.90	4.82	3.98	3.51	3.21	2.99	2.82	2.69	2.59	2.50	2.07	1.45
∞	0.10	2.71	2.31	2.09	1.95	1.85	1.78	1.72	1.68	1.64	1.61	1.43	1.08
∞	0.05	3.85	3.00	2.61	2.38	2.22	2.11	2.02	1.95	1.89	1.84	1.58	1.11
∞	0.01	6.66	4.63	3.80	3.34	3.04	2.82	2.66	2.53	2.43	2.34	1.90	1.16

Example. For an observed test statistic of $X = 5.1$ with 3 and 4 degrees of freedom, the tabular entries for α equal to 0.10, 0.05 and 0.01 are 4.19, 6.59 and 16.69, respectively. Hence $X = 5.1$ suggests a p-value between 0.10 and 0.05 or approximately 0.08.

Table T7 Number of subjects required for a range of the Cohen (1988) standardized effect size, Δ, for a continuous endpoint assuming a two-group comparison with equal numbers in each group.

	$\alpha = 0.05$	
Δ	$\beta = 0.2$	$\beta = 0.1$
0.2	788	1054
0.3	352	470
0.4	200	266
0.5	128	172
0.6	90	120
0.7	66	88
0.8	52	68
0.9	42	54
1.0	34	44
1.35	20	26

References

Numbers in parentheses after each entry are the chapters in which these are cited.

*Books indicated for further reading in Chapter 1.

*Altman DG (1991). *Practical Statistics for Medical Research*. London, Chapman and Hall. [1]

*Armitage P, Berry G and Matthews JNS (2002). *Statistical Methods in Medical Research*. (4th edn). Blackwell Science, Oxford. [1]

Altman DG, Lausen B, Sauerbrei W and Schumacher M (1994). Dangers of using "optimal" cutpoints in the evaluation of prognostic factors. *Journal of the National Cancer Institute*, **86**, 829–835 and 1798–1799. [7]

Altman DG, Machin D, Bryant TN and Gardner MJ (eds) (2000) *Statistics with Confidence*. (2nd edn) British Medical Journal, London. [4]

Altman DG and Royston P (2000). What do we mean by validating a prognostic model? *Statistics in Medicine*, **11**, 453–473. [7]

Bellary S, O'Hare JP, Raymond NT, Gumber A, Mughal S, Szczepura A, Kumar S and Barnett AH (2008). Enhanced diabetes care to patients of south Asian ethnic origin (the United Kingdom Asian Diabetes Study): a cluster randomised trial. *Lancet*, **371**, 1769–1776. [11]

Beyersmann J, Dettenkofer M, Bertz H and M Schumacher (2007). A competing risks analysis of bloodstream infection after stem-cell transplantation using subdistribution hazards and cause-specific hazards. *Statistics in Medicine*, **26**, 5360–5369. [10]

*Bland M (2000). *An Introduction to Medical Statistics*. (3rd edn). Oxford University Press, Oxford. [1]

Böhning D, Dietz E, Schlattman P, Mendoca L and Kirchner U (1999). The zero-inflated Poisson model and the decayed, missing and filled teeth index in dental epidemiology. *Journal of the Royal Statistical Society, (A)*, **162**, 195–209. [5]

Boos D and Stefanski L (2010). Efron's bootstrap. *Significance*, **7**, 186–188. [5]

Breiman L, Freedman JH, Olshen RA and Stone CJ (1984). *Classification and Regression Trees*. Wadsworth & Brooks/Cole Advanced Books and Software, Monterey, California. [9]

Busse WW, Lemanske Jr RF and Gern JE (2010). Role of viral infections in asthma exacerbations. *Lancet*, **376**, 826–834. [1, 2, 7, 11]

*Campbell MJ (2006). *Statistics at Square Two: Understanding Modern Statistical Applications in Medicine*. (2nd edn). Blackwell BMJ Books, Oxford. [1]

*Campbell MJ, Machin D and Walters SJ (2007). *Medical Statistics: A Commonsense Approach: A Text Book for the Health Sciences*, (4th edn) Wiley, Chichester. [1, 5]

Cassimally KA (2011). We come from one. *Significance*, **8**, 19–21. [3]

Chia B-H, Chia A, Ng W-Y and Tai B-C (2010). Suicide trends in Singapore: 1955–2004. *Archives of Suicide Research*, **14**, 276–283. [5]

Chinnaiya A, Venkat A, Chia D, Chee WY, Choo KB, Gole LA and Meng CT (1998). Intrahepatic vein fetal sampling: Current role in prenatal diagnosis. *Journal of Obstetrics and Gynaecology*, **24**, 239–246. [1, 4, 7]

Chong S-A, Tay JAM, Subramaniam M, Pek E and Machin D (2009). Mortality rates among patients with schizophrenia and tardive dyskinesia. *Journal of Clinical Psychopharmacology*, **29**, 5–8. [1, 5, 6, 7, 9, 11]

*Clayton D and Hills M (1993). *Statistical Models in Epidemiology*, Oxford University Press, Oxford. [1]

Cnattingius S, Hultman CM, Dahl M and Sparén P (1999). Very preterm birth, birth trauma, and the risk of anorexia nervosa among girls. *Archives of General Psychiatry*, **56**, 634–638. [4]

Cohen J (1988). *Statistical Power Analysis for the Behavioral Sciences*, 2nd edn. Lawrence Earlbaum, New Jersey. [7]

Cohn SL, Pearson ADJ, London WB, Monclair T, Ambros PF, Brodeur GM, Faldum A, Hero B, Iehara T, Machin D, Mosseri V, Simon T, Garaventa A, Castel V and Matthau KK (2009). The International Neuroblastoma Risk Group (INRG) Classification System: An INRG Task Force Report. *Journal of Clinical Oncology*, **27**, 289–297. [1, 9]

*Collett D (2002). *Modelling Binary Data*, (2nd edn) Chapman and Hall/CRC, London. [1]

*Collett D (2003). *Modelling Survival Data in Medical Research*, (2nd edn), Chapman and Hall/CRC, London. [1]

Contoli M, Message SD, Laza-Stanca V, Edwards MR, Wark PA, Bartlett NW, Kebadze T, Malia P, Stanciu LA, Parker HL, Slater L, Lewis-Antes A, Kon OM, Holgate ST, Davies DE, Kotenko SV, Papi A and Johnston SL (2006). Role of deficient type III interferon-lambda production in asthma exacerbations. *Nature Medicine*, **12**, 1023–1026. [1]

Cox DR (1972). Regression models and life tables (with discussion). *Journal of the Royal Statistical Society*, **B34**, 187–220. [6]

Diggle PJ (1990). *Time Series: A Biostatistical Introduction*. Oxford University Press, Oxford. [8]

*Diggle PJ, Liang K-Y and Zeger SL (1994). *Analysis of Longitudinal Data*. Oxford Science Publications, Clarendon Press, Oxford. [1, 8]

*Dobson AJ and Barnett AG (2008). *Introduction to Generalized Linear Models*. (3rd edn), Chapman and Hall/CRC, London. [1]

Everitt BS (2003) *Modern Medical Statistics: A Practical Guide*. Arnold Publishers, London. [9]

*Everitt BS and Rabe-Hesketh S (2006). *A Handbook of Statistical Analysis using Stata*. (4th edn), Chapman and Hall/CRC, London. [1]

Feinstein AR (1996). *Multivariable Analysis: An Introduction*. Yale University Press, New Haven and London. [9]

Fine JP and Gray RJ (1999). A proportional hazards model for the subdistribution of a competing risk. *Journal of the American Statistical Association*, **94**, 496–509. [10]

*Freeman JV, Walters SJ and Campbell MJ (2008). *How to Display Data*. BMJ Books, Blackwell Publishing, Oxford. [1]

Frison L and Pocock SJ (1992). Repeated measures in clinical trials: analysing mean summary statistics and its implications for design. *Statistics in Medicine*, **11**, 1685–1704. [11]

Grundy RH, Wilne SH, Robinson KJ, Ironside JW, Cox T, Chong WK, Michalski A, Campbell RHA, Bailey CC, Thorpe N, Pizer B, Punt J, Walker DA, Ellison DW and Machin D (2010). Primary postoperative chemotherapy without radiotherapy for treatment of brain tumours other than ependymoma in children under 3 years: Results of the first UKCCSG/SIOP CNS 9204 trial. *European Journal of Cancer*, **46**, 120–133. [10]

Grundy RG, Wilne SH, Weston CL, Robinson K, Lashford LS, Ironside J, Cox T, Chong WK, Campbell RHA, Bailey CC, Gattamaneni R, Picton S, Thorpe N, Mallucci C, English MW, Punt JAG, Walker DA, Ellison DW and Machin D (2007). Primary postoperative chemotherapy without radiotherapy for intracranial ependymoma in children: the UKCCSG/SIOP prospective study. *Lancet Oncology*, **8**, 696–705. [10]

Husain R, Liang S, Foster PJ, Gazzard G, Bunce C, Chew PTK, Oen FTS, Khaw PT, Seah SKL and Aung T (2012). Cataract surgery after trabulectomy: The effect of trabulectomy function. *Archives of Ophthalmology*, **130**, 165–170. [10]

ICH E9 Expert Working Group (1999). Statistical principles for clinical trials: ICH Harmonised Tripartite Guideline. *Statistics in Medicine*, **18**, 1905–1942. [7]

Ince D (2011). The Duke University scandal – what can be done? *Significance*, **8**, 113–115. [7]

Jackson DJ, Gangnon RE, Evans MD, Roberg KA, Anderson EL, Pappas TE, Printz MC, Lee W-M, Shult PA, Reisdorf E, Carlson-Dakes KT, Salazar LP, DaSilva DF, Tisler CJ, Gern JE and Lemanske RF (2008). Wheezing rhinovirus illnesses in early life predict asthma development in high-risk children. *American Journal of Respiratory and Critical Care Medicine*, **178**, 667–672. [4, 7]

*Kleinbaum G, Kupper LL, Muller KE and Nizam E (2007). *Applied Regression Analysis and Other Multivariable Methods*. (4th edn), Duxbury Press, Florence, Kentucky. [1]

Korenman S, Goldman N, Fu H (1997). Misclassification bias in estimates of bereavement effects. *American Journal of Epidemiology*, **145**, 995–1002. [10]

LeBlanc M and Crowley J (1993). Survival trees by goodness of split. *Journal of the American Statistical Association*, **88**, 457–467. [9]

Lee CH, Tai BC, Soon CY, Low AF, Poh KK, Yeo TC, Lim GH, Yip J, Omar AR, Teo SG and Tan HC (2010). A new set of intravascular ultrasound-derived anatomical criteria for defining functionally significant stenoses in small coronary arteries: results from Intravascular Ultrasound Diagnostic Evaluation of Atherosclerosis in Singapore (IDEAS) study. *American Journal of Cardiology*, **105**, 1378–1384. [7, 9]

Levitan EB, Yang AZ, Wolk W and Mittleman MA (2009). Adiposity and incidence of heart failure hospitalization and mortality: a population-based prospective study. *Circulation: Heart Failure*, **2**, 203–208. [7]

Levy HL, Milanowski A , Chakrapani A, Cleary M, Lee P, Trefz FK, Whitley CB, Feillet F, Feigenbaum AS, Bebchuk JD, Christ-Schmidt H and Dorenbaum A (2007). Efficacy of sapropterin dihydrochloride (tetra-hydrobiopterin, 6R-BH4) for reduction of phenylalanine concentration in patients with phenylketonuria: a phase III randomised placebo-controlled study. *Lancet*, **370**, 504–510. [11]

Little RJ, Cohen ML, Dickersin K, Emerson SS, Farrar JT, Neaton JD, Shih W, Siegel JP and Stern H (2012). The design and conduct of clinical trials to limit missing data. *Statistics in Medicine*, **31**, 3433 – 3443. [10]

*Machin D and Campbell MJ (2005). *Design of Studies for Medical Research*. Wiley, Chichester. [1]

*Machin D, Campbell MJ, Tan SB and Tan SH (2009). *Sample Size Tables for Clinical Studies*. (3rd edn). Wiley-Blackwell, Chichester. [1, 7]

*Machin D, Cheung Y-B and Parmar MKB (2006). *Survival Analysis: A Practical Approach*. (2nd edn). Wiley, Chichester. [1]

Maheswaran R, Pearson T, Hoysal N and Campbell MJ (2010). Evaluation of the impact of a health forecast alert service on admissions for chronic obstructive pulmonary disease in Bradford and Airedale. *Journal of Public Health*, **32**, 97–102. [1, 5]

Marshall RJ (2001). The use of classification and regression trees in clinical epidemiology. *Journal of Clinical Epidemiology*, **54**, 603–609. [9]

Marubini E and Valsecchi MG (1995). *Analysing Survival Data from Clinical Trials and Observational Studies*. Wiley, Chichester. [6]

*Mitchell MN (2012). *Interpreting and Visualizing Regression Models Using Stata*. Stata Press, College Station, TX. [1]

Nejadnik H, Hui JH, Choong EP-F, Tai B-C and Lee E-H (2010) Autologous bone marrow-derived mesenchymal cells versus autologous chondrocyte implantation: An observational cohort study. *American Journal of Sports Medicine*, **38**, 1110–1116. [8, 11]

Ng DPK, Fukushima M, Tai B-C, Koh D, Leong H, Imura H and Lim XL (2008). Reduced GFR and albuminuria in Chinese type 2 diabetes mellitus patients are both independently associated with activation of the TNF-α system. *Diabetologia*, **51**, 2318–2324. [1, 7]

Pearson ADJ, Pinkerton CR, Lewis IJ, Ellershaw C and Machin D (2008). High-dose rapid and standard induction chemotherapy for patients aged over 1 year with stage 4 neuroblastoma: a randomized trial. *Lancet Oncology*, **9**, 247–256. [6, 7, 10]

Poole-Wilson PA, Uretsky BF, Thygesen K, Cleland JGF, Massie BM and Rydén L (2003). Mode of death in heart failure: findings from the ATLAS trial. *Heart*, **89**: 42–48. [10]

Poon C-Y, Goh B-T, Kim M-J, Rajaseharan A, Ahmed S, Thongprasom K, Chaimusik M, Suresh S, Machin D, Wong H-B and Seldrup J (2006). A randomised controlled trial to compare steroid with cyclosporine for the topical treatment of oral lichen planus. *Oral Surgery, Oral Pathology, Oral Radiology and Endodontology*, **102**, 47–55. [1, 8, 11]

Pregibon (1981). Logistic regression diagnostics. *Annals of Statistics*, **9**, 705–724. [4]

*Rabe-Hesketh S and Skrondal A (2008). *Multilevel and Longitudinal Modeling Using Stata* (2nd edn), Stata Press, College Station, TX. [1, 8]

Richards SH, Bankhead C, Peters TJ, Austoker J, Hobbs FDR, Brown J, Tydeman C, Roberts L, Formby J, Redman V, Wilson S and Sharp DJ (2001). Cluster randomized controlled trial comparing the effectiveness and cost-effectiveness of two primary care interventions aimed at improving attendance for breast screening. *Journal of Medical Screening*, **8**, 91–98. [11]

Rothman KJ (2002). *Epidemiology: An Introduction*. Oxford University Press, New York, page 194. [7]

Royston P, Reitz M and Atzpodien J (2006). An approach to estimating prognosis using fractional polynomials in metastatic renal carcinoma. *British Journal of Cancer*, **94**, 1785–1788. [11]

Sackley CM, van den Berg ME, Lett K, Patel S, Hollands K, Wright CC and Hoppitt TJ (2009). Effects of a physiotherapy and occupational therapy intervention on mobility and activity in care home residents: a cluster randomized controlled trial. *British Medical Journal*, 2009 Sep 1, 339:b3123.doi: 10.1136bmj.b3123. [11]

SAS Institute (2012). *SAS Enterprise Miner (EM): Version* 12.1. SAS Institute, Cary, NC. [9]

Schoenfeld D (1982). Partial residuals for the proportional hazards regression model. *Biometrika*, **69**, 239–241. [6]

Sridhar T, Gore A, Boiangiu I, Machin D and Symonds RP (2009). Concomitant (without adjuvant) temozolomide and radiation to treat glioblastoma: A retrospective study. *Clinical Oncology*, **21**, 19–22 [6, 7, 10].

StataCorp (2007a). *Stata Base Reference Manual, Volume 2: A-H, Release 10*, College Station, TX. [11]

StataCorp (2007b). *Stata Base Reference Manual, Volume 2: I-P, Release 10*, College Station, TX. [4]

StataCorp (2007c). *Stata Base Reference Manual, Volume 2: Q-Z, Release 10*, College Station, TX. [7]

*Swinscow TV and Campbell MJ (2002). *Statistics at Square One*. (10th edn), Blackwell, BMJ Books, Oxford. [1]

Tai BC, Grundy R and Machin D (2011). On the importance of accounting for competing risks in paediatric cancer trials designed to delay or avoid radiotherapy. II. Adjustment for covariates and sample size issues. *International Journal of Radiation Oncology, Biology and Physics*, **79**, 1139–1146 [10]

Tai B-C, Peregoudov A and Machin D (2001). A competing risk approach to the analysis of trials of alternative intrauterine devices (IUDs) for fertility regulation. *Statistics in Medicine*, **20**, 3589–3600. [10]

Tan C-K, Law N-M, Ng H-S and Machin D (2003). Simple clinical prognostic model for hepatocellular carcinoma in developing countries and its validation. *Journal of Clinical Oncology*, **21**, 2294–2298. [7, 9]

Therneau T and Atkinson E (2011). An introduction to recursive partitioning using the RPART routines. Technical report, Mayo Foundation, Rochester. http://CRAN.R-project.org/package=rpart. [9]

Viardot-Foucault V, Prasath EB, Tai B-C, Chan JKY and Loh SF (2011). Predictive factors of success for Intra-Uterine Insemination: a single centre retrospective study. *Human Reproduction*, **26 (Suppl 1)**, 1232–1233. [5, 8]

Vuong Q (1989). Likelihood ratio tests for model selection and non-nested hypotheses. *Econometrica*, **57**, 307–334. [5]

Wee J, Tan E-H, Tai B-C, Wong H-B, Leong S-S, Tan T, Chua E-T, Yang E, Lee K-M, Fong K-W, Tan HSK, Lee K-S, Loong S, Sethi V, Chua E-J and Machin D (2005). Randomized trial of radiotherapy versus concurrent chemoradiotherapy followed by adjuvant chemotherapy in patients with American Joint Committee on Cancer/International Union against cancer stage III and IV nasopharyngeal cancer of the endemic variety. *Journal of Clinical Oncology*, **23**, 6730–6738. [1, 7, 10]

Whitehead J (1993). Sample size calculations for ordered categorical data. *Statistics in Medicine*, **12**, 2257–2272. [4]

Wight J, Jakubovic M, Walters S, Maheswaran R, White P and Lennon V (2004). Variation in cadaveric organ donor rates in the UK. *Nephrology Dialysis Transplantation*; **19**, 963–968. [5]

Young SS and Karr A (2011). Deming, data and observational studies: A process out of control and needing fixing. *Significance*, **8**, 116–119. [7]

Zhang H, Crowley J, Sox HC and Olshen RA (1999). Tree-structured statistical methods. In Armitage P and Colton T (eds). *Encyclopedia of Biostatistics*, **6**, 4561–4573. [9]

Zhang H, Holford T and Bracken MB (1996). A tree-based method of analysis for prospective studies. *Statistics in Medicine*, **15**, 37–49. [9]

Index

Regression Methods for Medical Research, First Edition. Bee Choo Tai and David Machin.
© 2014 Bee Choo Tai and David Machin. Published 2014 by John Wiley & Sons, Ltd.